Neutrophil Extracellular Traps

Neutrophil Extracellular Traps: Mechanisms and Role in Health and Disease

Editors

Hans-Joachim Anders
Shrikant R. Mulay

MDPI • Basel • Beijing • Wuhan • Barcelona • Belgrade • Manchester • Tokyo • Cluj • Tianjin

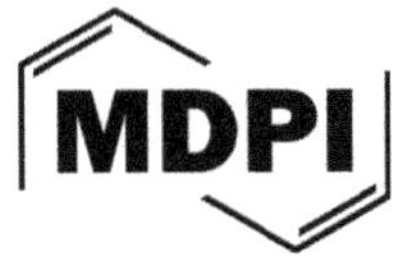

Editors
Hans-Joachim Anders
Klinikum der Universitat Munchen
Germany

Shrikant R. Mulay
CSIR-Central Drug Research Institute
India

Editorial Office
MDPI
St. Alban-Anlage 66
4052 Basel, Switzerland

This is a reprint of articles from the Special Issue published online in the open access journal *Cells* (ISSN 2073-4409) (available at: https://www.mdpi.com/journal/cells/special_issues/NETs).

For citation purposes, cite each article independently as indicated on the article page online and as indicated below:

LastName, A.A.; LastName, B.B.; LastName, C.C. Article Title. *Journal Name* **Year**, *Article Number*, Page Range.

ISBN 978-3-03943-519-7 (Hbk)
ISBN 978-3-03943-520-3 (PDF)

Cover image courtesy of Prof. Helen Liapis.

Contents

About the Editors

Hans-Joachim Anders was trained as a nephrologist and leads the Division of Nephrology at the inner city campus at the Ludwig Maximilians University of Munich, Germany. His research focuses on translational aspects of kidney disease. He is the recipient of the renowned award for "Outstanding Basic Science Contributions to Nephrology" from the European Renal Association (ERA-EDTA). He has authored more than 350 publications. He is currently Associate Editor of the Journal of the American Society of Nephrology and Nephrology Dialysis Transplantation, and has served or serves as a member of the Editorial Boards of the Clinical Journal of the American Society of Nephrology, Kidney International, BMC Nephrology, and Nature Reviews Nephrology.

Shrikant R. Mulay works as a Scientist at the Division of Pharmacology at CSIR-Central Drug Research Institute, Lucknow, India. He completed habilitation, as well as post-doctoral and Ph.D. training, at the Ludwig Maximilians University of Munich, Germany. His research interests are to understand the contribution of regulated necrosis and inflammation in the pathophysiology of kidney diseases. He is recipient of the renowned "Stanley Shaldon Young Investigators Award 2018" from the European Renal Association (ERA-EDTA). He has published more than 70 articles, including original research, invited reviews, and book chapters. He serves as an Ex-Officio Board Member of Young Nephrology Platform (YNP) of ERA-EDTA and an Editorial Board Member of the Frontiers in Pharmacology.

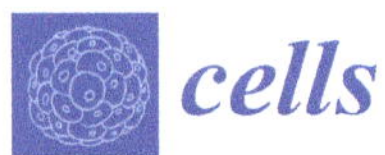 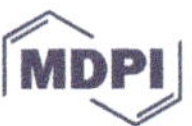

Editorial

Neutrophils and Neutrophil Extracellular Traps Regulate Immune Responses in Health and Disease

Shrikant R. Mulay [1,*] and Hans-Joachim Anders [2,*]

1 Division of Pharmacology, CSIR-Central Drug Research Institute, Lucknow 226031, India
2 Division of Nephrology, Department of Medicine IV, Hospital of the LMU Munich, 80336 Munich, Germany
* Correspondence: shrikant.mulay@cdri.res.in (S.R.M.); hjanders@med.uni-muenchen.de (H.-J.A.);
   Tel.: +91-522-2772450 (ext. 4863) (S.R.M.); +49-89-440053583 (H.-J.A.)

Received: 16 September 2020; Accepted: 17 September 2020; Published: 20 September 2020

1. Introduction

Neutrophils are first responders of antimicrobial host defense and sterile inflammation, and therefore, play important roles during health and disease. Almost 16 years after the first description of neutrophil extracellular traps (NETs) as an alternative mode of pathogen killing, it has become clear that NETs also largely contribute to sterile forms of inflammation [1]. Indeed, NETs contribute to all forms of thrombosis, microparticle-induced inflammation, autoimmune vasculitis, auto-inflammatory disorders, and secondary inflammation due to ischemic, toxic, or traumatic tissue injury [1]. Recently, NETs have also been found to be an essential component of the multi-organ complications of COVID-19 [2].

In this Special Issue in *Cells*, we selected a series of articles that highlight the role of neutrophils and NETs in various sterile and non-sterile, acute and chronic inflammatory conditions affecting both human and animal health. We hope that this Special Issue will instigate novel research questions in the minds of our readers and will be instrumental in the further development of the field.

2. Neutrophils and NETs in Infection

Neutrophils play crucial roles in innate and adaptive immune responses. They control the invading pathogens, e.g., bacteria, fungi, and viruses, via multiple mechanisms, e.g., phagocytosis and NET formation. Phagocytosis of pathogens kills by exposing them to intracellular bactericidal compounds, whereas NET formation results in trapping and killing pathogens outside the cell.

In this Special Issue, Manda-Handzlik and Demkow discuss the emerging role of NETs in central nervous system infections [3]. They suggested netting neutrophils as the main causative factor for disruption of the blood–brain barrier integrity, subsequently leading to neuroinflammation and cell death [3]. Likewise, Appelgren et al. found the presence of NETs to strongly correlate with the presence of pleocytosis and neutrophil-stimulating cytokines/chemokines in cerebrospinal fluid samples collected from pediatric and adult patients with Lyme neuroborreliosis, Lyme disease, tick-borne encephalitis, enteroviral meningitis, and other viral infections [4].

Infection by *Plasmodium* during malaria results in the formation of the insoluble crystalline pigment hemozoin by digestion of hemoglobin in red blood cells. Rupture of red blood cells releases hemozoin crystals into the circulation from where it is usually cleared by neutrophils. A wide range of crystalline particles have been demonstrated to induce NETs formation [5–7]. In this issue, Lautenschlager et al. demonstrate that engulfment of hemozoin crystals by neutrophils is regulated by crystal–platelet interactions as well as plasma proteins such as fibrinogen, where the latter inhibits crystal uptake and clearance from the extracellular space [8]. Surprisingly, unlike many other crystalline particles, the ingestion of hemozoin crystals by neutrophils does not induce NETs formation [8]. Next, Estúa-Acosta et al. challenge the idea that the eye is an immune-privileged organ and provide evidence

of NETs and their implication in pathophysiology in infectious keratitis, the leading cause of monocular blindness as well as non-infectious eye diseases [9]. Meanwhile, Magán-Fernández et al. summarize the current knowledge about the role of NETs in the pathogenesis of periodontitis [10]. Infection of the periodontium starts with the accumulation of a complex bacterial biofilm that induces dysbiosis between the gingival microbiome and the immune response of the host, which involves impaired NET formation and/or elimination [10]. Furthermore, the formation of biofilms promotes the efficient growth of pathogenic bacteria and fungi by providing optimal local environmental conditions and increased protection against the immune system [11]. The functional properties of the biofilm are regulated by a cell-to-cell communication system, called quorum sensing, which involves numerous quorum sensing-related molecules [11]. In this issue, Zawrotniak et al. define one quorum sensing molecule of *Candida albicans*, i.e., farnesol, that is capable of inducing NET formation, a process sensing the infection to the host immune system early and to limit spreading of the fungal infection [12].

The novel severe acute respiratory syndrome coronavirus (SARS-CoV)-2 infection, named COVID-19, is characterized by neutrophilia and increased neutrophil-to-lymphocyte ratio [13]. In this issue, we propose that continuous infiltration of neutrophils and NETs formation to the site of infection and at sites of organ injury drive necroinflammation and contribute to organ failure such as acute respiratory distress syndrome. NETs also contribute to cytokine storm and sepsis development as well as to the formation of endothelial injury and microvascular thrombosis during COVID-19 [14].

3. Neutrophils and NETs in Sterile Inflammation

Besides infections, neutrophils and NETs also play a critical role in the development of sterile inflammation in several chronic inflammatory conditions. In this issue, Manda-Handzlik and Demkow discuss the contribution of NETs in different pathological conditions affecting the central nervous system, e.g., trauma, neurodegeneration, and autoimmune diseases [3]. Estúa-Acosta et al. discuss the contribution of NETs in eye physiology, e.g., eye rheum formation as well as pathophysiological conditions, e.g., dry eye disease, corneal injuries like alkali burn, uveitis, diabetic retinopathy, and age-related macular degeneration [9]. Interestingly, the same mechanism was found to be responsible for uveitis in large animals. Fingerhut et al. demonstrate the presence of NETs in the vitreous body fluids derived from the eyes of horses with recurrent uveitis [15].

Furthermore, Bonaventura et al. emphasize the pathogenic roles of NETs in the initiation and progression of cardiovascular diseases e.g., acute myocardial infarction, diabetes, and obesity involving activation of the NLRP3 inflammasome and thrombosis [16]. They also highlight the need for standardized nomenclature and standardized techniques for NET assessment and novel therapies targeting NETs [16]. Neutrophils and NETs also contribute to the development of liver diseases [17,18]. In this issue, Zhou et al. decipher the molecular mechanisms of neutrophil chemotaxis and NETosis in murine chronic liver injury. They demonstrate that the cannabinoid receptor 1 mediates neutrophil chemotaxis and NETosis via the $G\alpha_{i/o}$/ROS/p38 MAPK signaling pathway in liver inflammation [19]. Above and beyond, cancer cells have been shown to induce NETs formation to support metastasis [20]. Decker et al., in this issue, evaluated the correlation between NETosis and disease progression during head and neck cancer [21]. They observe neutrophils from head and neck cancer patients and show increased NETosis in patients at an early stage compared to that of late-stage or healthy controls. Therefore, elevated NETosis can be used as a biomarker for the prognosis of the disease [21]. Consistent with this, Fousert et al. also propose NETs as promising biomarkers for autoimmune diseases since they contribute to the development of autoimmunity by breaking self-tolerance [22]. They further conclude that therapeutics targeted at neutrophils and NETs will be beneficial for the treatment of inflammatory autoimmune diseases [22].

4. Perspective

It is becoming evident that studying NETs reveals novel insights into the pathogenesis of many diseases. Whether or not NETs can also be a potential therapeutic target remains unclear at this

point. Animal studies have demonstrated that inhibiting certain signaling pathways can prevent NETs formation, can enhance NETs clearance, or at least, cleave the externalized chromatin, which accounts for many of the pathogenic effects of NETs. However, whether such interventions will prove efficacious and safe in human disease settings remains to be demonstrated. The first clinical trials are testing the effects of nebulized Dornase, a recombinant form of DNAse I that cleaves extracellular NETs chromatin, in mechanically ventilated patients with severe COVID-19 (NCT04432987, NCT04359654, NCT04402970) or severe trauma (NCT03368092) as an attempt to reduce NETs-related respiratory failure. Positive data of such trials may encourage clinical trials with NETs-targeting interventions also in other clinical domains. We hope that the readers of this *Cells* issue enjoy the scientific content and feel inspired to continue research in this evolving domain for a better understanding of disease and hopefully also, for better treatment options for NETs-related disorders in the future.

Author Contributions: Both authors have made a substantial, direct, and intellectual contribution to the work, and approved it for publication. All authors have read and agreed to the published version of the manuscript.

Funding: S.R.M. acknowledges the financial support from the Ramalingaswami Fellowship of the Department of Biotechnology, Government of India (BT/RLF/Re-entry/01/2017), and the Council of Scientific and Industrial Research (CSIR)—Central Drug Research Institute (CDRI). H.-J.A. acknowledges the financial support from the Deutsche Forschungsgemeinschaft (DFG) (AN372/16-2, 20-2, 23-1, 24-1).

Conflicts of Interest: The authors declare no conflict of interest.

References

1. Papayannopoulos, V. Neutrophil extracellular traps in immunity and disease. *Nat. Rev. Immunol.* **2018**, *18*, 134–147. [CrossRef]
2. Skendros, P.; Mitsios, A.; Chrysanthopoulou, A.; Mastellos, D.C.; Metallidis, S.; Rafailidis, P.; Ntinopoulou, M.; Sertaridou, E.; Tsironidou, V.; Tsigalou, C.; et al. Complement and tissue factor-enriched neutrophil extracellular traps are key drivers in COVID-19 immunothrombosis. *J. Clin. Investig.* **2020**. [CrossRef]
3. Manda-Handzlik, A.; Demkow, U. The Brain Entangled: The Contribution of Neutrophil Extracellular Traps to the Diseases of the Central Nervous System. *Cells* **2019**, *8*, 1477. [CrossRef]
4. Appelgren, D.; Enocsson, H.; Skogman, B.H.; Nordberg, M.; Perander, L.; Nyman, D.; Nyberg, C.; Knopf, J.; Munoz, L.E.; Sjowall, C.; et al. Neutrophil Extracellular Traps (NETs) in the Cerebrospinal Fluid Samples from Children and Adults with Central Nervous System Infections. *Cells* **2019**, *9*, 43. [CrossRef]
5. Mulay, S.R.; Anders, H.J. Crystallopathies. *N. Engl. J. Med.* **2016**, *374*, 2465–2476. [CrossRef]
6. Desai, J.; Foresto-Neto, O.; Honarpisheh, M.; Steiger, S.; Nakazawa, D.; Popper, B.; Buhl, E.M.; Boor, P.; Mulay, S.R.; Anders, H.J. Particles of different sizes and shapes induce neutrophil necroptosis followed by the release of neutrophil extracellular trap-like chromatin. *Sci. Rep.* **2017**, *7*, 15003. [CrossRef]
7. Mulay, S.R.; Steiger, S.; Shi, C.; Anders, H.J. A guide to crystal-related and nano- or microparticle-related tissue responses. *FEBS J.* **2020**, *287*, 818–832. [CrossRef] [PubMed]
8. Lautenschlager, S.O.S.; Kim, T.; Bidoia, D.L.; Nakamura, C.V.; Anders, H.J.; Steiger, S. Plasma Proteins and Platelets Modulate Neutrophil Clearance of Malaria-Related Hemozoin Crystals. *Cells* **2019**, *9*, 93. [CrossRef] [PubMed]
9. Estua-Acosta, G.A.; Zamora-Ortiz, R.; Buentello-Volante, B.; Garcia-Mejia, M.; Garfias, Y. Neutrophil Extracellular Traps: Current Perspectives in the Eye. *Cells* **2019**, *8*, 979. [CrossRef] [PubMed]
10. Magan-Fernandez, A.; Rasheed Al-Bakri, S.M.; O'Valle, F.; Benavides-Reyes, C.; Abadia-Molina, F.; Mesa, F. Neutrophil Extracellular Traps in Periodontitis. *Cells* **2020**, *9*, 1494. [CrossRef] [PubMed]
11. Dal Co, A.; Brenner, M.P. Tracing cell trajectories in a biofilm. *Science* **2020**, *369*, 30–31. [CrossRef] [PubMed]
12. Zawrotniak, M.; Wojtalik, K.; Rapala-Kozik, M. Farnesol, a Quorum-Sensing Molecule of Candida Albicans Triggers the Release of Neutrophil Extracellular Traps. *Cells* **2019**, *8*, 1611. [CrossRef] [PubMed]
13. Huang, C.; Wang, Y.; Li, X.; Ren, L.; Zhao, J.; Hu, Y.; Zhang, L.; Fan, G.; Xu, J.; Gu, X.; et al. Clinical features of patients infected with 2019 novel coronavirus in Wuhan, China. *Lancet* **2020**, *395*, 497–506. [CrossRef]
14. Tomar, B.; Anders, H.J.; Desai, J.; Mulay, S.R. Neutrophils and Neutrophil Extracellular Traps Drive Necroinflammation in COVID-19. *Cells* **2020**, *9*, 1383. [CrossRef] [PubMed]

15. Fingerhut, L.; Ohnesorge, B.; von Borstel, M.; Schumski, A.; Strutzberg-Minder, K.; Morgelin, M.; Deeg, C.A.; Haagsman, H.P.; Beineke, A.; von Kockritz-Blickwede, M.; et al. Neutrophil Extracellular Traps in the Pathogenesis of Equine Recurrent Uveitis (ERU). *Cells* **2019**, *8*, 1528. [CrossRef] [PubMed]

16. Bonaventura, A.; Vecchie, A.; Abbate, A.; Montecucco, F. Neutrophil Extracellular Traps and Cardiovascular Diseases: An Update. *Cells* **2020**, *9*, 231. [CrossRef] [PubMed]

17. Xu, R.; Huang, H.; Zhang, Z.; Wang, F.S. The role of neutrophils in the development of liver diseases. *Cell Mol. Immunol.* **2014**, *11*, 224–231. [CrossRef]

18. Meijenfeldt, F.A.V.; Jenne, C.N. Netting Liver Disease: Neutrophil Extracellular Traps in the Initiation and Exacerbation of Liver Pathology. *Semin. Thromb. Hemost.* **2020**, *46*, 724–734. [CrossRef]

19. Zhou, X.; Yang, L.; Fan, X.; Zhao, X.; Chang, N.; Yang, L.; Li, L. Neutrophil Chemotaxis and NETosis in Murine Chronic Liver Injury via Cannabinoid Receptor 1/ Galphai/o/ ROS/ p38 MAPK Signaling Pathway. *Cells* **2020**, *9*, 373. [CrossRef]

20. Park, J.; Wysocki, R.W.; Amoozgar, Z.; Maiorino, L.; Fein, M.R.; Jorns, J.; Schott, A.F.; Kinugasa-Katayama, Y.; Lee, Y.; Won, N.H.; et al. Cancer cells induce metastasis-supporting neutrophil extracellular DNA traps. *Sci. Transl. Med.* **2016**, *8*, 361ra138. [CrossRef]

21. Decker, A.S.; Pylaeva, E.; Brenzel, A.; Spyra, I.; Droege, F.; Hussain, T.; Lang, S.; Jablonska, J. Prognostic Role of Blood NETosis in the Progression of Head and Neck Cancer. *Cells* **2019**, *8*, 946. [CrossRef] [PubMed]

22. Fousert, E.; Toes, R.; Desai, J. Neutrophil Extracellular Traps (NETs) Take the Central Stage in Driving Autoimmune Responses. *Cells* **2020**, *9*, 915. [CrossRef] [PubMed]

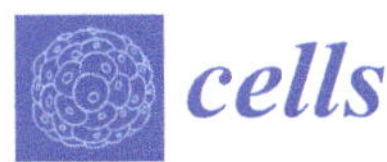 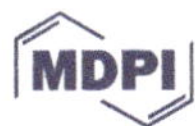

Review

The Brain Entangled: The Contribution of Neutrophil Extracellular Traps to the Diseases of the Central Nervous System

Aneta Manda-Handzlik [1,2,*] and Urszula Demkow [1]

1   Department of Laboratory Diagnostics and Clinical Immunology of Developmental Age, Medical University of Warsaw, 02-091 Warsaw, Poland; urszula.demkow@litewska.edu.pl
2   Postgraduate School of Molecular Medicine, Medical University of Warsaw, 02-091 Warsaw, Poland
*   Correspondence: aneta.manda-handzlik@wum.edu.pl

Received: 30 October 2019; Accepted: 18 November 2019; Published: 21 November 2019

Abstract: Under normal conditions, neutrophils are restricted from trafficking into the brain parenchyma and cerebrospinal fluid by the presence of the brain–blood barrier (BBB). Yet, infiltration of the central nervous system (CNS) by neutrophils is a well-known phenomenon in the course of different pathological conditions, e.g., infection, trauma or neurodegeneration. Different studies have shown that neutrophil products, i.e., free oxygen radicals and proteolytic enzymes, play an important role in the pathogenesis of BBB damage. It was recently observed that accumulating granulocytes may release neutrophil extracellular traps (NETs), which damage the BBB and directly injure surrounding neurons. In this review, we discuss the emerging role of NETs in various pathological conditions affecting the CNS.

Keywords: neutrophil extracellular traps (NETs); Alzheimer's disease; multiple sclerosis; ischemic stroke; meningitis; central nervous system; brain; neurons; brain–blood barrier; neutrophils

---

1. Neutrophils in the Central Nervous System (CNS)

Neutrophils, crucial cells of innate immunity, are scarce in the central nervous system (CNS) under normal conditions. They are restricted from trafficking into the brain parenchyma and cerebrospinal fluid (CSF) by the presence of the brain–blood barrier (BBB). Tight junctions between brain endothelial cells ensure barrier integrity and high selectivity [1–3]. Yet, the infiltration of the CNS by neutrophils in various pathological conditions, e.g., infection, trauma, brain ischemia, neurodegeneration or autoimmunity, is a well-known phenomenon. Different studies have shown that neutrophil products, i.e., free oxygen radicals and proteolytic enzymes including matrix metalloproteinase 9 (MMP-9), play an important role in the pathogenesis of BBB damage [4,5]. It was recently observed that accumulating granulocytes may also release extracellular web-like structures composed of DNA and proteins called neutrophil extracellular traps (NETs), which damage the BBB and account for subsequent injury of surrounding neurons and other cells of the brain [1,6].

2. Neutrophil Extracellular Traps (NETs) in Physiology and Pathology

Although the term "NETs" was coined, and their biological relevance was discovered, by the Zychlinsky group in 2004 [7], it is worth noting that an atypical form of neutrophil death following stimulation with phorbol 12-myristate 13-acetate was identified almost a decade earlier by Takei et al. [8]. Current consensus is that NET release is a highly variable phenomenon, either accompanied by cell survival or ultimately eliciting lytic cell death [9]. Furthermore, the NET backbone can be composed of DNA of nuclear, mitochondrial or both origins [9,10]. An abundance of studies has revealed a broad spectrum of NET targets—including bacteria, parasites, fungi and viruses [11]. Currently, it is widely accepted that the major role of NETs is to entrap and immobilize pathogens, preventing an infection from spreading [7], but much more controversy has arisen around the pathogen-killing properties of NETs [12]. Regardless of the direct effect of NETs on pathogens' viability, the release of these structures constitutes an efficient antimicrobial strategy. However, it should be underlined that an overabundance of lytic, cytotoxic proteins (including histones, neutrophil elastase (NE) and defensins) and autoantigens (such as DNA, histones, myeloperoxidase (MPO) and proteinase 3) in NETs may have dramatic consequences for the host. The disturbance between NET formation and clearance has thus been implicated in a number of various diseases, both systemic and limited to a certain organ or tissue. For example, excessive formation of NETs contributes to the pathogenesis of psoriasis, systemic lupus erythematosus, diabetes, cystic fibrosis, and cancer [13–17]. As mentioned above, it has been also recognized that NETs can be implicated in brain disorders and other pathological conditions affecting the CNS. In this review, we summarize the current state-of-the-art regarding the role of NETs in neurological pathologies.

3. NETs in Ischemic Stroke

Acute brain injury, including ischemic stroke, always initiates local inflammation in the CNS. A key hallmark of neuroinflammation is damage of the BBB and transmigration of immune cells into the brain, leading to neuronal death. Animal studies proved that ischemic areas of the brain are infiltrated by neutrophils within a few hours after the onset of experimental ischemia [18–21]. Neutrophils are attracted by chemical mediators and damage-associated molecular patterns arising from sterile inflammation invoked by ischemia–reperfusion. Locally produced interleukin (IL)-1 plays a crucial role in this process. IL-1 is responsible for the recruitment and transmigration of neutrophils across damaged BBB [6] (Figure 1). Further activation of these cells in inflamed tissues of the brain is connected with profound changes of their phenotype and release of decondensed DNA threads decorated with extracellular proteases [6]. Accordingly, Perez-Puig et al. described the presence of citrullinated histone 3, a hallmark of NET formation, in the ischemic brain after 24 h ischemia [22]. Positive staining for citrullinated histone 3 was observed in neutrophils expressing typical features of cells undergoing NET release (decondensation of nuclear chromatin) [22]. Neutrophils with characteristic phenotypic changes were found in the lumen of capillaries, in perivascular spaces, in the brain parenchyma nearby blood vessels, and surrounding pericytes, suggesting that NETs might contribute to the damage of the BBB. Additional examination of brain tissue from patients who died from stroke revealed co-localization of MPO and NE in neutrophils found in perivascular spaces [22]. Other authors described the presence of decondensed DNA released from neutrophils in the inflammatory brain lesions of experimental animals [23].

On the one hand, local NETs formation is believed to protect injured brain from further bacterial attack. On the other hand, the inflammatory milieu exerts direct neurotoxic effects. Allen et al. observed that transmigrated neutrophils co-locate with neurons [6]. A number of highly significant associations were found between neuronal loss after ischemic stroke and neutrophil transmigration. Allen et al. [6] showed in vitro that transmigrated neutrophils cultured with neurons for 3 h significantly decreased neuronal viability. This effect was not abrogated by DNase treatment of conditioned medium from transmigrated granulocytes; thus, a decrease of neuronal viability was not attributable to extracellular DNA. Furthermore, the inhibition of neutrophil-derived extracellular proteases associated with NETs significantly decreased neutrophil-mediated neurotoxicity. Interestingly, the key neutrophilic proteases, cathepsin-G, NE, proteinase-3 and MMP-9, seem to collectively attack neurons as shown in experiments when a mixture of their inhibitors, but not any single specific inhibitor, nearly completely reversed the neutrophil-dependent neurotoxic effect [6]. Altogether, these authors identified a novel neuroinflammatory mechanism: the development of rapid neurotoxicity of neutrophils initiated by IL-1–induced cerebrovascular transmigration. Consistently, Allen et al. proved that rapidly developed (30 min) neutrophil-dependent neurotoxicity is mediated by neutrophil-derived proteases released upon degranulation or associated with NETs. Accordingly, these authors proposed a new therapeutic strategy against neuronal death in the course of brain injury, based on blockade of IL-1. Such an approach is believed to protect the brain from NET-dependent neurotoxicity [6].

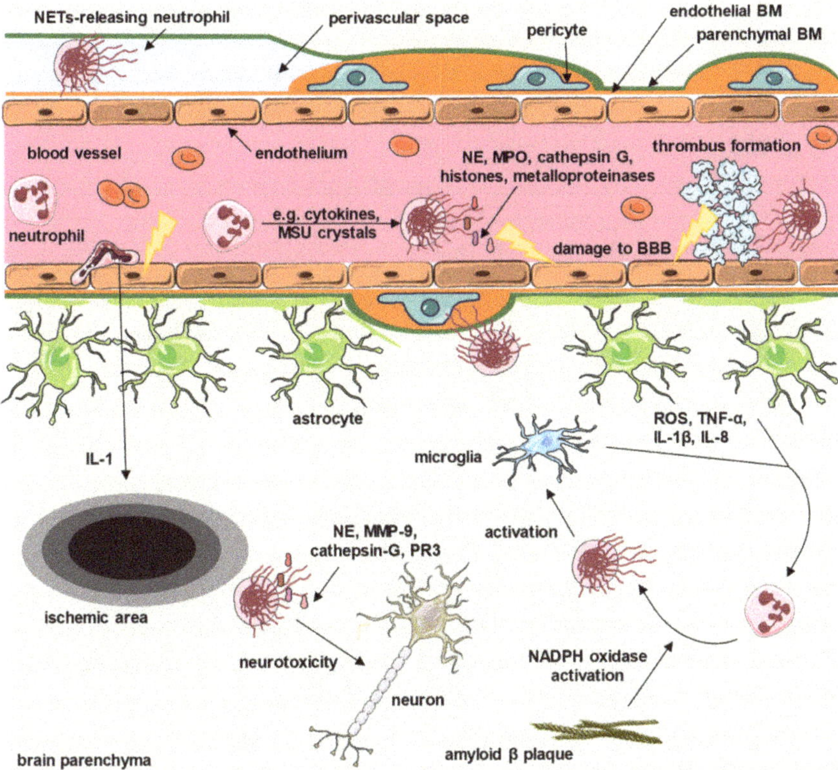

Figure 1. Proposed contribution of neutrophil extracellular traps (NETs) to central nervous system diseases. Depending on the underlying disease, various factors (cytokines, amyloid β plaques, reactive oxygen species (ROS), monosodium urate (MSU) crystals and others) activate granulocytes to release NETs. Intravascular NETs activate the coagulation cascade and enhance formation of thrombi, and also carry cytotoxic proteins that directly damage the brain–blood barrier (BBB). Extravasated granulocytes release NETs within perivascular spaces, as well as within brain parenchyma. NETs exert neurotoxic effects and activate microglia, which further enhances NET release. BM—basement membrane, PR3—proteinase 3, MMP-9—matrix metalloproteinase 9, TNF-α—tumor necrosis factor α, IL—interleukin, NE—neutrophil elastase, MPO—myeloperoxidase, NADPH—the reduced form of nicotinamide adenine dinucleotide phosphate. This figure contains elements available at Servier Medical Art repository, licensed under a Creative Commons Attribution 3.0 Unported License.

Further, it was proven that in the course of brain ischemia, web-like structures formed inside and around capillaries enhance thrombus formation (Figure 1). We can hypothesize that histones are crucial thrombogenic components of NETs because it was shown that extracellular histones are potent stimuli for thrombin generation in vitro [24,25]. Examination of thrombi retrieved from the brain circulation of ischemic stroke patients revealed the presence of DNA and citrullinated histone 3 scaffold [22,26,27]. This secondary thrombosis further contributes to the prolongation of the period of ischemia. It is believed that NET formation may be responsible for the no-reflow phenomenon, closing the time window for thrombolytic therapy [22]. This result suggests that intravascular decondensed DNA fibers may play a previously unanticipated role in the resistance to fibrinolytic therapy. Recanalization in patients with acute ischemic stroke is achieved only in less than a half of the patients who receive tissue plasminogen activator (t-PA) within hours of the onset of symptoms. In accord with these observations, t-PA resistance may be attributed to the formation of NET scaffolds enclosing platelets and activating the intrinsic coagulation pathway. Therefore, it has been speculated that NETs promote secondary microthrombosis [22]. It was reported that older thrombi are rich in citrullinated histone 3 and positive for NE, the key hallmarks of NETs, compared to fresh thrombi [28]. These observations may help to devise novel approaches to widen the therapeutic window for fibrinolysis in order to prevent permanent neurological damage of patients with stroke. This conclusion corresponds with the findings that DNase 1 improved the therapeutic efficacy of t-PA [28]. Given the low-cost and safety of DNase 1, which is already FDA-approved for cystic fibrosis therapy, it could, in combination with fibrinolytic therapy, significantly improve the outcome of ischemic stroke patients [28].

Finally NETs are believed to account for the development of stroke-induced systemic immunosuppression [5,29]. Activated granulocytes releasing NETs decrease the T lymphocyte activation threshold in vitro [30]. Even though NETs play a role in the upregulation of CD25 and CD69, and the phosphorylation of the TCR-associated signaling kinase ZAP70, these effects are not associated with the proliferation of CD4+ T cells [30]. Further studies are warranted to discern alternative links between NETs and systemic immunosuppression in the course of ischemic stroke [5].

4. Neurodegeneration

Chronic neurodegenerative diseases including Alzheimer's disease (AD), Parkinson's disease (PD) and the prion-associated diseases (PAS) are not typically assigned to neuroinflammatory conditions, however some specialists consistently highlight the links between these disorders and the local innate immune response [1]. For example, Zenaro et al. provided evidence that netting neutrophils contribute to the pathogenesis of Alzheimer's disease (AD) [31]. AD is a neurodegenerative disease characterized by progressive cognitive impairment and memory loss. The most consistent neuropathological feature of an AD brain is the presence of neuritic plaques consisting of amyloid-β and neurofibrillary tangles formed by aggregates of hyperphosphorylated tau-protein. A convincing body of evidence supports the inflammatory background of AD and several subpopulations of blood-derived white blood cells, including neutrophils, have been found in the brains of these patients [32–35]. Recent studies by Prof. Constantin's group highlighted that neutrophils transmigrated into brain parenchyma accumulate in close proximity to amyloid-β plaques, as amyloid-β triggers neutrophils' adhesion to the endothelium and provides a stop signal to crawling cells [31]. Both intravascular adhesion and migration of neutrophils inside the parenchyma in the areas with amyloid-β plaques are controlled by LFA-1 integrin. Strikingly, neutrophils inside the cortical vessels and brain parenchyma released NETs both in transgenic mouse models of AD as well as in individuals with AD. This observation suggested that neuronal injury and damage to the BBB in AD can be at least partially caused by the detrimental effect of NETs on the vessel wall and surrounding tissues. Same authors, in a comprehensive review paper, proposed plausible explanations for the role of NETs in AD pathology [36]. Pietronigro et al. provided evidence for the presence of NETs in the brain capillaries and tissue of AD mice. These results point to the fact that local NET formation may contribute to local BBB damage and loss of neurons in AD [36]. Importantly, endothelial cortical cells in AD subjects are characterized by increased expression of adhesion molecules and production of pro-inflammatory cytokines, such as tumor necrosis factor (TNF-α), IL-8 and IL-1β [37,38]. Adhesion of granulocytes to activated vasculature may stimulate neutrophils to produce reactive oxygen species (ROS) and favour the release of NETs, presumably with the contribution of activated platelets via intercellular adhesion molecule (ICAM)-2 and the lymphocyte function-associated antigen (LFA)-1 interaction. As previously described, intravascular NETs promote thrombosis, which further exacerbates brain microvessel pathology [36]. Furthermore, intravascular NETs can cause direct toxic effects to the endothelium due to the release of proteolytic proteins, such as NE, metalloproteinases (MMPs) and cathepsin G (Figure 1). NE and MMPs are implicated in the disruption of junctional complexes and endothelial cell retraction. NE itself increases endothelial cell permeability, whilst MPO and histones induce endothelial cell death [39–41]. Above all, histones have been identified as major NET-associated proteins that induce cell death [24]. Altogether, NETs may represent an important player involved in the loss of BBB integrity. On the other hand, activated glial cells within the parenchyma initiate a vicious cycle, encompassing neutrophils crawling towards amyloid-β plaques. It is suggested that mediators produced by microglial cells and astrocytes, such as ROS, TNFα, IL-1β and IL-8, can easily activate neutrophils to form NETs, which in turn further activate glial cells [36,42]. What is more, amyloid-β activates NADPH oxidase, a key enzyme participating in NET release [43]. Amyloid-β plaques in line with netting neutrophils are postulated to constitute another feedback loop amplifying neuroinflammation [36]. NET constituents can be harmful to neural cells within brain parenchyma, as they proteolytically cleave extracellular matrix proteins, activate inflammasome pathways and the mitochondrial apoptosis pathway [36,44–46].

Although NET release seems to provide a sound explanation for many aspects of AD neuroinflammation, the role of NETs in this disease has been recently acknowledged and requires further rooting in experimental data before NETs can be used as a target of AD therapy. It would also be interesting to identify whether NETs induce the generation of autoantibodies in AD and whether they could constitute an AD biomarker [36].

5. Autoimmune Diseases

As early as in the very first report on the phenomenon of NET release, it was recognized that NETs expose intracellular antigens and may contribute to the development of autoimmune diseases [7]. Indeed, NETs have been implicated in numerous autoimmune conditions, including systemic autoimmune diseases that may affect the central and peripheral nervous system, as well as neural antigen-specific autoimmunity [11]. For example, elevated levels of circulating NET formation markers were identified in multiple sclerosis (MS). MS is a progressive neurodegenerative disorder with a strong autoinflammatory background, characterized by spatiotemporally separated multifocal demyelination and perivascular inflammation within the CNS [47]. Early studies on circulating NET markers in MS patients argued against a key role of NETs in the pathogenesis of this disease, since only a subset of relapsing remitting MS patients exhibited significant formation of NETs in vivo [48]. Intriguingly, although the level of MPO-DNA complexes did not correlate with disease activity in MS patients, they were more abundant in males than in females, suggesting that the variability in NET release may account for sex-specific differences in MS pathogenesis. NETs were not detected in CSF samples of MS patients, which corresponds with previous reports pointing to the absence of neutrophils within the CNS of MS patients. Yet, it was suggested that cytotoxic components of NETs may contribute to BBB damage in this disease [48] (Figure 1). The putative role of neutrophils and NETs in MS pathogenesis is further supported by data from experimental autoimmune encephalomyelitis (EAE), a model for MS [49,50]. As an example, it has been well documented that NETs activate inflammatory T helper 17 (Th17) cells to produce their signature, neutrophil-recruiting cytokine, interleukin-17 (IL-17) [51,52]. Notably, interfering with neutrophil–IL-17 interactions significantly reduces severity and delays the onset of EAE [53]. Similarly, the IL-17 level is elevated in CSF in MS patients and correlates with neutrophil expansion in CSF as well as with damage to the BBB [54]. Furthermore, EAE is alleviated and BBB function is re-established by depleting NET-associated proteins such as MPO and NE [55,56]. Rodent models of autoimmune CNS disorders provide data that corresponds well with observations in humans. Strikingly, the increased plasma levels of NE in MS patients are associated with clinical disability and lesion burden [57]. All aforementioned premises constitute a solid background for the proposed contribution of NET release to MS pathogenesis, but the functional link between these two phenomena is still far from being elucidated [58]. Accordingly, current studies focus on an in-depth analysis of the role of NETs and their constituents in MS-related inflammation [58,59].

NETs have been also implicated in neuropsychiatric manifestations of SLE. Tay et al. suggested a model of cognitive dysfunction in SLE that assumes that neutrophil activation, transmigration and subsequent intrathecal NET release could be a consequence of cerebral endothelium activation by anti-NR2A/B (anti-*N*-methyl-D-aspartate receptor subunit NR2A/B) autoantibodies. As a consequence, NETs formed within the brain parenchyma promote neuronal cell death, leading to cognitive impairment in SLE patients [60].

Finally, it should be noted that although previous research has focused primarily on NET formation within the CNS, these structures were also identified in histological material from peripheral nerves of patients with other systemic autoimmune diseases [61].

6. CNS Infections

CNS infections, such as meningitis or encephalitis, can be caused by various pathogens including bacteria, viruses, parasites and fungi. These devastating conditions, resulting from a local failure of the immune response mechanism, may ultimately lead to irreversible brain damage. Although the contribution of neutrophils to brain infections has been investigated for decades, the discovery of NETs provided new insights in the field by identification of a new player with a previously unanticipated role in these disorders. Nevertheless, a clear role of NETs in the infected CSF compartment and in brain tissue is still far from being elucidated. Lumbar puncture followed by the examination of CSF from patients with bacterial meningitis reveals massive transmigration of neutrophils across the BBB [62]. Other authors observed intensive infiltration of neutrophils in leptomeningitis and intraparenchymal vasculitis [63–65]. Recent literature reports that NETs are formed in the CSF of patients with pneumococcal meningitis, but not in viral meningitis, CNS borreliosis and subarachnoid haemorrhage [65,66]. In vitro culture of human neutrophils with bacteria isolated from meningitis patients (*S. pneumoniae, N. meningitidis, L. monocytogenes, S. aureus, E. coli, A. baumanii, S. oralis, S. capitis* and *S. epidermidis*) revealed that all except *L. monocytogenes* induced NETs [66]. Shotgun proteomic analysis of the CSF from patients with meningitis confirmed the presence of NET-related proteins, such as MPO, NE, proteinase-3 (PR3), cathelicidin LL-37, MMP-9, heparin binding protein (HBP), neutrophil gelatinase-associated lipocalin (NGAL), and histones [66]. Mohanty et al. also detected the presence of NETs in the CSF from rats with pneumococcal meningitis [66]. In order to shed light on the role of NETs in the pathogenesis of meningitis, these authors performed a set of experiments using a rat meningitis and an in vitro model, attempting to degrade NETs with DNase I. They discovered that DNase I significantly cleared bacteria in affected organs (lungs, brain, spleen) and decreased bacterial viability in the presence of neutrophils in vitro. The eradication of bacteria from the brain of DNase-treated rats correlated with the decrease of IL-1β levels. This effect was abrogated by inhibitors of phagocytosis, NADPH oxidase and MPO, confirming the role of phagocytosis and oxidative stress as bactericidal mechanisms in meningitis. Accordingly, NETs participate in the detrimental response to *S. pneumonia* infection, promoting pneumococcal survival in the brain by protecting them from phagocytosis and killing by bactericidal factors. Previously Beiter et al. also observed that pneumococci are entrapped but not killed by NETs [67]. These observations correspond with the findings of the clinical study performed by Tillet et al., who noted a 26% decline in mortality from pneumococcal meningitis after addition of DNase to penicillin therapy [68]. Studies detailing the NET-evading mechanisms proved that pneumococci can produce nucleases or modify the cell surface to avoid NET-mediated killing and to further disseminate to other organs [67,69,70]. Another strain of bacteria with the ability to survive in NETs is methicillin-resistant *S. aureus* [71]. Studies by Mohanty et al. [66] highlighted the complex interplay between various inflammatory mechanisms, including NETs, during pneumococcal meningitis.

In the course of bacterial sepsis, the presence of NETs has been demonstrated in the blood. As described previously, circulating NETs activate the coagulation system, increasing viscosity and changing the rheological properties of the blood [72]. Accordingly, changes in CSF hydrodynamics, as a consequence of NET generation in the CSF compartment, may hinder CSF circulation leading to the development of oedema and increased intracranial pressure [73].

Further study addressing the major role of NETs and NET-degrading DNAses in meningitis was undertaken by de Buhr et al. [65]. These authors demonstrated the presence of NETs in *S. suis* meningitis despite the activity of both host and bacterial DNases in the CSF of infected piglets. Furthermore, de Buhr et al. used an in vitro model of *S. suis*-infected human choroid plexus epithelial cells to examine NET formation and degradation. They found that transmigrated granulocytes vigorously released NETs in the "CSF compartment" to entrap *S. suis* bacteria. These web-like structures were not degraded by two pathogen DNases: SsnA and EndAsuis, previously shown to degrade NETs in vitro [74,75]. In line with these observations, the authors identified two host antimicrobial proteins: human and porcine cathelicidins (respectively, LL-37 and PR-39), which may stabilize NETs and protect them from degradation.

Like many other mechanisms of the immune response, NETs can be both detrimental and protective. Aforementioned studies by de Buhr et al. and Mohanty et al. highlight the diverging effects of NET release in CNS [65,66]. Remarkably, some pathogens become entrapped in NETs to prevent an infection from spreading [65], while others benefit from spatial support provided by these three-dimensional structures and easily become disseminated [66].

Besides meningitis, NETs exert a detrimental effect on BBB integrity and toxicity towards neurons in other infectious diseases affecting CNS. For example, NETs have been proposed to contribute to the loss of BBB integrity in the course of cerebral malaria [76]. Infected red blood cells rupture and release precipitated uric acid (monosodium urate, MSU) crystals, which constitute a potent inducer of NETs [77,78] (Figure 1). Importantly, circulating NETs entrapping parasites were identified in the vasculature of children infected with *Plasmodium falciparum* [79]. As mentioned before, NET fibers may provide a scaffold for the activation of the coagulation cascade, which on one hand protects endothelial cells from damage by MSU crystals, but on the other hand reduces blood flow to end organs, or, in the worst-case scenario, completely abrogates perfusion or triggers disseminated intravascular coagulation. Concurrent processes of NET release and thrombus formation result in the production of inflammatory factors, which compromise BBB integrity and lead to the development of cerebral malaria, being the most severe neurological complication of malaria infection [76,80].

7. Peripheral Diseases with Infiltration of Central Nervous System by Neutrophils

Several lines of evidence have indicated that peripheral (e.g., cancer outside the CNS) or systemic diseases, such as sepsis, may result in neuroinflammation and accumulation of myeloid cells in the CNS [81–84]. Furthermore, diseases primary affecting organs other than the brain, might present with neurological manifestations. For example, cancer patients with a tumor localized outside the CNS, are often characterized by fatigue, tremors, gait disorders, visual disturbances, motor and sensory deficits, as well as cognitive dysfunction, developing prior to cancer diagnosis/therapy [84–86]. Yet, exact mechanisms of CNS-mediated cancer symptoms have not been well understood so far. The importance of the aforementioned observations has been recently underscored by Burfeind et al., who identified neutrophils as key role players promoting neuroinflammation and the occurrence of neurological symptoms in a murine model of pancreatic ductal adenocarcinoma (PDAC) [84]. The authors demonstrated that myeloid cells (with neutrophils as the predominant type of infiltrating cells) were recruited to the brain early in the course of malignancy and this was mediated by the chemokine receptor type 2 (CCR2)/C-C motif chemokine ligand 2 (CCL2) axis. Granulocytes accumulated in the velum interpositum, meninges adjacent to regions regulating behavior, appetite and body composition, degranulated and released NETs identified as threads co-locating MPO and citrullinated histone 3. Furthermore, disturbance of CCR2–CCL2 signaling attenuated neutrophil accumulation and alleviated CNS-driven disorders, such as anorexia and muscle catabolism, observed in mice inoculated with cancer cells [84]. Although the exact role of NET release as a mechanism contributing to neurological disorders in PDAC has not been investigated, future studies are warranted to shed new light on these issues.

8. May NETs Play a Role in the Development of Brain Tumors?

The CNS is a frequent site for different kinds of primary tumors and metastases from distant organs (i.e., lung cancer, breast cancer and melanoma). The most common primary CNS malignancies encompass a wide spectrum of over 150 histologically, molecularly and clinically distinct conditions, including gliomas and non-glial tumors (meningiomas, medulloblastomas) [87]. The brain tumor microenvironment (TME), crucial for the growth and progression of a tumor, is composed of extracellular matrix components, various mediators and cells: endothelial cells, pericytes, fibroblasts and immune cells including neutrophils [88]. TME is a critical regulator of cancer progression and the response to therapy, thus it may exert a pro-or anti-tumorigenic effect [89]. The observations of both human and animal brain tumors showed that neutrophils are crucial players in TME. These cells are able to cross the BBB and brain-tumor barrier (BTB) to infiltrate the tumor [90,91]. They are attracted to the TME by numerous chemotactic factors, such as IL-8, TNF and CCL2, released by malignant or surrounding cells [92]. Tumor-associated neutrophils (TANs) in the brain release mediators that further attract new populations of neutrophils. These cells have been shown to become activated and to modulate tumor cell motility, migration and invasion [88,93]. For example, TANs show enhanced NADPH (reduced nicotinamide adenine dinucleotide phosphate) oxidase activity, which leads to the production of ROS, especially hydrogen peroxide, which are cytotoxic to tumor cells [94]. Notably, depending on the environmental setting, NET generation may sharply rely on the function of active NADPH oxidase [95,96]. Even though there is no direct experimental evidence on the link between NETs and CNS malignancies, consistent with numerous studies highlighting the prominent role of NETs in tumor growth and metastasis formation in all kind of malignancies, it can be anticipated that NETs in the brain mediate the same effects. Some preliminary evidence indicates that NET-related proteins such as elastase, proteinase-3 and cathepsin G enable invasion of brain tumors by degradation of the extracellular matrix structures [97,98]. Furthermore, the presence of extracellular citrullinated H3 was confirmed in the circulation of cancer patients, including 129 patients with brain tumors. In the case of many other tumors, it was proved that NETs prepare the metastatic niche by entrapping circulating tumor cells [99]. Additionally, NETs promote adhesion of tumor cells to distant organ sites and the presence of NETs in the capillaries of the liver enables the formation of micrometastases in this organ [100,101]. These lines of evidence can indirectly support the hypothesis that NETs may confer similar effects for both primary brain tumors and metastases. A number of highly significant associations were found between neutrophils and the response to therapy of brain malignancies [91,102]. Furthermore, numerous reports point to the negative prognostic value of neutrophil presence and their participation in neuroinflammation in the milieu of brain tumors [91,93,102–105]. As noted above, current evidence only indirectly points to the participation of NETs in the biology of primary and secondary brain tumors, and we must acknowledge that this issue has not been thoroughly studied yet. Accordingly, further intensive studies are warranted in order to explore this issue and to open new possibilities for therapeutic interventions in those detrimental conditions.

9. Conclusions

An increasing body of evidence suggests that NET formation in the CNS might be a common phenomenon, occurring in many brain disorders of various origin. In the present paper, we aimed to describe the role of NETs across a variety of brain disorders driven by a complex of interacting mechanisms. We consider NETs as an element of disease-specific mechanisms; however, in parallel, we have revealed the underlying unity of mechanisms across different brain diseases. A universal, over-arching machinery gives rise to the disruption of BBB integrity and the increase of its permeability, microcirculatory disturbances, vascular leakage, thrombosis, release of proinflammatory cytokines, oxidative stress, neuronal injury and death as well as neuroinflammation. Netting neutrophils have the capacity to actively participate in these cellular and molecular cascades, leading to inflammation and cell death by releasing metalloproteinases, proteases, cytokines, extracellular histones, DNA and ROS. The essentially similar pathogenic mechanisms can diversify over time depending on the initial insult, nature and location of the injury. Further efforts will hopefully address the question of whether this newly recognized relationship between the CNS disorders and NET formation can influence future diagnostic strategies and open novel therapeutic avenues for individuals suffering from the aforementioned conditions.

Author Contributions: A.M.-H.: conception, literature search, figure preparation, writing the initial draft and revising it critically for important intellectual content, final approval of the version to be published; U.D.: conception, literature search, writing the initial draft and revising it critically for important intellectual content, final approval of the version to be published.

Funding: This research received no external funding.

Acknowledgments: AMH is a recipient of a START 2019 Stipend by the Foundation for Polish Science. Figure 1 contains elements available at Servier Medical Art repository, licensed under a Creative Commons Attribution 3.0 Unported License. http://smart.servier.com/.

Conflicts of Interest: The authors declare no conflict of interest.

References

1. Perry, V.H.; Anthony, D.C.; Bolton, S.J.; Brown, H.C. The blood-brain barrier and the inflammatory response. *Mol. Med. Today* **1997**, *3*, 335–341. [CrossRef]

2. Gemechu, M.J.; Bentivoglio, M. T Cell recruitment in the brain during normal aging. *Front. Cell Neurosci.* **2012**, *6*, 38. [CrossRef] [PubMed]

3. Daneman, R.; Prat, A. The blood-brain barrier. *Cold Spring Harb. Perspect. Biol.* **2015**, *7*, a020412. [CrossRef] [PubMed]

4. Matsuo, Y.; Onodera, H.; Shiga, Y.; Nakamura, M.; Ninomiya, M.; Kihara, T.; Kogure, K. Correlation between myeloperoxidase-quantified neutrophil accumulation and ischemic brain injury in the rat: Effects of neutrophil depletion. *Stroke* **1994**, *25*, 1469–1475. [CrossRef]

5. Strecker, K.J.; Schmidt, A.; Schabitz, W.R.; Minnerup, J. Neutrophil granulocytes in cerebral ischemia—Evolution from killers to key players. *Neurochem. Int.* **2017**, *107*, 117–126. [CrossRef]

6. Allen, C.; Thornton, P.; Denes, A.; McColl, B.W.; Pierozynski, A.; Monestier, M.; Pinteaux, E.; Rothwell, N.J.; Allan, S.M. Neutrophil cerebrovascular transmigration triggers rapid neurotoxicity through release of proteases associated with decondensed DNA. *J. Immunol.* **2012**, *189*, 381–392. [CrossRef]

7. Brinkmann, V.; Reichard, U.; Goosmann, C.; Fauler, B.; Uhlemann, Y.; Weiss, D.S.; Weinrauch, Y.; Zychlinsky, A. Neutrophil extracellular traps kill bacteria. *Science* **2004**, *303*, 1532–1535. [CrossRef]

8. Takei, H.; Araki, A.; Watanabe, H.; Ichinose, A.; Sendo, F. Rapid killing of human neutrophils by the potent activator phorbol 12-myristate 13-acetate (PMA) accompanied by changes different from typical apoptosis or necrosis. *J. Leukoc. Biol.* **1996**, *59*, 229–240. [CrossRef]

9. Boeltz, S.; Amini, P.; Anders, H.J.; Andrade, F.; Bilyy, R.; Chatfield, S.; Cichon, I.; Clancy, D.M.; Desai, J.; Dumych, T.; et al. To NET or not to NET: Current opinions and state of the science regarding the formation of neutrophil extracellular traps. *Cell Death Differ.* **2019**, *26*, 395–408. [CrossRef]

10. Manda, A.; Pruchniak, M.P.; Arazna, M.; Demkow, U. Neutrophil extracellular traps in physiology and pathology. *Cent. Eur. J. Immunol.* **2014**, *39*, 116–121. [CrossRef]

11. Papayannopoulos, V. Neutrophil extracellular traps in immunity and disease. *Nat. Rev. Immunol.* **2018**, *18*, 134–147. [CrossRef] [PubMed]

12. Menegazzi, R.; Decleva, E.; Dri, P. Killing by neutrophil extracellular traps: Fact or folklore? *Blood* **2012**, *119*, 1214–1216. [CrossRef] [PubMed]

13. Abdol Razak, N.; Elaskalani, O.; Metharom, P. Pancreatic cancer-induced neutrophil extracellular traps: A potential contributor to cancer-associated thrombosis. *Int. J. Mol. Sci.* **2017**, *18*, 487. [CrossRef] [PubMed]

14. Bryk, A.H.; Prior, S.M.; Plens, K.; Konieczynska, M.; Hohendorff, J.; Malecki, M.T.; Butenas, S.; Undas, A. Predictors of neutrophil extracellular traps markers in type 2 diabetes mellitus: Associations with a prothrombotic state and hypofibrinolysis. *Cardiovasc. Diabetol.* **2019**, *18*, 49. [CrossRef] [PubMed]

15. Skrzeczynska-Moncznik, J.; Wlodarczyk, A.; Zabieglo, K.; Kapinska-Mrowiecka, M.; Marewicz, E.; Dubin, A.; Potempa, J.; Cichy, J. Secretory leukocyte proteinase inhibitor-competent DNA deposits are potent stimulators of plasmacytoid dendritic cells: Implication for psoriasis. *J. Immunol.* **2012**, *189*, 1611–1617. [CrossRef] [PubMed]

16. Law, S.M.; Gray, R.D. Neutrophil extracellular traps and the dysfunctional innate immune response of cystic fibrosis lung disease: A review. *J. Inflamm.* **2017**, *14*, 29. [CrossRef]

17. Leffler, J.; Martin, M.; Gullstrand, B.; Tyden, H.; Lood, C.; Truedsson, L.; Bengtsson, A.A.; Blom, A.M. Neutrophil extracellular traps that are not degraded in systemic lupus erythematosus activate complement exacerbating the disease. *J. Immunol.* **2012**, *188*, 3522–3531. [CrossRef]

18. Zhang, R.L.; Chopp, M.; Chen, H.; Garcia, J.H. Temporal profile of ischemic tissue damage, neutrophil response, and vascular plugging following permanent and transient (2H) middle cerebral artery occlusion in the rat. *J. Neurol. Sci.* **1994**, *125*, 3–10. [CrossRef]

19. Garcia, J.H.; Liu, K.F.; Yoshida, Y.; Lian, J.; Chen, S.; del Zoppo, G.J. Influx of leukocytes and platelets in an evolving brain infarct (Wistar rat). *Am. J. Pathol.* **1994**, *144*, 188–199.

20. Chu, H.X.; Kim, H.A.; Lee, S.; Moore, J.P.; Chan, C.T.; Vinh, A.; Gelderblom, M.; Arumugam, T.V.; Broughton, B.R.; Drummond, G.R.; et al. Immune cell infiltration in malignant middle cerebral artery infarction: Comparison with transient cerebral ischemia. *J. Cereb. Blood. Flow. Metab.* **2014**, *34*, 450–459. [CrossRef]

21. Shi, Y.; Zhang, L.; Pu, H.; Mao, L.; Hu, X.; Jiang, X.; Xu, N.; Stetler, R.A.; Zhang, F.; Liu, X.; et al. Rapid endothelial cytoskeletal reorganization enables early blood-brain barrier disruption and long-term ischaemic reperfusion brain injury. *Nat. Commun.* **2016**, *7*, 10523. [CrossRef] [PubMed]

22. Perez-de-Puig, I.; Miro-Mur, F.; Ferrer-Ferrer, M.; Gelpi, E.; Pedragosa, J.; Justicia, C.; Urra, X.; Chamorro, A.; Planas, A.M. Neutrophil recruitment to the brain in mouse and human ischemic stroke. *Acta Neuropathol.* **2015**, *129*, 239–257. [CrossRef] [PubMed]

23. Denes, A.; Humphreys, N.; Lane, T.E.; Grencis, R.; Rothwell, N. Chronic systemic infection exacerbates ischemic brain damage via a CCL5 (regulated on activation, normal T-cell expressed and secreted)-mediated proinflammatory response in mice. *J. Neurosci.* **2010**, *30*, 10086–10095. [CrossRef] [PubMed]

24. Hoeksema, M.; van Eijk, M.; Haagsman, H.P.; Hartshorn, K.L. Histones as mediators of host defense, inflammation and thrombosis. *Future Microbiol.* **2016**, *11*, 441–453. [CrossRef]

25. Semeraro, F.; Ammollo, C.T.; Morrissey, J.H.; Dale, G.L.; Friese, P.; Esmon, N.L.; Esmon, C.T. Extracellular histones promote thrombin generation through platelet-dependent mechanisms: Involvement of platelet TLR2 and TLR4. *Blood* **2011**, *118*, 1952–1961. [CrossRef]

26. Massberg, S.; Grahl, L.; von Bruehl, M.L.; Manukyan, D.; Pfeiler, S.; Goosmann, C.; Brinkmann, V.; Lorenz, M.; Bidzhekov, K.; Khandagale, A.B.; et al. Reciprocal coupling of coagulation and innate immunity via neutrophil serine proteases. *Nat. Med.* **2010**, *16*, 887–896. [CrossRef]

27. Fuchs, T.A.; Brill, A.; Duerschmied, D.; Schatzberg, D.; Monestier, M.; Myers, D.D., Jr.; Wrobleski, S.K.; Wakefield, T.W.; Hartwig, J.H.; Wagner, D.D. Extracellular DNA traps promote thrombosis. *Proc. Natl. Acad. Sci. USA* **2010**, *107*, 15880–15885. [CrossRef]

28. Laridan, E.; Denorme, F.; Desender, L.; Francois, O.; Andersson, T.; Deckmyn, H.; Vanhoorelbeke, K.; de Meyer, S.F. Neutrophil extracellular traps in ischemic stroke thrombi. *Ann. Neurol.* **2017**, *82*, 223–232. [CrossRef]

29. Ruhnau, J.; Schulze, K.; Gaida, B.; Langner, S.; Kessler, C.; Broker, B.; Dressel, A.; Vogelgesang, A. Stroke alters respiratory burst in neutrophils and monocytes. *Stroke* **2014**, *45*, 794–800. [CrossRef]

30. Tillack, K.; Breiden, P.; Martin, R.; Sospedra, M. T lymphocyte priming by neutrophil extracellular traps links innate and adaptive immune responses. *J. Immunol.* **2012**, *188*, 3150–3159. [CrossRef]

31. Zenaro, E.; Pietronigro, E.; della Bianca, V.; Piacentino, G.; Marongiu, L.; Budui, S.; Turano, E.; Rossi, B.; Angiari, S.; Dusi, S.; et al. Neutrophils promote Alzheimer's disease-like pathology and cognitive decline via LFA-1 integrin. *Nat. Med.* **2015**, *21*, 880–886. [CrossRef] [PubMed]

32. Savage, M.J.; Iqbal, M.; Loh, T.; Trusko, S.P.; Scott, R.; Siman, R. Cathepsin G: Localization in human cerebral cortex and generation of amyloidogenic fragments from the beta-amyloid precursor protein. *Neuroscience* **1994**, *60*, 607–619. [CrossRef]

33. Czirr, E.; Wyss-Coray, T. The immunology of neurodegeneration. *J. Clin. Invest.* **2012**, *122*, 1156–1163. [CrossRef] [PubMed]

34. Wyss-Coray, T. Inflammation in Alzheimer disease: Driving force, bystander or beneficial response? *Nat. Med.* **2006**, *12*, 1005–1015. [CrossRef] [PubMed]

35. Szekely, C.A.; Zandi, P.P. Non-Steroidal anti-inflammatory drugs and Alzheimer's disease: The epidemiological evidence. *CNS Neurol. Disord. Drug Targets* **2010**, *9*, 132–139. [CrossRef] [PubMed]

36. Pietronigro, E.C.; della Bianca, V.; Zenaro, E.; Constantin, G. NETosis in Alzheimer's Disease. *Front. Immunol.* **2017**, *8*, 211. [CrossRef]

37. Grammas, P.; Ovase, R. Inflammatory factors are elevated in brain microvessels in Alzheimer's disease. *Neurobiol. Aging* **2001**, *22*, 837–842. [CrossRef]

38. Grammas, P.; Samany, P.G.; Thirumangalakudi, L. Thrombin and inflammatory proteins are elevated in Alzheimer's disease microvessels: Implications for disease pathogenesis. *J. Alzheimers Dis.* **2006**, *9*, 51–58. [CrossRef]

39. Rodrigues, S.F.; Granger, D.N. Blood cells and endothelial barrier function. *Tissue Barriers* **2015**, *3*, e978720. [CrossRef]

40. Suttorp, N.; Nolte, A.; Wilke, A.; Drenckhahn, D. Human neutrophil elastase increases permeability of cultured pulmonary endothelial cell monolayers. *Int. J. Microcirc. Clin. Exp.* **1993**, *13*, 187–203.

41. Saffarzadeh, M.; Juenemann, C.; Queisser, M.A.; Lochnit, G.; Barreto, G.; Galuska, S.P.; Lohmeyer, J.; Preissner, K.T. Neutrophil extracellular traps directly induce epithelial and endothelial cell death: A predominant role of histones. *PLoS ONE* **2012**, *7*, e32366. [CrossRef] [PubMed]

42. Heneka, M.T.; Carson, M.J.; el Khoury, J.; Landreth, G.E.; Brosseron, F.; Feinstein, D.L.; Jacobs, A.H.; Wyss-Coray, T.; Vitorica, J.; Ransohoff, R.M.; et al. Neuroinflammation in Alzheimer's disease. *Lancet Neurol.* **2015**, *14*, 388–405. [CrossRef]

43. Abramov, A.Y.; Duchen, M.R. The role of an astrocytic NADPH oxidase in the neurotoxicity of amyloid beta peptides. *Philos. Trans. R Soc. Lond. B Biol. Sci.* **2005**, *360*, 2309–2314. [CrossRef] [PubMed]

44. Allam, R.; Kumar, S.V.; Darisipudi, M.N.; Anders, H.J. Extracellular histones in tissue injury and inflammation. *J. Mol. Med.* **2014**, *92*, 465–472. [CrossRef]

45. Peppin, G.J.; Weiss, S.J. Activation of the endogenous metalloproteinase, gelatinase, by triggered human neutrophils. *Proc. Natl. Acad. Sci. USA* **1986**, *83*, 4322–4326. [CrossRef]

46. Gilthorpe, J.D.; Oozeer, F.; Nash, J.; Calvo, M.; Bennett, D.L.; Lumsden, A.; Pini, A. Extracellular histone H1 is neurotoxic and drives a pro-inflammatory response in microglia. *F1000Research* **2013**, *2*, 148. [CrossRef]

47. Yoshii, F.; Shinohara, Y. Autoimmune neurological diseases. *J. Jpn. Med. Assoc.* **2004**, *47*, 425–430.

48. Tillack, K.; Naegele, M.; Haueis, C.; Schippling, S.; Wandinger, K.P.; Martin, R.; Sospedra, M. Gender differences in circulating levels of neutrophil extracellular traps in serum of multiple sclerosis patients. *J. Neuroimmunol.* **2013**, *261*, 108–119. [CrossRef]

49. Croxford, A.L.; Kurschus, F.C.; Waisman, A. Mouse models for multiple sclerosis: Historical facts and future implications. *Biochim. Biophys. Acta* **2011**, *1812*, 177–183. [CrossRef]

50. Afraei, S.; Sedaghat, R.; Zavareh, F.T.; Aghazadeh, Z.; Ekhtiari, P.; Azizi, G.; Mirshafiey, A. Therapeutic effects of pegylated-interferon-alpha2a in a mouse model of multiple sclerosis. *Cent. Eur. J. Immunol.* **2018**, *43*, 9–17. [CrossRef]

51. Lambert, S.; Hambro, C.A.; Johnston, A.; Stuart, P.E.; Tsoi, L.C.; Nair, R.P.; Elder, J.T. Neutrophil extracellular traps induce human Th17 cells: Effect of psoriasis-associated *TRAF3IP2* genotype. *J. Invest. Derm.* **2019**, *139*, 1245–1253. [CrossRef] [PubMed]

52. Warnatsch, A.; Ioannou, M.; Wang, Q.; Papayannopoulos, V. Inflammation: Neutrophil extracellular traps license macrophages for cytokine production in atherosclerosis. *Science* **2015**, *349*, 316–320. [CrossRef] [PubMed]

53. Komiyama, Y.; Nakae, S.; Matsuki, T.; Nambu, A.; Ishigame, H.; Kakuta, S.; Sudo, K.; Iwakura, Y. IL-17 plays an important role in the development of experimental autoimmune encephalomyelitis. *J. Immunol.* **2006**, *177*, 566–573. [CrossRef] [PubMed]

54. Kostic, M.; Dzopalic, T.; Zivanovic, S.; Zivkovic, N.; Cvetanovic, A.; Stojanovic, I.; Vojinovic, S.; Marjanovic, G.; Savic, V.; Colic, M. IL-17 and glutamate excitotoxicity in the pathogenesis of multiple sclerosis. *Scand. J. Immunol.* **2014**, *79*, 181–186. [CrossRef] [PubMed]

55. Zhang, H.; Ray, A.; Miller, N.M.; Hartwig, D.; Pritchard, K.A.; Dittel, B.N. Inhibition of myeloperoxidase at the peak of experimental autoimmune encephalomyelitis restores blood-brain barrier integrity and ameliorates disease severity. *J. Neurochem.* **2016**, *136*, 826–836. [CrossRef] [PubMed]

56. Yu, G.; Zheng, S.; Zhang, H. Inhibition of myeloperoxidase by N-acetyl lysyltyrosylcysteine amide reduces experimental autoimmune encephalomyelitis-induced injury and promotes oligodendrocyte regeneration and neurogenesis in a murine model of progressive multiple sclerosis. *Neuroreport* **2018**, *29*, 208–213. [CrossRef] [PubMed]

57. Rumble, J.M.; Huber, A.K.; Krishnamoorthy, G.; Srinivasan, A.; Giles, D.A.; Zhang, X.; Wang, L.; Segal, B.M. Neutrophil-Related factors as biomarkers in EAE and MS. *J. Exp. Med.* **2015**, *212*, 23–35. [CrossRef]

58. Woodberry, T.; Bouffler, S.E.; Wilson, A.S.; Buckland, R.L.; Brustle, A. The emerging role of neutrophil granulocytes in multiple sclerosis. *J. Clin. Med.* **2018**, *7*, 511. [CrossRef]

59. MS Research Australia. NETS: A New Target for Treating MS. Available online: https://msra.org.au/project/neutrophil-extracellular-traps-new-target-treating-ms/ (accessed on 10 October 2019).

60. Tay, S.H.; Mak, A. Anti-NR2A/B antibodies and other major molecular mechanisms in the pathogenesis of cognitive dysfunction in systemic lupus erythematosus. *Int. J. Mol. Sci.* **2015**, *16*, 10281–10300. [CrossRef]

61. Takeuchi, H.; Kawasaki, T.; Shigematsu, K.; Kawamura, K.; Oka, N. Neutrophil extracellular traps in neuropathy with anti-neutrophil cytoplasmic autoantibody-associated microscopic polyangiitis. *Clin. Rheumatol.* **2017**, *36*, 913–917. [CrossRef]

62. Conly, J.M.; Ronald, A.R. Cerebrospinal fluid as a diagnostic body fluid. *Am. J. Med.* **1983**, *75*, 102–108. [CrossRef]

63. Hutchings, M.; Weller, R.O. Anatomical relationships of the pia mater to cerebral blood vessels in man. *J. Neurosurg.* **1986**, *65*, 316–325. [CrossRef] [PubMed]

64. Malipiero, U.; Koedel, U.; Pfister, H.W.; Leveen, P.; Burki, K.; Reith, W.; Fontana, A. TGFbeta receptor II gene deletion in leucocytes prevents cerebral vasculitis in bacterial meningitis. *Brain* **2006**, *129*, 2404–2415. [CrossRef] [PubMed]

65. De Buhr, N.; Reuner, F.; Neumann, A.; Stump-Guthier, C.; Tenenbaum, T.; Schroten, H.; Ishikawa, H.; Muller, K.; Beineke, A.; Hennig-Pauka, I.; et al. Neutrophil extracellular trap formation in the *Streptococcus suis*-infected cerebrospinal fluid compartment. *Cell Microbiol.* **2017**, *19*. [CrossRef]

66. Mohanty, T.; Fisher, J.; Bakochi, A.; Neumann, A.; Cardoso, J.F.P.; Karlsson, C.A.Q.; Pavan, C.; Lundgaard, I.; Nilson, B.; Reinstrup, P.; et al. Neutrophil extracellular traps in the central nervous system hinder bacterial clearance during pneumococcal meningitis. *Nat. Commun.* **2019**, *10*, 1667. [CrossRef] [PubMed]

67. Beiter, K.; Wartha, F.; Albiger, B.; Normark, S.; Zychlinsky, A.; Henriques-Normark, B. An endonuclease allows *Streptococcus pneumoniae* to escape from neutrophil extracellular traps. *Curr. Biol.* **2006**, *16*, 401–407. [CrossRef] [PubMed]

68. Johnson, A.J.; Ayvazian, J.H.; Tillett, W.S. Crystalline pancreatic desoxyribonuclease as an adjunct to the treatment of pneumococcal meningitis. *N. Engl. J. Med.* **1959**, *260*, 893–900. [CrossRef]

69. Jhelum, H.; Sori, H.; Sehgal, D. A novel extracellular vesicle-associated endodeoxyribonuclease helps *Streptococcus pneumoniae* evade neutrophil extracellular traps and is required for full virulence. *Sci. Rep.* **2018**, *8*, 7985. [CrossRef]

70. Storisteanu, D.M.; Pocock, J.M.; Cowburn, A.S.; Juss, J.K.; Nadesalingam, A.; Nizet, V.; Chilvers, E.R. Evasion of neutrophil extracellular traps by respiratory pathogens. *Am. J. Respir. Cell. Mol. Biol.* **2017**, *56*, 423–431. [CrossRef]

71. Bhattacharya, M.; Berends, E.T.M.; Chan, R.; Schwab, E.; Roy, S.; Sen, C.K.; Torres, V.J.; Wozniak, D.J. *Staphylococcus aureus* biofilms release leukocidins to elicit extracellular trap formation and evade neutrophil-mediated killing. *Proc. Natl. Acad. Sci. USA* **2018**, *115*, 7416–7421. [CrossRef]

72. Alhamdi, Y.; Toh, C.H. Recent advances in pathophysiology of disseminated intravascular coagulation: The role of circulating histones and neutrophil extracellular traps. *F1000Research* **2017**, *6*, 2143. [CrossRef] [PubMed]

73. Liu, Y.W.; Li, S.; Dai, S.S. Neutrophils in traumatic brain injury (TBI): Friend or foe? *J. Neuroinflamm.* **2018**, *15*, 146. [CrossRef] [PubMed]

74. De Buhr, N.; Neumann, A.; Jerjomiceva, N.; von Kockritz-Blickwede, M.; Baums, C.G. *Streptococcus suis* DNase SsnA contributes to degradation of neutrophil extracellular traps (NETs) and evasion of NET-mediated antimicrobial activity. *Microbiology* **2014**, *160*, 385–395. [CrossRef] [PubMed]

75. De Buhr, N.; Stehr, M.; Neumann, A.; Naim, H.Y.; Valentin-Weigand, P.; von Kockritz-Blickwede, M.; Baums, C.G. Identification of a novel DNase of Streptococcus suis (EndAsuis) important for neutrophil extracellular trap degradation during exponential growth. *Microbiology* **2015**, *161*, 838–850. [CrossRef]

76. Boeltz, S.; Munoz, L.E.; Fuchs, T.A.; Herrmann, M. Neutrophil extracellular traps open the Pandora's box in severe malaria. *Front. Immunol.* **2017**, *8*, 874. [CrossRef] [PubMed]

77. Schorn, C.; Janko, C.; Latzko, M.; Chaurio, R.; Schett, G.; Herrmann, M. Monosodium urate crystals induce extracellular DNA traps in neutrophils, eosinophils, and basophils but not in mononuclear cells. *Front. Immunol.* **2012**, *3*, 277. [CrossRef] [PubMed]

78. Schorn, C.; Janko, C.; Krenn, V.; Zhao, Y.; Munoz, L.E.; Schett, G.; Herrmann, M. Bonding the foe—NETting neutrophils immobilize the pro-inflammatory monosodium urate crystals. *Front. Immunol.* **2012**, *3*, 376. [CrossRef]

79. Baker, V.S.; Imade, G.E.; Molta, N.B.; Tawde, P.; Pam, S.D.; Obadofin, M.O.; Sagay, S.A.; Egah, D.Z.; Iya, D.; Afolabi, B.B.; et al. Cytokine-Associated neutrophil extracellular traps and antinuclear antibodies in *Plasmodium falciparum* infected children under six years of age. *Malar. J.* **2008**, *7*, 41. [CrossRef]

80. Idro, R.; Marsh, K.; John, C.C.; Newton, C.R. Cerebral malaria: Mechanisms of brain injury and strategies for improved neurocognitive outcome. *Pediatr. Res.* **2010**, *68*, 267–274. [CrossRef]

81. He, H.; Geng, T.; Chen, P.; Wang, M.; Hu, J.; Kang, L.; Song, W.; Tang, H. NK cells promote neutrophil recruitment in the brain during sepsis-induced neuroinflammation. *Sci. Rep.* **2016**, *6*, 27711. [CrossRef]

82. D'Mello, C.; Le, T.; Swain, M.G. Cerebral microglia recruit monocytes into the brain in response to tumor necrosis factoralpha signaling during peripheral organ inflammation. *J. Neurosci.* **2009**, *29*, 2089–2102. [CrossRef] [PubMed]

83. D'Mello, C.; Riazi, K.; Le, T.; Stevens, K.M.; Wang, A.; McKay, D.M.; Pittman, Q.J.; Swain, M.G. P-selectin-mediated monocyte-cerebral endothelium adhesive interactions link peripheral organ inflammation to sickness behaviors. *J. Neurosci.* **2013**, *33*, 14878–14888. [CrossRef] [PubMed]

84. Burfeind, K.G.; Zhu, X.; Norgard, M.A.; Levasseur, P.R.; Olson, B.; Michaelis, K.A.; Torres, E.R.S.; Patel, E.M.; Jeng, S.; McWeeney, S.; et al. A distinct neutrophil population invades the central nervous system during pancreatic cancer. *bioRxiv* **2019**, 659060. [CrossRef]

85. Miller, A.H.; Ancoli-Israel, S.; Bower, J.E.; Capuron, L.; Irwin, M.R. Neuroendocrine-immune mechanisms of behavioral comorbidities in patients with cancer. *J. Clin. Oncol.* **2008**, *26*, 971–982. [CrossRef]

86. Meyers, C.A. Neurocognitive dysfunction in cancer patients. *Oncology* **2000**, *14*, 75–79.

87. Louis, D.N.; Ohgaki, H.; Wiestler, O.D.; Cavenee, W.K.; Burger, P.C.; Jouvet, A.; Scheithauer, B.W.; Kleihues, P. The 2007 WHO classification of tumours of the central nervous system. *Acta Neuropathol.* **2007**, *114*, 97–109. [CrossRef]

88. Quail, D.F.; Joyce, J.A. The microenvironmental landscape of brain tumors. *Cancer. Cell.* **2017**, *31*, 326–341. [CrossRef]

89. Schulz, M.; Salamero-Boix, A.; Niesel, K.; Alekseeva, T.; Sevenich, L. Microenvironmental regulation of tumor progression and therapeutic response in brain metastasis. *Front. Immunol.* **2019**, *10*, 1713. [CrossRef]

90. Uehara, T.; Baba, I.; Nomura, Y. Induction of cytokine-induced neutrophil chemoattractant in response to various stresses in rat C6 glioma cells. *Brain Res.* **1998**, *790*, 284–292. [CrossRef]

91. Fossati, G.; Ricevuti, G.; Edwards, S.W.; Walker, C.; Dalton, A.; Rossi, M.L. Neutrophil infiltration into human gliomas. *Acta Neuropathol.* **1999**, *98*, 349–354. [CrossRef]

92. Coffelt, S.B.; Wellenstein, M.D.; de Visser, K.E. Neutrophils in cancer: Neutral no more. *Nat. Rev. Cancer* **2016**, *16*, 431–446. [CrossRef] [PubMed]

93. Gabrusiewicz, K.; Rodriguez, B.; Wei, J.; Hashimoto, Y.; Healy, L.M.; Maiti, S.N.; Thomas, G.; Zhou, S.H.; Wang, Q.H.; Elakkad, A.; et al. Glioblastoma-Infiltrated innate immune cells resemble M0 macrophage phenotype. *JCI Insight* **2016**, *1*. [CrossRef] [PubMed]

94. Granot, Z.; Henke, E.; Comen, E.A.; King, T.A.; Norton, L.; Benezra, R. Tumor entrained neutrophils inhibit seeding in the premetastatic lung. *Cancer Cell* **2011**, *20*, 300–314. [CrossRef] [PubMed]

95. Douda, D.N.; Khan, M.A.; Grasemann, H.; Palaniyar, N. SK3 channel and mitochondrial ROS mediate NADPH oxidase-independent NETosis induced by calcium influx. *Proc. Natl. Acad. Sci. USA* **2015**, *112*, 2817–2822. [CrossRef] [PubMed]

96. Kenny, E.F.; Herzig, A.; Kruger, R.; Muth, A.; Mondal, S.; Thompson, P.R.; Brinkmann, V.; Bernuth, H.V.; Zychlinsky, A. Diverse stimuli engage different neutrophil extracellular trap pathways. *Elife* **2017**, *6*. [CrossRef]

97. Dumitru, C.A.; Lang, S.; Brandau, S. Modulation of neutrophil granulocytes in the tumor microenvironment: Mechanisms and consequences for tumor progression. *Semin. Cancer Biol.* **2013**, *23*, 141–148. [CrossRef]

98. Shamamian, P.; Schwartz, J.D.; Pocock, B.J.Z.; Monea, S.; Whiting, D.; Marcus, S.G.; Mignatti, P. Activation of progelatinase A (MMP-2) by neutrophil elastase, cathepsin G, and proteinase-3: A role for inflammatory cells in tumor invasion and angiogenesis. *J. Cell Physiol.* **2001**, *189*, 197–206. [CrossRef]

99. Wu, C.F.; Andzinski, L.; Kasnitz, N.; Kroger, A.; Klawonn, F.; Lienenklaus, S.; Weiss, S.; Jablonska, J. The lack of type I interferon induces neutrophil-mediated pre-metastatic niche formation in the mouse lung. *Int. J. Cancer* **2015**, *137*, 837–847. [CrossRef]

100. Cools-Lartigue, J.; Spicer, J.; McDonald, B.; Gowing, S.; Chow, S.; Giannias, B.; Bourdeau, F.; Kubes, P.; Ferri, L. Neutrophil extracellular traps sequester circulating tumor cells and promote metastasis. *J. Clin. Investig.* **2013**, *123*, 3446–3458. [CrossRef]

101. Spicer, J.D.; McDonald, B.; Cools-Lartigue, J.J.; Chow, S.C.; Giannias, B.; Kubes, P.; Ferri, L.E. Neutrophils promote liver metastasis via mac-1-mediated interactions with circulating tumor cells. *Cancer Res.* **2012**, *72*, 3919–3927. [CrossRef]

102. Liang, J.; Piao, Y.; Holmes, L.; Fuller, G.N.; Henry, V.; Tiao, N.; de Groot, J.F. Neutrophils promote the malignant glioma phenotype through S100A4. *Clin. Cancer Res.* **2014**, *20*, 187–198. [CrossRef] [PubMed]

103. Bambury, R.M.; Teo, M.Y.; Power, D.G.; Yusuf, A.; Murray, S.; Battley, J.E.; Drake, C.; O'Dea, P.; Bermingham, N.; Keohane, C.; et al. The association of pre-treatment neutrophil to lymphocyte ratio with overall survival in patients with glioblastoma multiforme. *J. Neurooncol.* **2013**, *114*, 149–154. [CrossRef] [PubMed]

104. McNamara, G.M.; Templeton, A.J.; Maganti, M.; Walter, T.; Horgan, A.M.; McKeever, L.; Min, T.; Amir, E.; Knox, J.J. Neutrophil/lymphocyte ratio as a prognostic factor in biliary tract cancer. *Eur. J. Cancer.* **2014**, *50*, 1581–1589. [CrossRef] [PubMed]

105. Mitsuya, K.; Nakasu, Y.; Kurakane, T.; Hayashi, N.; Harada, H.; Nozaki, K. Elevated preoperative neutrophil-to-lymphocyte ratio as a predictor of worse survival after resection in patients with brain metastasis. *J. Neurosurg.* **2017**, *127*, 433–437. [CrossRef] [PubMed]

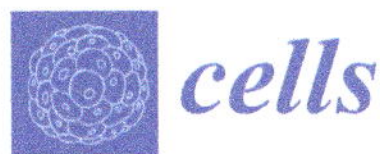 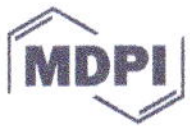

Article

Neutrophil Extracellular Traps (NETs) in the Cerebrospinal Fluid Samples from Children and Adults with Central Nervous System Infections

Daniel Appelgren [1], Helena Enocsson [2], Barbro H. Skogman [3], Marika Nordberg [4],
Linda Perander [4], Dag Nyman [5], Clara Nyberg [4], Jasmin Knopf [6], Luis E. Muñoz [6],
Christopher Sjöwall [2] and Johanna Sjöwall [7,8,*]

[1] Division of Drug Research, Department of Medical and Health Sciences, Linköping University,
    SE-581 85 Linköping, Sweden; daniel.appelgren@liu.se
[2] Division of Neuro and Inflammation Sciences, Department of Clinical and Experimental Medicine,
    Linköping University, SE-581 85 Linköping, Sweden; helena.enocsson@liu.se (H.E.);
    christopher.sjowall@liu.se (C.S.)
[3] Center for Clinical Research Dalarna-Uppsala University, Region Dalarna and Faculty of Medicine and
    Health Sciences, Örebro University, SE-702 81 Örebro, Sweden; barbro.hedinskogman@regiondalarna.se
[4] Åland Central Hospital, Department of Infectious Diseases, AX-22 100 Mariehamn, Åland, Finland;
    marika.nordberg@ahs.ax (M.N.); linda.perander@ahs.ax (L.P.); clara.nyberg@aland.net (C.N.)
[5] Bimelix AB, AX-22 100 Mariehamn, Åland, Finland; dag.nyman@aland.net
[6] Department of Internal Medicine 3-Rheumatology and Immunology, Universitätsklinikum Erlangen,
    Friedrich-Alexander-University Erlangen-Nürnberg (FAU), DE-91 054 Erlangen, Germany;
    jasmin.knopf@uk-erlangen.de (J.K.); luis.munoz@uk-erlangen.de (L.E.M.)
[7] Clinic of Infectious Diseases, Linköping University Hospital, SE-581 85 Linköping, Sweden
[8] Department of Clinical and Experimental Medicine, Linköping University, SE-581 85 Linköping, Sweden
[*] Correspondence: johanna.sjowall@liu.se

Received: 28 October 2019; Accepted: 17 December 2019; Published: 23 December 2019

Abstract: Neutrophils operate as part of the innate defence in the skin and may eliminate the *Borrelia* spirochaete via phagocytosis, oxidative bursts, and hydrolytic enzymes. However, their importance in Lyme neuroborreliosis (LNB) is unclear. Neutrophil extracellular trap (NET) formation, which is associated with the production of reactive oxygen species, involves the extrusion of the neutrophil DNA to form traps that incapacitate bacteria and immobilise viruses. Meanwhile, NET formation has recently been studied in pneumococcal meningitis, the role of NETs in other central nervous system (CNS) infections has previously not been studied. Here, cerebrospinal fluid (CSF) samples from clinically well-characterised children ($N = 111$) and adults ($N = 64$) with LNB and other CNS infections were analysed for NETs (DNA/myeloperoxidase complexes) and elastase activity. NETs were detected more frequently in the children than the adults ($p = 0.01$). NET presence was associated with higher CSF levels of CXCL1 ($p < 0.001$), CXCL6 ($p = 0.007$), CXCL8 ($p = 0.003$), CXCL10 ($p < 0.001$), MMP-9 ($p = 0.002$), TNF ($p = 0.02$), IL-6 ($p < 0.001$), and IL-17A ($p = 0.03$). NETs were associated with fever ($p = 0.002$) and correlated with polynuclear pleocytosis ($r_s = 0.53$, $p < 0.0001$). We show that neutrophil activation and active NET formation occur in the CSF samples of children and adults with CNS infections, mainly caused by *Borrelia* and neurotropic viruses. The role of NETs in the early phase of viral/bacterial CNS infections warrants further investigation.

Keywords: neutrophil extracellular traps; cerebrospinal fluid; adults; children; central nervous system; infection; chemokines; cytokines; borrelia; virus

---

1. Introduction

Lyme neuroborreliosis (LNB), which is caused by a complex of Gram-negative spirochaetes called *Borrelia burgdorferi sensu lato* and transmitted to humans by the *Ixodes ricinus* tick, is the most serious manifestation of Lyme disease (LD) [1]. *Borrelia* constitutes a common cause of bacterial infection of the central nervous system (CNS) among children and adults in Sweden [2–5] and Finland [6]. According to the diagnostic criteria for LNB [7], mononuclear pleocytosis must be present in the cerebrospinal fluid (CSF), and this is an indicator of an active infection. Despite being a bacterial CNS infection, LNB is characterised by a distinct mononuclear predominance in the CSF. The reason for the relatively low proportion of polynuclear cells, such as neutrophils, not only in the CSF [8] but also in the skin of patients with *erythema migrans* [9]—the earliest manifestation of a borrelia infection—remains unclear. However, as the neutrophils may be present at an early stage prior to lumbar puncture or skin biopsy, they might be overlooked.

Neutrophils are an essential component of the innate immune system, in that they limit locally the pathogen load through phagocytosis and the production of hydrolytic enzymes and chemokines, thereby orchestrating the subsequent adaptive immune response against the bacteria [10]. Beyond this, neutrophils create extracellular traps (NETs), which consist of the neutrophil's own DNA in the form of de-condensed chromatin, histones, peptides including neutrophil elastase (NE), and myeloperoxidase (MPO). Thus, they entrap extracellular pathogens, causing bacterial death, in a process that was first described in 2004 and termed 'NETosis' [11–13]. NETs are capable of binding both Gram-negative and Gram-positive bacteria, and their activities not only result in bacterial death but also prevent further spread of the infection and maintain homeostasis at the point of entry, even in unexpected body compartments [14–16]. NETs can also ensnare and immobilise viruses, thereby preventing viral entry into cells and spreading [17].

The activities and roles of NETs are mostly unknown in the context of LD and human CNS infections overall. Nevertheless, NETs have been detected in the skin samples of Borrelia-infected, tick-bitten mice and have been shown to entrap and kill the spirochaetes despite a tick saliva-mediated decrease in the production of reactive oxygen species by the neutrophils [18]. In addition, NETs were detected in the CSF in a porcine model of *Streptococcus suis* meningitis [19] and in a human study of acute bacterial meningitis caused by pneumococci, in which the NETs were shown to play a harmful role in hinder the clearance of bacteria from the rat brain. However, in the same study, NETs were not detected in the CSF samples of patients with LNB (*N* = 3) and acute viral meningitis (*N* = 4) [20].

Neutrophils and their activation products are important early during infection, and they most likely affect the course and outcome of many diseases. With LNB, children tend to seek medical care earlier than adults owing to their having higher frequencies of meningeal symptoms and facial nerve palsy [3,4,21]. Therefore, we systematically evaluated whether NETs could be detected (using two different assays) in the CSF samples of children and adults with LNB, as well as in CSF samples from other infections and disorders affecting the CNS. NETs play a complex role in inflammation, although in general they are more stable than cytokines/chemokines and are thus more suitable for analyses of innate immune activation, especially in the sensitive environment of the CNS [22].

2. Patients and Methods

2.1. Paediatric Patients

The clinical characteristics of the children are shown in Table 1. CSF samples from 111 well-characterised children (64 girls, 47 boys; median age, 10 years; interquartile range [IQR], 5–15 years) with definitive or possible LNB (*N* = 28), tick-borne encephalitis (TBE; *N* = 3), enteroviral meningitis (EVM; *N* = 7), other viral infection (OVI, *N* = 4), and other non-infectious disorders with neurological or CNS symptoms without pleocytosis (*N* = 69; as described in Table 1) were obtained by lumbar puncture prospectively during the period 2010–2014 as part of a multi-centre study evaluating children with suspected LNB in Sweden, as previously reported [23]. LNB was diagnosed according to European guidelines [7]. Definite LNB ($N = 20$) was defined as the presence of: (i) symptoms attributable to LNB, (ii) mononuclear pleocytosis in the CSF, and (iii) intrathecally produced anti-Borrelia antibodies. All the children in the 'possible LNB' group ($N = 8$) had symptoms that were attributable to LNB and pleocytosis in the CSF but had neither detectable intrathecally produced anti-Borrelia antibodies nor clinical signs or laboratory evidence of other infections. These children all responded well to antibiotic treatment. Definite and possible LNB ($N = 28$) were referred to collectively as 'LNB patients'. All samples were drawn before the initiation of antibiotic treatment, and the CSF samples for evaluation of NETs were frozen at $-70\ ^\circ$C until analysis. All the children were evaluated for intrathecal anti-Borrelia antibody production (*Borrelia burgdorferi*-specific IgG and/or IgM), using the flagella antigen-based, enzyme-linked immunosorbent assay (ELISA, for serum and CSF) in the IDEIA Lyme Neuroborreliosis Kit (Oxoid Ltd., Hampshire, UK) [24]. An index >0.3 was considered as positive, indicating intrathecal production of anti-Borrelia antibodies according to the manufacturer's instructions. Pleocytosis in the CSF was defined as $\geq 5 \times 10^6$ cells/L. The children were followed for assessment of recovery 2 months after admittance to hospital.

Table 1. Characteristics of paediatric patients.

On Admission		LNB ($N = 28$)	TBE ($N = 3$)	EVM ($N = 7$)	OVI ($N = 4$)	Other Disorder ($N = 69$)
Age	Median (range)	10 (3–15)	10 (3–15)	10 (4–15)	4 (1–14)	13 (0–19)
Sex	Female, N (%)	14 (50)	0	2 (30)	3 (75)	44 (64)
Duration of symptoms	<1 week, N (%)	16 (59)	1 (50)	5 (83)	1 (100)	9 (22)
	1–4 weeks, N (%)	9 (33)	1 (50)	1 (17)	0	11 (27)
	1–2 months, N (%)	1 (4)	0	0	0	5 (12)
	>2 months, N (%)	1 (4)	0	0	0	16 (39)
Clinical features	Facial nerve palsy, N (%)	22 (79)	0 (0)	0 (0)	1 (25)	17 (25)
	Meningeal symptoms [°], N (%)	22 (79)	2 (67)	7 (100)	1 (25)	50 (72)
	Fever >38 °C, N (%)	13 (46)	2 (67)	7 (100)	2 (50)	7 (10)
	Fatigue, N (%)	23 (82)	3 (100)	6 (86)	4 (100)	38 (55)
Laboratory findings	Pleocytosis *, median (range)	157 (20–486)	100 (0–130)	156 (20–634)	0 (0–6)	0 (0–74)
	CSF mono, median (range)	149 (8–484)	77 (0–116)	86 (16–610)	6	0 (0–40)
	CSF poly, median (range)	4 (0–30)	14 (0–28)	24 (4–164)	0	0 (0–34)
Recovery at follow-up: 2 *months*	Yes, N (%)	25 (89)	2 (67)	7 (100)	2 (50)	45 (65)

CSF, cerebrospinal fluid; LNB, Lyme neuroborreliosis; LD, Lyme disease; TBE, tick-borne encephalitis; EVM, enteroviral meningitis; OVI, other viral infection; Other disorders (Demyelinating polyneuropathy, Idiopathic peripheral facial nerve palsy, Idiopathic intracranial hypertension, Epilepsy, Head trauma, Myasthenia, Infantile spasm, Autoimmune encephalitis, Guillan-Barré syndrome, Narcolepsy, Optic neuritis, Fatigue, Microcephaly, Mycoplasma infection, Voice hallucinations, Periodic fever aphthous stomatitis pharyngitis cervical adenitis (PFAPA), Papillary oedema, Multiple sclerosis). * $\geq 5 \times 10^6$ cells /L; [°] Meningeal symptoms: Headache, Neck pain, Neck stiffness.

2.2. Adult Patients

The clinical characteristics of the adult patients are shown in Table 2. CSF samples from 64 well-characterised adults (36 women, 28 men; median age, 55 years; IQR, 43–63 years) with LNB ($N = 32$), unspecified LD ($N = 6$), TBE ($N = 3$), other viral meningitides (OVM, $N = 2$), and other non-infectious disorders with neurological or CNS symptoms ($N = 21$; as described in Table 2) were prospectively collected by lumbar puncture as part of the clinical routine for patients who were being evaluated for suspected tick-borne CNS infection at Åland Central Hospital (Mariehamn, Finland) [7]. Definite LNB ($N = 29$) was defined as the presence of: (i) symptoms attributable to LNB; (ii) mononuclear pleocytosis in the CSF; and (iii) intrathecally produced anti-Borrelia antibodies. In addition, the level of CSF-CXCL13 was high (>100 pg/mL) in all the patients, supporting the diagnosis [25]. Patients in the possible LNB group ($N = 3$) had symptoms attributable to LNB and mononuclear pleocytosis in the CSF, and they showed neither clinical signs nor laboratory evidence of other infections. Increased levels of CSF-CXCL13 supported the diagnosis. The patients with definite and possible LNB ($N = 31$) were collectively referred to as the 'LNB patients'. Unspecified LD is a common manifestation in the highly Borrelia-endemic Åland Islands (personal communication, the Åland Borrelia Research Group, Åland Islands), where a large proportion of the population has anti-Borrelia antibodies in the serum and in the CSF due to previous exposure. Unspecified LD is defined as the presence of: (i) new symptoms suggestive of LD (headache, radiating pain, myalgia, arthralgia and fatigue); (ii) significantly increased anti-Borrelia antibody levels in the serum; (iii) a clear effect of antibiotic treatment for *B. burgdorferi* on current symptoms; (iv) a lack of pleocytosis and no increase in CSF-CXCL13; and (v) neither clinical signs nor laboratory evidence of other infections. Pleocytosis in the CSF was defined as $\geq 5 \times 10^6$ cells/L. The CSF samples from adults were handled in the same manner as those from the children, i.e., frozen at $-70\ ^\circ$C until analysis. CSF samples were analysed for anti-Borrelia IgG antibodies using the recomBead Luminex-based assay (Mikrogen, Germany). An index >0.3 was considered as positive, indicating intrathecal production of anti-Borrelia antibodies, in line with the manufacturer's instructions. The adult patients were followed for the assessment of recovery 3 weeks and 6 months after admittance to hospital.

Table 2. Characteristics of adult patients.

On Admission		LNB (N = 32)	LD Unspec. (N = 6)	TBE (N = 3)	OVM (N = 2)	Other Disorders (N = 21)
Age	Median (range)	58 (18–82)	52 (30–80)	50 (46–57)	60 (50–69)	51 (24–88)
Sex	Female, N (%)	15 (47)	6 (100)	1 (33)	1 (50)	13 (62)
Duration of symptoms	<1 week, N (%)	4 (13)	0 (0)	0	0	1 (5)
	1–4 weeks, N (%)	7 (23)	1 (20)	3 (100)	1 (50)	1 (5)
	1–2 months, N (%)	10 (31)	1 (20)	0	0	1 (5)
	>2 months, N (%)	11 (34)	3 (60)	0	1 (50)	18 (86)
Clinical features	Facial nerve palsy, N (%)	5 (16)	1 (17)	0	0	0
	Meningeal symptoms °, N (%)	15 (47)	3 (50)	2 (67)	2 (100)	10 (48)
	Fever >38 °C, N (%)	3 (9)	0	3 (100)	1 (50)	3 (14)
	Fatigue, N (%)	17 (53)	5 (83)	3 (100)	1 (50)	9 (43)
	Radiating pain, N (%)	22 (69)	2 (33)	0	1 (50)	9 (43)
Laboratory findings	Pleocytosis *, median (range)	43 (6–390)	5 (4–5)	82 (51–131)	33 (18–47)	6 (0–292)
	CSF mono, median (range)	67 (5–355)	NA	62 (49–118)	26 (6–45)	54 (17–91) [&]
	CSF poly, median (range)	3 (0–45)	NA	13 (2–20)	7 (2–12)	106 (10–202) [&]
Recovery at follow-up:						
3 weeks	Yes, N (%)	12 (38)	3 (50)	0	1 (50)	4 (20)
6 months	Yes, N (%)	24 (77)	6 (100)	2 (67)	1 (50)	8 (42)

CSF, cerebrospinal fluid; LNB, Lyme neuroborreliosis; LD, Lyme disease; TBE, tick-borne encephalitis; OVM, other viral meningitis; Other disorders (Guillan-Barré syndrome, Spinal disk hernia, Trigeminal neuralgia, Sinusitis, Hypermobility syndrome, Depression, Chronic fatigue syndrome, Benign intracranial hypertension, Dementia, Recurrent iridocyclitis, Cerebral ischemia, Subarachnoidal haemorrhage, Chronic musculoskeletal pain, Meningeal inflammation of unknown origin). NA, not analysed. * $\geq 5 \times 10^6$/L; [&] Based on 2 samples (cell count $<10 \times 10^6$ not diff in mono/poly); ° Meningeal symptoms: Headache, Neck pain, Neck stiffness.

2.3. NET Remnant Assay (NETs)

Phorbol-12-myristate-13-acetate (PMA; Sigma-Aldrich, St Louis, MO, USA)-induced NETs were used to create the standard curve for the ELISA. To induce NETs, neutrophils were isolated through Percoll density centrifugation, as described previously [26]. The neutrophils were re-suspended in culture media [RPMI 1640 plus 2% foetal bovine serum (FBS)], seeded onto a 12-well plate at 1.5×10^6 cells per well, and stimulated with 20 nM PMA for 3 h. The wells were then washed twice with culture medium before incubation with 20 U/mL of the restriction enzyme *Alu*I (New England Biolabs Inc., Ipswich, MA, USA) at 37 °C for 20 min to cleave the NETs. The samples were centrifuged at 300× *g* for 5 min and NET-rich supernatants were pooled, aliquoted, and stored at $-80\ ^\circ$C.

The NET remnant ELISA was performed as previously described [27], although with PBS plus 0.05% Tween 20 used as the blocking and washing solution. A 96-well Nunc MediSorp immunoplate was coated with a monoclonal mouse anti-human MPO antibody (DAKO, Carpinteria, CA, USA) at 4 °C overnight. Blocking solution was added for 1 h at room temperature before incubation with standards (PMA-induced NETs), CSF samples, and a peroxidase-labelled anti-DNA antibody (detection antibody of the Human Cell Death Detection ELISA[PLUS]; Roche Diagnostics GmbH, Mannheim, Germany) for 2 h. Standards and samples were run in duplicate. For the standard curve, an 8-point dilution series with 2-fold dilutions of the PMA-induced NETs was used, and two plasma samples (high and low values) served as positive controls. After incubation, a substrate for peroxidase (ABTS; Roche Diagnostics) was added for 40 min before the plate was read at 405 nm in a VersaMax ELISA microplate reader (Molecular Devices, Sunnyvale, CA, USA). All the samples were interpolated from the standard curve using the sigmoidal 4-parameter logistic regression equation and reported as arbitrary units (a.u.). Non-detectable samples were given the value of 0 a.u. Analysis of NETs in the 175 CSF samples, which originated from the 111 children and 64 adults, was performed at the Division of Drug Research, Linköping University (Linköping, Sweden) [28].

2.4. Neutrophil Elastase (NE) Activity Assay

To confirm NET formation, 28 representative CSF samples (from 26 children and 2 adults) were also analysed for NE activity at the Friedrich-Alexander-Universität Erlangen-Nürnberg (Erlangen, Germany). For measurement of NE activity in the CSF, 100 μL of CSF were added to 100 μL PBS plus 25 μL of 1 M fluorogenic substrate MeOSuc-AAPV-AMC (sc-201163; Santa Cruz Biotechnology) plus 25 μL of 3.3 mM sivelestat (S7198; Sigma-Aldrich) or PBS in black 96-well plates (137101; ThermoFischer Scientific), as previously described [28]. Fluorescence readings were acquired on a TECAN Infinite 200 Pro using the filter set (excitation 360 nm, emission 465 nm) after 51 h of incubation at 37 °C. Assays were performed with technical duplicates and the results are expressed as mean fluorescence intensity (m.f.i.).

2.5. Cytokine and Chemokine Assays

CSF samples from 13 NET remnant-positive children (54% girls; mean age, 9 years; IQR, 5–13 years) and 25 age- and sex-matched NET remnant-negative children (52% girls; mean age, 9 years; IQR, 4.5–12 years) were analysed for chemokines and cytokines using two different magnetic Luminex® assays (both from R&D Systems, Abingdon, UK). The Human Magnetic Luminex® assay was used to measure the levels of CXCL1, CXCL6, CXCL8 (IL-8), CXCL10, and MMP-9, whereas a high-sensitivity assay (Luminex® Performance Assay) was used for the quantification of TNF, IL-6, and IL-17A. The m.f.i. value of the respective analyte was obtained using FLEXMAP 3D (Luminex Inc., Austin, TX, USA), and the Bio-Plex Manager ver. 6.2 software (Bio-Rad Laboratories, Hercules, CA, USA) was used for data analysis. One of the 11 NET-positive samples was not available for the high-sensitivity assay. The samples were run in two different dilutions at a minimum, and the concordance between dilutions was checked carefully when concentrations had to be determined from different dilutions. Concentrations above the range of quantification were assigned the value of the expected concentration of the highest standard. An m.f.i. value below the lowest standard concentration was assigned a value of 0. The cytokines and chemokines were selected based on their associations with neutrophils and/or NETosis [29–32].

2.6. Statistics

Data were analysed using the GraphPad Prism ver. 8.01 software (GraphPad Software Inc., San Diego, CA, USA). Chi-square or Fisher's exact test was used to compare discrete variables in 2 × 2 contingency tables. D'Agostino and Pearson omnibus normality tests were used to determine whether or not the data for continuous variables had a Gaussian distribution. For a non-Gaussian distribution of the data, the Mann–Whitney U-test was applied in comparisons between two groups with independent observations. The Kruskal–Wallis test was used for comparisons of more than two groups and if the Kruskal–Wallis test result was significant, Dunn's *post hoc* test was performed. For correlation analyses, Spearman's rank correlation coefficient (r_s) was employed. In all the analyses, a *p*-value < 0.05 was considered statistically significant.

2.7. Ethics

The study protocol was approved by the Regional Ethics Review Board in Uppsala (Dnr 2010/106, children) and the local Ethics Committee of the Åland Health Care, Finland (2/2010, 1/2011, adults).

3. Results

3.1. CSF-NETs in Relation to Patient Diagnoses

NETs were detected in the CSF samples of significantly more children than adults (p = 0.01); in 14 (13%) children, whereof 7 (6%) with LNB, 4 (4%) with EVM, 2 (2%) with TBE, and 1 (1%) with idiopathic peripheral facial nerve palsy (IPFP) without pleocytosis (belonged to the OVI group). Only one adult patient, with meningitis and mononuclear pleocytosis caused by Varicella zoster virus (VZV), had detectable NETs (5 a.u.). The range of NETs levels were as follows: NET-positive patients with LNB, 2–18 a.u. (IQR, 3.2–12.7); NET-positive patients with EVM, 38–2643 a.u. (IQR, 56–2023); in the two NET-positive patients with TBE, 39–74 a.u.; and in the single NET-positive patient with IPFP, the level was 17 a.u. The proportions of NET-positive patients in the LNB (25%), TBE (67%), EVM (57%), and OVI (25%) groups did not differ significantly. Higher levels of NETs were observed among patients with fever (p = 0.002). The NETs levels correlated significantly with the total white blood cell counts in the CSF samples (r_s = 0.43, p < 0.001) (Figure 1A), and with polynuclear pleocytosis (r_s = 0.53, p < 0.0001) (Figure 1B) as well as mononuclear pleocytosis (r_s = 0.41, p < 0.0001) (Figure 1C), although not with age, gender or duration of symptoms. However, when the 14 NET-positive children were analysed separately, the levels of NETs were shown to correlate with polynuclear but not with mononuclear pleocytosis (r_s = 0.58, p = 0.03 and r_s = −0.10, p = 0.72, respectively) (Figure 1D,E). Children with EVM displayed a significantly shorter disease duration than the children with LNB (p = 0.03); and the number of polynuclear cells in CSF among paediatric patients showed an inverse significant correlation with the duration of neurological symptoms (data available for 77 of the 111 cases; r_s = −0.45, p < 0.0001).

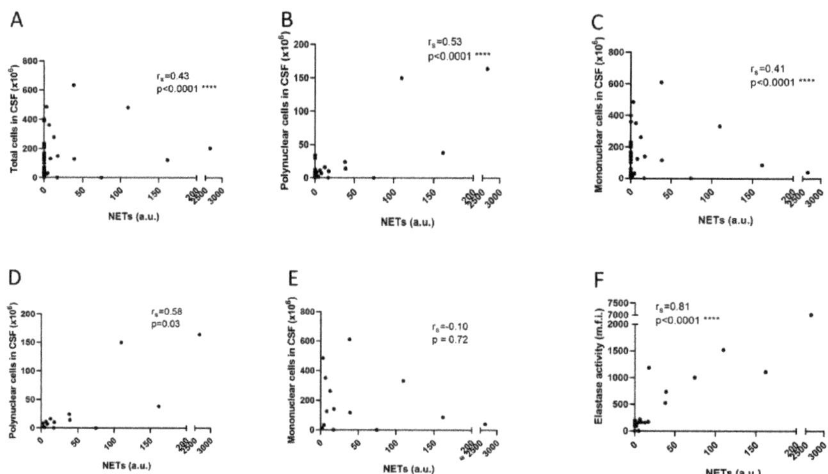

Figure 1. Correlations between cell counts in the CSF and NET remnants: (**A–C**) (*N* = 111 children) and (**D–E**) (*N* = 14 children). Correlation between NET remnants and elastase activity: (**F**) (*N* = 28; 13 NET-positive and 15 NET-negative cases).

3.2. CSF-NE Activity

NE activity was detected in 13/13 NET-positive children but was not detected in the NET-positive adult patient (overall concordance between methods: 93%). The levels of NETs and NE activity correlated significantly ($r_s = 0.81$, $p < 0.0001$) (Figure 1F).

3.3. NETs in Relation to Clinical Outcome in Children

As we only found one NET-positive adult patient, we focused on evaluating NETs in relation to the disease prognosis for children (Table 1). The vast majority of the LNB cases (25/28; 89%) had recovered at the two-month follow-up. Two of the non-recovered children were NET-negative and one had low levels of NETs (2 a.u.). Accordingly, the occurrence of NETs in the CSF was not associated with recovery among the children with LNB ($p = 0.72$). All seven children with EVM were fully recovered at the two-month follow-up, four of whom were NET-positive. Among the three patients with TBE, one of the two patients who recovered was NET-positive, as was the patient who did not recover. Two of the four OVI cases had recovered at follow-up, whereas none had detectable NETs in the CSF. Only two patients in the group with other neurological and non-neurological disorders with CNS symptoms were NET-positive, and they had not recovered at follow-up.

3.4. Cytokines and Chemokines

All eight cytokines/chemokines were detected in at least one sample among the NET-positive ($N = 13$) and NET-negative ($N = 24$ or 25) CSF samples, respectively. The total number of samples within the range of quantification is shown in Table 3. The levels of all the cytokines/chemokines were significantly higher among children with NETs: IL-6 ($p < 0.001$), CXCL8 ($p = 0.003$), IL-17A ($p = 0.03$), TNF ($p = 0.02$), MMP-9 ($p = 0.002$), CXCL1 ($p < 0.001$), CXCL6 ($p = 0.007$) and CXCL10 ($p < 0.001$) (Figure 2A–H) and fever ($N = 16$); IL-6 ($p < 0.001$), CXCL8 ($p = 0.001$), IL-17A ($p = 0.028$), TNF ($p < 0.001$), MMP-9 ($p = 0.009$), CXCL1 ($p = 0.002$), CXCL6 ($p = 0.002$), and CXCL10 ($p = 0.001$). Furthermore, all the cytokines/chemokines, with the exception of IL-17A, were detected at significantly higher levels in the CSF samples from children with pleocytosis ($N = 24$) ($p < 0.001$). A strong and significant correlation was noted between the CSF levels of IL-6, CXCL8, TNF, MMP-9, CXCL1, CXCL6, CXCL10 and NETs, NE, and total CSF cell count, as well as mononuclear and polynuclear pleocytosis, respectively (Table 3). The levels of IL-6, CXCL8, TNF, MMP-9, CXCL1 and CXCL10 in the CSF samples obtained from the different patient groups, respectively, are shown in Figure 3A–H. All the cytokines, with the exception of IL-17A, were present at significantly higher levels in the patients with EVM compared to the patients with "other neurological and non-neurological disorders". Furthermore, all the cytokines/chemokines, with the exceptions of CXCL1, CXCL6, and IL-17A, were detected at higher levels in the patients with LNB, as compared to the patients with "other neurological and non-neurological disorders". CXCL6 was the only cytokine that was detected at significantly different levels when comparing the LNB group with the EVM patient group.

Table 3. Spearman's correlation between cytokines, chemokines, cells and NETs in CSF.

Analyte	Quantified *	NETs (Remnants)		NETs (Elastase) [†]		Cells (Total)		Polynuclear Cells		Mononuclear Cells	
		r_s	*p*-Value	r_s	*p*-Value	r_s	*p*-Value	r_s	*p*-Value	r_s	*p*-Value
CXCL1	21/38	0.61	<0.001	0.76	<0.001	0.52	0.006	0.69	<0.001	0.48	0.02
CXCL6	14/38	0.52	0.007	0.65	0.002	0.72	<0.001	0.74	<0.001	0.67	<0.001
CXCL8	38/38	0.53	0.006	0.64	0.003	0.60	<0.001	0.65	<0.001	0.57	0.002
CXCL10	32/38	0.56	0.002	0.66	0.002	0.79	<0.001	0.81	<0.001	0.76	<0.001
MMP9	25/38	0.53	0.006	N/A	n.s.	0.70	<0.001	0.65	<0.001	0.68	<0.001
TNF	22/37	N/A	n.s.	N/A	n.s.	0.81	<0.001	0.65	<0.001	0.80	<0.001
IL-6	28/37	0.70	<0.001	0.81	<0.001	0.63	<0.001	0.73	<0.001	0.59	<0.001
IL-17A	4/37	N/A	n.s.	N/A	n.s.	N/A	n.s.	0.46	0.03	N/A	n.s.

* Samples within range of quantification (*N*)/total number of samples analysed (*N*). All samples outside the range of quantification were below the range of quantification, except for CXCL10; [†] Data on NETs by elastase assay was only available in 26 samples (CXCL1, CXCL6, CXCL8, CXCL10, MMP9) or 25 samples (TNF, IL-6 and IL-17A); *p*-values have been multiplied by the number of analytes (i.e. 8) to adjust for multiple testing. Grey shading indicates $r_s \geq 0.70$. n.s. = non-significant, N/A = Not applicable.

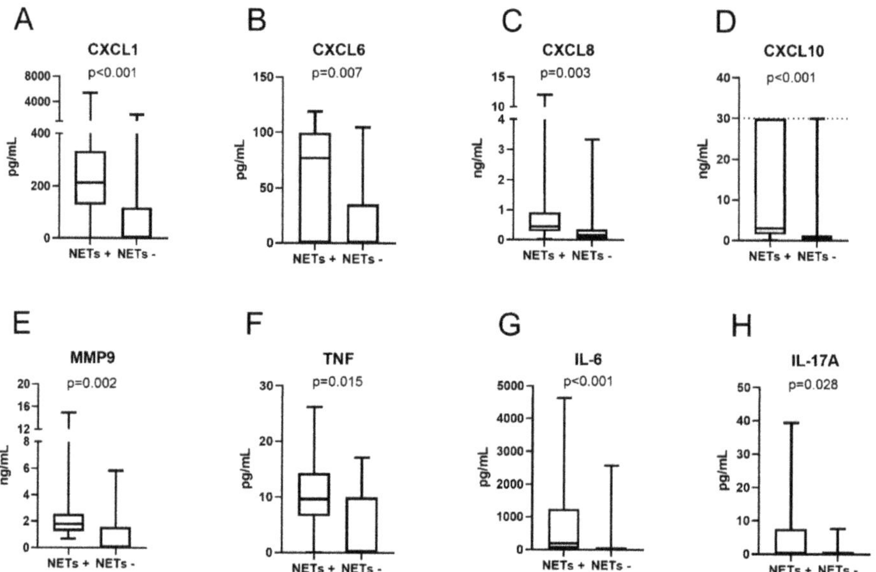

Figure 2. Concentrations of chemokines (**A–D**), MMP9 (**E**) and cytokines (**F–H**) in the CSF samples from the NET remnant-positive and NET remnant-negative children. Whiskers indicate the min-max values. The *p*-values are derived from the Mann–Whitney *U*-test. CXCL10 concentrations above the range of quantification (>30 ng/mL, *N* = 5) were assigned a value of 30 ng/mL (upper range of quantification is indicated by a dashed line). NETs: neutrophil extracellular traps.

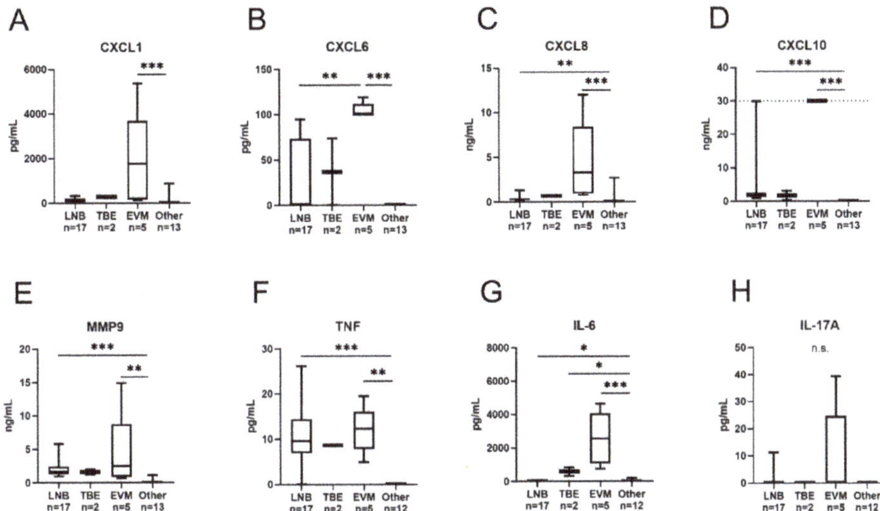

Figure 3. Concentrations of chemokines (**A–D**), MMP9 (**E**) and cytokines (**F–H**) in the CSF samples from the different patient groups. Whiskers indicate the min-max values. CXCL10 concentrations above the range of quantification (>30 ng/mL, $N = 5$) were assigned a value of 30 ng/mL (upper range of quantification is indicated by a dashed line). Only one child (rotavirus infection, no pleocytosis) belonged to the OVI group and is not included in the figure. LNB. Lyme neuroborreliosis; TBE, tick-borne encephalitis; EVM, enteroviral meningitis; Other, other non-infectious neurological and non-neurological disorders with CNS symptoms. * $p < 0.05$, ** $p < 0.01$, *** $p < 0.001$

4. Discussion

In recent years, interest in NETs has shifted from their roles in innate immune defence to their pathogenic importance in several clinical conditions, such as autoimmune diseases, cancer, cardio-vascular morbidity, and most recently, in infections [14,33]. In the present study, we present, for the first time, evidence of NETs in the CSF of patients with LNB with meningeal inflammation, consisting of both mononuclear and polynuclear pleocytosis, as well as in patients with viral infections of the CNS. NETs are defined as complexes of DNA and MPO, although NE constitutes an additional NET component [34]. All but two of the CSF samples with detectable NETs displayed NE activity also, supporting the actual presence of NETs in the samples (concordance between methods: 93%).

The levels of NETs showed strong variability between the different patient groups, ranging from 2 to 2000 a.u. Interestingly, the highest levels of NETs were detected in children with EVM and TBE, who also had the highest median levels of polynuclear cells. Children with EVM also had the highest median levels of NETs/neutrophil-associated cytokines and chemokines in their CSF samples (among the 38 patients in whom cytokines and chemokines were analysed). In addition, the levels of NETs correlated significantly with the numbers of polynuclear cells, i.e., including neutrophils, which were absent in the paediatric controls (Other disorders) and were overall present at lower levels in the adult patients with longer disease duration, which might explain the absence of NETs in these samples. The only adult who possessed detectable NETs had VZV meningitis with a symptom duration of several weeks and few polynuclear cells in the CSF.

The median pleocytosis values were comparable among children with LNB and EVM, although the proportion of polynuclear cells was higher in the latter group. This may be due to the fact that all the patients with EVM had meningeal signs and, consequently, a significantly shorter disease duration before admittance to hospital, as compared to the patients with LNB. In line with this, the numbers of polynuclear cells in the CSF were found to be inversely correlated with the duration of symptoms.

The finding of neutrophil activation in both LNB and EVM is intriguing, since these infections have similarities with respect to both clinical presentation and CSF cellular profile, which may include neutrophil predominance in the early phase [35]. Several studies have de facto shown the presence of neutrophil-activating cytokines and chemokines in the CSF samples of patients with LNB [36–39] and EVM [40,41], and the production of neutrophil chemo-attractants, such as CXCL1, CXCL8 and CXCL10 after *in vitro* stimulation of neuronal cells in response to *B. burgdorferi* spirochaetes [42]. Thus, there appears to be a prerequisite for neutrophil recruitment into the CNS in infections caused by *B. burgdorferi* and enterovirus. To clarify further the presence of neutrophils in these CNS infections, we analysed several potent neutrophil-activating cytokines and chemokines in the NET-positive samples. The results showed increased levels of almost all the measured cytokines/chemokines, and these levels strongly correlated with both poly- and mononuclear pleocytosis.

The chemokine CXCL10, also called interferon (IFN) γ-inducible protein 10 (IP-10), is produced by innate immune cells, such as neutrophils, and it stimulates chemotaxis of mononuclear cells into the CNS in response to meningitis/encephalitis caused by, for instance, enterovirus [43], *B. burgdorferi* [44], and TBE virus [45]. Furthermore, IP-10 has been proposed as a potential discriminator between bacterial and viral CNS infections [41]. Interestingly, CXCL10 was particularly increased in the EVM group, in which the proportion of polynuclear cells was highest. We also found especially increased levels of the fever-inducing cytokines TNF and IL-6 [46] in the EVM group, in which all the patients reported having fever. The chemokines CXCL1, CXCL6 and CXCL8 bind to the CXC-receptor 2 on neutrophils [47], activating them and enabling their entry into the CNS during infections [48]. The highest levels of these cytokines were, as expected, detected in the EVM patients. IL-17A, which is produced by Th17 cells, is a potent activator of neutrophils through stimulation of CXCL1 and CXCL8. Its pathogenic role in the CNS has been studied in LNB [36] and in other bacterial as well as viral CNS infections [49].

The paucity of NETs in the CSF of the adult patients in general, and in the adult LNB patients in particular, might be attributable to a delay between innate immune activation and CSF analysis through lumbar puncture, since the adult patients had longer duration of symptoms at admittance. While the reason for the modest neutrophil activation in LNB is unknown, it might involve an inhibitory effect of the spirochaetes on early pathogen recognition and elimination. Indeed, outer surface proteins (Osp), which are major virulence factors expressed on the surface of *B. burgdorferi* in the early phase of LD, are required for the spirochaetes to establish infection. OspB have been shown to inhibit the phagocytosis and oxidative burst of human neutrophils and may interfere with complement activation [50]. OspC is known to protect *Borrelia sp.* from phagocytosis by mononuclear phagocytes, and also to some extent by neutrophils [51].

Since extracellular traps are not produced exclusively by neutrophils, being also produced by mononuclear cells, termed monocyte or macrophage extracellular traps (METs) [52,53], we calculated the proportions of polynuclear and mononuclear cells in the NET-positive samples. It proved to be specifically the polynuclear cells, rather than the cause of the pleocytosis (i.e., the diagnosis), that correlated with the levels of NETs. Moreover, the NET levels and NE activity showed a high degree of correlation. Therefore, we conclude that the NET structures detected were primarily of neutrophil origin. Despite measuring the NET components with two different methods, we cannot affirm unambiguously that the presence of these components is exclusively the result of NET formation, which is always a limitation when one is not studying the actual cellular processes. To investigate this aspect further, cells from the CSF need to be monitored in detail.

We are unable to draw firm conclusions regarding the levels of NETs in relation to disease recovery in any of the patient groups, except in the paediatric LNB group, in which the occurrence of NETs at admission was shown not to be associated with poor clinical outcome at the two-month follow-up. The strengths of the present study are that it is hypothesis driven and has a systematic design, in addition to having well-characterised patients and concordant results. However, the uneven distribution of patients in the different groups and the heterogeneity within the group of other disorders are limitations that made comparisons of the results between patients more difficult.

5. Conclusions

We demonstrate the presence of NETs in the CSF samples collected from patients with LNB and viral CNS infections and show that NETs strongly correlate with the presence of pleocytosis and neutrophil-stimulating cytokines/chemokines in the CSF. Further studies of human neutrophils and their activation products are warranted, so as to elucidate their pathogenic and prognostic roles in acute bacterial and viral infections of the CNS.

Author Contributions: All authors have read and agree to the published version of the manuscript. Conceptualization, J.S., C.S. and D.A.; methodology, D.A., H.E., J.S., J.K. and L.E.M.; software, D.A. and H.E.; validation, D.A., H.E., M.N., L.P., D.N., C.S. and J.S.; formal analysis, D.A., H.E., C.S. and J.S.; investigation, D.A., H.E., B.H.S., M.N., L.P., D.N., C.N., J.K., L.E.M. and J.S.; resources, D.A., H.E., B.H.S., M.N., L.P., D.N., C.N., J.K., L.E.M., C.S. and J.S.; data curation, D.A., H.E. and L.E.M., writing—original draft preparation, D.A., H.E., J.K., L.E.M. and J.S.; writing—review and editing, D.A., H.E., B.H.S., M.N., L.P., D.N., C.N., J.K., L.E.M., C.S. and J.S.; visualization, D.A., H.E., C.S. and J.S.; supervision, C.S., D.N. and L.E.M.; project administration, J.S.; funding, D.A., B.H.S., D.N., L.E.M. and C.S.; acquisition, D.A., L.E.M., C.S. and J.S. All authors have read and agreed to the published version of the manuscript.

Funding: This study was funded by grants from Region Östergötland (ALF grants), the Swedish Rheumatism Association, the Ingrid Asp Foundation, the Center for Clinical Research Dalarna, the King Gustaf V and Queen Victoria's Freemasons Foundations, the Åland Cultural Foundation, the Wilhelm & Else Stockmann Foundation, the German Research Foundation (project GRK1660), the European Commission (H2020-MSCA-RISE-2015; project 690836 PANG) and the VolkswagenStiftung (grant 90361).

Acknowledgments: We thank Susanne Olausson at Bimelix, Mariehamn, the Åland Islands, and Karin Elving at Clinical Microbiology, Region Dalarna, Sweden for invaluable assistance with the CSF samples. The authors thank all the patients and their parents/guardians for participating in the study, as well as the staff at the paediatric units in Linköping, Norrköping, Jönköping, Skövde, Lidköping, Västerås and Falun for patient recruitment.

References

1. Halperin, J.J. Lyme neuroborreliosis. *Curr. Opin. Infect. Dis.* **2019**, *32*, 259–264. [CrossRef] [PubMed]
2. Henningsson, A.J.; Malmvall, B.E.; Ernerudh, J.; Matussek, A.; Forsberg, P. Neuroborreliosis-An epidemiological, clinical and healthcare cost study from an endemic area in the south-east of Sweden. *Clin. Microbiol. Infect.* **2010**, *16*, 1245–1251. [CrossRef] [PubMed]
3. Skogman, B.H.; Croner, S.; Nordwall, M.; Eknefelt, M.; Ernerudh, J.; Forsberg, P. Lyme neuroborreliosis in children: A prospective study of clinical features, prognosis, and outcome. *Pediatr. Infect. Dis. J.* **2008**, *27*, 1089–1094. [CrossRef] [PubMed]
4. Sodermark, L.; Sigurdsson, V.; Nas, W.; Wall, P.; Trollfors, B. Neuroborreliosis in Swedish Children: A Population-based Study on Incidence and Clinical Characteristics. *Pediatr. Infect. Dis. J.* **2017**, *36*, 1052–1056. [CrossRef] [PubMed]
5. Dahl, V.; Wisell, K.T.; Giske, C.G.; Tegnell, A.; Wallensten, A. Lyme neuroborreliosis epidemiology in Sweden 2010 to 2014: Clinical microbiology laboratories are a better data source than the hospital discharge diagnosis register. *Euro Surveill.* **2019**, *24*, 20. [CrossRef]
6. Pietikainen, A.; Oksi, J.; Hytonen, J. Point-of-care testing for CXCL13 in Lyme neuroborreliosis. *Diagn Microbiol. Infect. Dis.* **2018**, *91*, 226–228. [CrossRef]
7. Mygland, A.; Ljostad, U.; Fingerle, V.; Rupprecht, T.; Schmutzhard, E.; Steiner, I.; European Federation of Neurological Societies. EFNS guidelines on the diagnosis and management of European Lyme neuroborreliosis. *Eur. J. Neurol.* **2010**, *17*, 8–16. [CrossRef]
8. Shah, S.S.; Zaoutism, T.E.; Turnquist, J.; Hodinka, R.L.; Coffin, S.E. Early differentiation of Lyme from enteroviral meningitis. *Pediatr. Infect. Dis. J.* **2005**, *24*, 542–545. [CrossRef]
9. Salazar, J.C.; Pope, C.D.; Sellati, T.J.; Feder, H.M.; Jr Kiely, T.G.; Dardick, K.R.; Buckman, R.L.; Moore, M.W.; Caimano, M.J.; Pope, J.G.; et al. Coevolution of markers of innate and adaptive immunity in skin and peripheral blood of patients with erythema migrans. *J. Immunol.* **2003**, *171*, 2660–2670. [CrossRef]

10. Liew, P.X.; Kubes, P. The Neutrophil's Role During Health and Disease. *Physiol. Rev.* **2019**, *99*, 1223–1248. [CrossRef]

11. Kruger, P.; Saffarzadeh, M.; Weber, A.N.; Rieber, N.; Radsak, M.; von Bernuth, H.; Benarafa, C.; Roos, D.; Skokowa, J. Hartl DNeutrophils: Between host defence immune modulation,, tissue, injury. *PLoS Pathog.* **2015**, *11*, e1004651. [CrossRef] [PubMed]

12. Papayannopoulos, V. Neutrophil extracellular traps in immunity and disease. *Nat. Rev. Immunol.* **2018**, *18*, 134–147. [CrossRef]

13. Brinkmann, V.; Reichard, U.; Goosmann, C.; Fauler, B.; Uhlemann, Y.; Weiss, D.S.; Weinrauch, Y.; Zychlinsky, A. Neutrophil extracellular traps kill bacteria. *Science* **2004**, *303*, 1532–1535. [CrossRef] [PubMed]

14. Brinkmann, V. Neutrophil Extracellular Traps in the Second Decade. *J. Innate Immun.* **2018**, *10*, 414–421. [CrossRef] [PubMed]

15. Mahajan, A.; Gruneboom, A.; Petru, L.; Podolska, M.J.; Kling, L.; Maueroder, C.; Dahms, F.; Christiansen, S.; Günter, L.; Krenn, V.; et al. Frontline Science: Aggregated neutrophil extracellular traps prevent inflammation on the neutrophil-rich ocular surface. *J. Leukoc. Biol.* **2019**, *105*, 1087–1098. [CrossRef]

16. Munoz, L.E.; Boeltz, S.; Bilyy, R.; Schauer, C.; Mahajan, A.; Widulin, N.; Grüneboom, A.; Herrmann, I.; Boada, E.; Rauh, M.; et al. Neutrophil Extracellular Traps Initiate Gallstone Formation. *Immunity* **2019**, *51*, 443–450. [CrossRef]

17. Schonrich, G.; Raftery, M.J. Neutrophil Extracellular Traps Go Viral. *Front. Immunol.* **2016**, *7*, 366. [CrossRef]

18. Menten-Dedoyart, C.; Faccinetto, C.; Golovchenko, M.; Dupiereux, I.; Van Lerberghe, P.B.; Dubois, S.; Desmet, C.; Elmoualij, B.; Baron, F.; Rudenko, N.; et al. Neutrophil extracellular traps entrap and kill Borrelia burgdorferi sensu stricto spirochetes and are not affected by Ixodes ricinus tick saliva. *J. Immunol.* **2012**, *189*, 5393–5401. [CrossRef]

19. De Buhr, N.; Reuner, F.; Neumann, A.; Stump-Guthier, C.; Tenenbaum, T.; Schroten, H.; Ishikawa, H.; Müller, K.; Beineke, A.; Hennig-Pauka, I.; et al. Neutrophil extracellular trap formation in the Streptococcus suis-infected cerebrospinal fluid compartment. *Cell Microbiol.* **2017**, *19*, 12649. [CrossRef]

20. Mohanty, T.; Fisher, J.; Bakochi, A.; Neumann, A.; Cardoso, J.F.P.; Karlsson, C.A.Q.; Pavan, C.; Lundgaard, I.; Nilson, B.; Peter, R.; et al. Neutrophil extracellular traps in the central nervous system hinder bacterial clearance during pneumococcal meningitis. *Nat. Commun.* **2019**, *10*, 1667. [CrossRef]

21. Knudtzen, F.C.; Andersen, N.S.; Jensen, T.G.; Skarphedinsson, S. Characteristics and Clinical Outcome of Lyme Neuroborreliosis in a High Endemic Area, 1995–2014: A Retrospective Cohort Study in Denmark. *Clin. Infect. Dis.* **2017**, *65*, 1489–1495. [CrossRef] [PubMed]

22. Schauer, C.; Janko, C.; Munoz, L.E.; Zhao, Y.; Kienhofer, D.; Frey, B. Aggregated neutrophil extracellular traps limit inflammation by degrading cytokines and chemokines. *Nat. Med.* **2014**, *20*, 511–517. [CrossRef] [PubMed]

23. Backman, K.; Skogman, B.H. Occurrence of erythema migrans in children with Lyme neuroborreliosis and the association with clinical characteristics and outcome—A prospective cohort study. *BMC Pediatr.* **2018**, *18*, 189. [CrossRef] [PubMed]

24. Hansen, K.; Lebech, A.M. Lyme neuroborreliosis: A new sensitive diagnostic assay for intrathecal synthesis of Borrelia burgdorferi-specific immunoglobulin GA. and M. *Ann. Neurol.* **1991**, *30*, 197–205. [CrossRef]

25. Rupprecht, T.A.; Manz, K.M.; Fingerle, V.; Lechner, C.; Klein, M.; Pfirrmann, M.; Koedel, U. Diagnostic value of cerebrospinal fluid CXCL13 for acute Lyme neuroborreliosis. A systematic review and meta-analysis. *Clin. Microbiol. Infect.* **2018**, *24*, 1234–1240. [CrossRef]

26. Soderberg, D.; Kurz, T.; Motamedi, A.; Hellmark, T.; Eriksson, P.; Segelmark, M. Increased levels of neutrophil extracellular trap remnants in the circulation of patients with small vessel vasculitis, but an inverse correlation to anti-neutrophil cytoplasmic antibodies during remission. *Rheumatolog (Oxf.)* **2015**, *54*, 2085–2094. [CrossRef]

27. Kessenbrock, K.; Krumbholz, M.; Schonermarck, U.; Back, W.; Gross, W.L.; Werb, Z.; Gröne, H.J.; Brinkmann, V.; Jenne, D.E. Netting neutrophils in autoimmune small-vessel vasculitis. *Nat. Med.* **2009**, *15*, 623–625. [CrossRef]

28. Appelgren, D.; Dahle, C.; Knopf, J.; Bilyy, R.; Vovk, V.; Sundgren, P.C.; Bengtsson, A.A.; Wetterö, J.; Muñoz, L.E.; Herrmann, M.; et al. Active NET formation in Libman-Sacks endocarditis without antiphospholipid antibodies: A dramatic onset of systemic lupus erythematosus. *Autoimmunity* **2018**, *51*, 310–318. [CrossRef]

29. Rumble, J.M.; Huber, A.K.; Krishnamoorthy, G.; Srinivasan, A.; Giles, D.A.; Zhang, X.; Wang, L.; Segal, B.M. Neutrophil-related factors as biomarkers in EAE and MS. *J. Exp. Med.* **2015**, *212*, 23–35. [CrossRef]

30. Michael, M.; Vermeren, S. A neutrophil-centric view of chemotaxis. *Essays Biochem.* **2019**, *63*, 607–618.

31. Isailovic, N.; Daigo, K.; Mantovani, A.; Selmi, C. Interleukin-17 and innate immunity in infections and chronic inflammation. *J. Autoimmun.* **2015**, *60*, 1–11. [CrossRef]

32. Hellberg, S.; Eklund, D.; Gawel, D.R.; Kopsen, M.; Zhang, H.; Nestor, C.E.; Kockum, I.; Olsson, T.; Skogh, T.; Kastbom, A.; et al. Dynamic Response Genes in CD4+ T Cells Reveal a Network of Interactive Proteins that Classifies Disease Activity in Multiple Sclerosis. *Cell Rep.* **2016**, *16*, 2928–2939. [CrossRef] [PubMed]

33. O'Neil, L.J.; Kaplan, M.J.; Carmona-Rivera, C. The Role of Neutrophils and Neutrophil Extracellular Traps in Vascular Damage in Systemic Lupus Erythematosus. *J. Clin. Med.* **2019**, *8*, 1325. [CrossRef] [PubMed]

34. Papayannopoulos, V.; Metzler, K.D.; Hakkim, A.; Zychlinsky, A. Neutrophil elastase and myeloperoxidase regulate the formation of neutrophil extracellular traps. *J. Cell Biol.* **2010**, *191*, 677–691. [CrossRef]

35. Makis, A.; Shipway, D.; Hatzimichael, E.; Galanakis, E.; Pshezhetskiy, D.; Chaliasos, N.; Stebbing, J.; Siamopoulou, A. Cytokine and adhesion molecule expression evolves between the neutrophilic and lymphocytic phases of viral meningitis. *J. Interferon Cytokine Res.* **2010**, *30*, 661–665. [CrossRef] [PubMed]

36. Gyllemark, P.; Forsberg, P.; Ernerudh, J.; Henningsson, A.J. Intrathecal Th17- and B cell-associated cytokine and chemokine responses in relation to clinical outcome in Lyme neuroborreliosis: A large retrospective study. *J. Neuroinflamm.* **2017**, *14*, 27. [CrossRef] [PubMed]

37. Pietikainen, A.; Maksimow, M.; Kauko, T.; Hurme, S.; Salmi, M.; Hytonen, J. Cerebrospinal fluid cytokines in Lyme neuroborreliosis. *J. Neuroinflamm.* **2016**, *13*, 273. [CrossRef]

38. Cerar, T.; Ogrinc, K.; Lotric-Furlan, S.; Kobal, J.; Levicnik-Stezinar, S.; Strle, F.; Ruzić-Sabljic, E. Diagnostic value of cytokines and chemokines in lyme neuroborreliosis. *Clin. Vaccine Immunol.* **2013**, *20*, 1578–1584. [CrossRef]

39. Eckman, E.A.; Pacheco-Quinto, J.; Herdt, A.R.; Halperin, J.J. Neuroimmunomodulators in Neuroborreliosis and Lyme Encephalopathy. *Clin. Infect. Dis.* **2018**, *67*, 80–88. [CrossRef]

40. Park, S.E.; Shin, K.; Song, D.; Nam, S.O.; Kim, K.M.; Lyu, S.Y. Comparison of Cerebrospinal Fluid Cytokine Levels in Children of Enteroviral Meningitis With Versus Without Pleocytosis. *J. Interferon Cytokine Res.* **2018**, *38*, 348–355. [CrossRef]

41. Maric, L.S.; Lepej, S.Z.; Gorenec, L.; Grgic, I.; Trkulja, V.; Rode, O.D.; Roglic, S.; Grmoja, T.; Barisic, N.; Tesovic, G. Chemokines CXCL10, CXCL11, and CXCL13 in acute disseminated encephalomyelitis, non-polio enterovirus aseptic meningitis, and neuroborreliosis: CXCL10 as initial discriminator in diagnostic algorithm? *Neurol Sci.* **2018**, *39*, 471–479. [CrossRef] [PubMed]

42. Brissette, C.A.; Kees, E.D.; Burke, M.M.; Gaultney, R.A.; Floden, A.M.; Watt, J.A. The multifaceted responses of primary human astrocytes and brain microvascular endothelial cells to the Lyme disease spirochete, Borrelia burgdorferi. *ASN Neuro* **2013**, *5*, 221–229. [CrossRef] [PubMed]

43. Cavcic, A.; Tesovic, G.; Gorenec, L.; Grgic, I.; Benic, B.; Lepej, S.Z. Concentration gradient of CXCL10 and CXCL11 between the cerebrospinal fluid and plasma in children with enteroviral aseptic meningitis. *Eur. J. Paediatr. Neurol.* **2011**, *15*, 502–507. [CrossRef] [PubMed]

44. Henningsson, A.J.; Tjernberg, I.; Malmvall, B.E.; Forsberg, P.; Ernerudh, J. Indications of Th1 and Th17 responses in cerebrospinal fluid from patients with Lyme neuroborreliosis: A large retrospective study. *J. Neuroinflamm.* **2011**, *8*, 36. [CrossRef]

45. Zajkowska, J.; Moniuszko-Malinowska, A.; Pancewicz, S.A.; Muszynska-Mazur, A.; Kondrusik, M.; Grygorczuk, S.; Swierzbińska-Pijanowska, R.; Dunaj, J.; Czupryna, P. Evaluation of CXCL10, CXCL11, CXCL12 and CXCL13 chemokines in serum and cerebrospinal fluid in patients with tick borne encephalitis (TBE). *Adv. Med. Sci.* **2011**, *56*, 311–317. [CrossRef]

46. Evans, S.S.; Repasky, E.A.; Fisher, D.T. Fever and the thermal regulation of immunity: The immune system feels the heat. *Nat. Rev. Immunol.* **2015**, *15*, 335–349. [CrossRef]

47. Sadik, C.D.; Kim, N.D.; Luster, A.D. Neutrophils cascading their way to inflammation. *Trends Immunol.* **2011**, *32*, 452–460. [CrossRef]

48. Simmons, S.B.; Liggitt, D.; Goverman, J.M. Cytokine-regulated neutrophil recruitment is required for brain but not spinal cord inflammation during experimental autoimmune encephalomyelitis. *J. Immunol.* **2014**, *193*, 555–563. [CrossRef]

49. Morichi, S.; Urabe, T.; Morishita, N.; Takeshita, M.; Ishida, Y.; Oana, S.; Yamanaka, G.; Kashiwagi, Y.; Kawashima, H. Pathological analysis of children with childhood central nervous system infection based on changes in chemokines and interleukin-17 family cytokines in cerebrospinal fluid. *J. Clin. Lab Anal.* **2018**, *32*, 521784686. [CrossRef]

50. Hartiala, P.; Hytonen, J.; Suhonen, J.; Lepparanta, O.; Tuominen-Gustafsson, H.; Viljanen, M.K. Borrelia burgdorferi inhibits human neutrophil functions. *Microbes Infect.* **2008**, *10*, 60–68. [CrossRef]

51. Carrasco, S.E.; Troxell, B.; Yang, Y.; Brandt, S.L.; Li, H.; Sandusky, G.E.; Condon, K.W.; Serezani, C.H.; Yang, X.F. Outer surface protein OspC is an antiphagocytic factor that protects Borrelia burgdorferi from phagocytosis by macrophages. *Infect. Immun.* **2015**, *83*, 4848–4860. [CrossRef] [PubMed]

52. Doster, R.S.; Rogers, L.M.; Gaddy, J.A.; Aronoff, D.M. Macrophage Extracellular Traps: A Scoping Review. *J. Innate Immun.* **2018**, *10*, 3–13. [CrossRef] [PubMed]

53. Granger, V.; Faille, D.; Marani, V.; Noel, B.; Gallais, Y.; Szely, N.; Flament, H.; Pallardy, M.; Chollet-Martin, S.; de Chaisemartin, L. Human blood monocytes are able to form extracellular traps. *J. Leukoc. Biol.* **2017**, *102*, 775–781. [CrossRef] [PubMed]

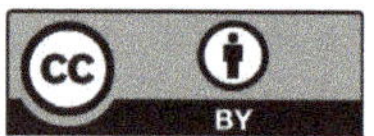

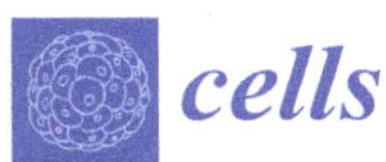 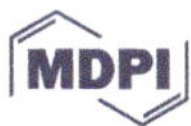

Article

Plasma Proteins and Platelets Modulate Neutrophil Clearance of Malaria-Related Hemozoin Crystals

Sueli de Oliveira Silva Lautenschlager [1], Tehyung Kim [2], Danielle Lazarim Bidóia [1], Celso Vataru Nakamura [1], Hans-Joachim Anders [2] and Stefanie Steiger [2,*]

[1]   Postgraduate Program in Pharmaceutical Sciences, State University of Maringá, Maringá, Paraná 5790, Brazil; lautenschlager@uem.br (S.d.O.S.L.); dlbidoia@gmail.com (D.L.B.); cvnakamura@uem.br (C.V.N.)

[2]   Division of Nephrology, Department of Medicine IV, Hospital of the LMU Munich, 80336 Munich, Germany; tehyung95@gmail.com (T.K.); hjanders@med.uni-muenchen.de (H.-J.A.)

*   Correspondence: stefanie.steiger@med.uni-muenchen.de; Tel.: +49-89-4400-52129

Received: 28 November 2019; Accepted: 20 December 2019; Published: 30 December 2019

Abstract: Hemozoin is an insoluble crystalline pigment produced by the malaria parasite *Plasmodia* upon digesting host hemoglobin inside red blood cells. Red blood cell rupture releases hemozoin crystals into the circulation from where they are cleared by phagocytes such as neutrophils. We speculated that plasma proteins would affect the ability of neutrophils to clear hemozoin crystals. To test this, we cultured human blood neutrophils with hemozoin ex vivo and found that neutrophils ingested hemozoin (0.1–1 µm crystal size) in a dose-dependent manner into phagosomes and vesicles/vacuoles, resulting in morphological changes including nuclear enlargement, and vesicle formation, but not cell membrane rupture or release of neutrophil extracellular traps. The presence of human plasma significantly inhibited the ability of neutrophils to ingest hemozoin crystals. Platelet-poor plasma further inhibited the uptake of hemozoin by neutrophils. Selective exposure to fibrinogen completely replicated the plasma effect. Taken together, neutrophils cleared hemozoin crystals from the extracellular space via endocytosis into phagosomes and vesicles without inducing the release of neutrophil extracellular traps. However, human plasma components such as fibrinogen limited hemozoin clearance, whereas the presence of platelets augmented this process. These factors may influence the pro-inflammatory potential of hemozoin crystals in malaria.

Keywords: hemozoin; neutrophils; plasma; fibrinogen; platelet; malaria

---

1. Introduction

Malaria is a life-threatening disease caused by the *Plasmodium* parasite [1]. Globally, approximately 216 million cases of malaria were reported in 2016 with an estimate of 445,000 deaths [1]. Upon parasite (called sporozoite) transmission to humans through the bites of infected mosquitoes, the parasites distribute via the bloodstream to the liver. Within the liver, each sporozoite multiplies into thousands of merozoites that reach back into the bloodstream, where they infect red blood cells for further replication. Parasite replication occurs in a cyclic fashion within red blood cells. During this erythrocytic cycle, the parasite degrades hemoglobin into amino acids and heme inside the digestive vacuole, where the heme monomer is further oxidized into a toxic inert biocrystalline form called malarial pigment or hemozoin (HZ) [2–4]. Upon red blood cell rupture, HZ as well as other parasite toxins including *Plasmodium* DNA and glycosylphosphatidylinositol are released into circulation and recognized by pattern recognition receptors expressed on phagocytes and other immune cells in the blood and tissues [5]. This erythrocytic cycle is responsible for most of the pathological symptoms of malaria such as fever through the induction of a pro-inflammatory pyrogenic immune response [6].

Among the phagocytes, neutrophils are the first line of defense to respond to pathogens by generating reactive oxygen species, and antimicrobial peptides and proteases, or by neutrophil extracellular trap (NET) formation [7,8]. Studies have linked neutrophil activation and circulating NETs to the pathogenesis of malaria, including parasite sequestration in the microvasculature and endothelial dysfunction, resulting in impaired tissue perfusion and organ dysfunction [9–11]. A previous report demonstrated the presence of NETs in children with uncomplicated falciparum malaria with parasites trapped within NETs [12] and in malaria patients with severe disease [13,14]. However, there is a paucity of data on the direct interaction of HZ crystals and neutrophils, but the severity of malaria is associated with the clearance capacity of circulating HZ crystals by neutrophils [15]. HZ can interact with serum/plasma molecules such as proteins, lipids, and DNA, even before they encounter immune cells [16,17]. Whether human plasma can affect the HZ crystal clearing capacity by neutrophils is currently not known. We hypothesized that human plasma proteins would impair the ability of neutrophils to internalize HZ crystals.

2. Material and Methods

2.1. Isolation of Human Blood Neutrophils

Blood from human healthy individuals was collected in S-Monovette with lithium heparin (Sarstedt, Germany), and plasma was separated and neutrophils were isolated using standard dextran sedimentation followed by Ficoll–Hypaque density centrifugation procedures [18]. Neutrophils were suspended in Roswell Park Memorial Institute (RPMI) medium (0.5×10^5 cells/200 μL or 2.5×10^5 cells/mL) and seeded into 96-well or 24-well plates in a 5% carbon dioxide atmosphere at 37 °C for 30 min before stimulation. The study to obtain whole blood samples from healthy volunteers was approved by the local Ethical Review Board of the Medical Faculty at the Hospital of the Ludwig-Maximilians-University (LMU) Munich. Informed consent was obtained from all subjects.

2.2. Fluorescence Microscopy of Hemozoin Uptake

Human blood neutrophils were cultured ex vivo in the presence or absence of synthetic HZ (50 and 100 μg/mL, Invivogen, San Diego, CA, USA) in RPMI medium with or without 10%, 30%, or 50% human plasma in 8-well chamber slides (7.5×10^5 cells/well, Nunc Lab-Tek, Sigma-Aldrich, Germany) for 1, 2, and 18 h. After incubation, cells were fixed using 4% paraformaldehyde for 10 min at room temperature, washed twice with Dulbecco's Phosphate-Buffered Saline (D-PBS), and stained with phalloidin green for 40 min (165 nM, Sigma-Aldrich, indicates actin filaments). After membrane staining, cells were mounted with 4′,6-Diamidin-2-phenylindol (DAPI) (Sigma-Aldrich, indicates cell nuclei). The uptake of HZ by neutrophils was visualized using a Leica TL Light-emitting diodes (LED) fluorescence or confocal microscope (Leica, Wetzlar, Germany).

2.3. Uptake of Hemozoin in Neutrophils Using Flow Cytometry

Human blood neutrophils were cultured ex vivo in 96-well plates (0.5×10^5 cells/200 μL) in the presence or absence of HZ (50 and 100 μg/mL) or silica crystals (200 μg/mL, Sigma-Aldrich, Germany) in RPMI medium without or with 10%, 30%, or 50% human plasma for 1, 2, and 18 h. In some experiments, cytochalasin D (10 μM, Sigma-Aldrich) was used to block phagocytosis of HZ crystals. To look at the effect of plasma proteins, HZ crystals were pre-incubated with or without fibrinogen (0.5 mg/mL, Sigma-Aldrich), albumin (3.25 mg/mL, Bethyl Labs, Montgomery, AL, USA), or Ringer's solution (30%, negative control, Fresenius Kabi, Germany) for 30 min prior to stimulation with neutrophils. After stimulation, culture supernatants were collected and stored at −20 °C until further use, and cells harvested to quantify the percentage of cells that had internalized HZ crystals (HZ crystal$^+$ neutrophils) were determined by flow cytometry using the BD FACSCalibur flow cytometer and FlowJo v7 software (Tree Star, Ashland, OR, USA).

To confirm intracellular uptake of HZ by neutrophils, human neutrophils were cultured with or without HZ (50 and 100 μg/mL) in RPMI medium for 2 h and then stained with the pHrodo red acetoxymethyl (AM) intracellular pH indicator (Thermo Fisher Scientific, Germany) for flow cytometry analysis as per the manufacturer's protocol. An increase in the mean fluorescence intensity (MFI) of pHrodo red indicates an intracellular pH drop following HZ uptake.

2.4. Preparation and Stimulation of Neutrophils with Platelet-Poor Plasma

Human blood was drawn and standard dextran sedimentation performed to remove red blood cells. The top layer was removed and transferred into a 15 mL FALCON tube prior to centrifugation at $1500\,g$ for 15 min. Using a new transfer pipette, the top layer was transferred into a new 15 mL FALCON tube and centrifuged at $1500\,g$ for 15 min. After centrifugation, the top $\frac{3}{4}$ of plasma was removed using a transfer pipette and transferred into a new 15 mL FALCON tube. Isolated human blood neutrophils were then cultured in the presence or absence of synthetic HZ (50 and 100 µg/mL) in RPMI medium with or without 10%, 30%, or 50% human platelet-poor plasma for 2 h. After stimulation, neutrophils were either stained for fluorescence microscopy or harvested for flow cytometry to determine the percentage of HZ crystal$^+$ neutrophils.

2.5. Morphological and Ultrastructural Analysis by Electron Microscopy

Blood neutrophils from healthy individuals were isolated and cultured (6.4×10^5 cell/mL) ex vivo in the presence or absence of HZ (50 and 100 µg/mL) in RPMI medium with or without 30% human plasma for 2 h, and processed for scanning electron microscopy (SEM) and transmission electron microscopy (TEM).

For SEM, the samples were fixed in 2.5% glutaraldehyde in 0.1 M sodium cacodylate buffer, pH 7.2 at 4 °C for 24 h. Afterwards, the samples were adhered to poly-L-lysine-coated glass slides, dehydrated with increasing concentrations of ethanol (30% to 100%), followed by critical point drying in carbon dioxide to remove any water trace. Samples were then mounted on a stub and coated with gold. The analysis was carried out on a FEI Scios SEM (Hillsboro, OR, USA).

For TEM, the samples were fixed with 2.5% glutaraldehyde in 0.1 M sodium cacodylate buffer (pH 7.2) at 4 °C for 24 h. Post-fixation was performed using a solution of 1% osmium tetroxide, 0.8% potassium ferrocyanide, and 10.0 mM CaCl2 in 0.1 M cacodylate buffer for 1 h. Afterwards, samples were dehydrated in an increasing acetone gradient (30% to 100%) and embedded in Polybed 812 resin. Ultrathin sections were obtained, mounted on copper grids, and stained with uranyl acetate and lead citrate. Analysis was performed on a JEOL JM 1400 TEM (Jeol, Tokyo, Japan).

2.6. Statistical Analysis

Statistical analysis was performed using GraphPad Prism 7.0 software (GraphPad, San Diego, CA, USA). Data were compared either by one-way ANOVA with Tukey's post-hoc test to calculate significance between three or more groups, or two-way ANOVA with Bonferroni's comparison post-hoc test was carried out when using two parameters with multiple groups. Data are presented as mean ± SD. Differences were considered significant if $p < 0.05$. ns indicates not significant. Sample sizes are indicated in each corresponding figure legend.

3. Results

3.1. Neutrophils Took up Hemozoin Crystals under Serum/Plasma-Free Condition

HZ is thermally stable and insoluble, and can be visualized as a crystalline purple-black pigment, which is birefringent under polarized light (Figure S1A). Scanning electron microscopy (SEM) illustrated that HZ crystals had a size of 0.1–1 µm and were quite uniform in shape (Figure S1B) compared to other crystalline particles, including crystals of monosodium urate, calcium oxalate, and cholesterol, as well as asbestos fibers [19,20].

To investigate the capacity of neutrophils to internalize HZ, we cultured human blood neutrophils in the presence or absence of HZ crystals in RPMI medium for 2 h, and performed fluorescence microscopy using the actin stain phalloidin (green) and the nuclear marker DAPI (blue). As illustrated in Figure 1A,A′, the uptake of HZ resulted in morphological changes in neutrophils, in particular in size/shape, as indicated by phalloidin, and in deformed nuclei/granules, as indicated by DAPI. Flow cytometry analysis revealed that neutrophils increased in size and granularity following uptake of HZ, as shown by an increase in side scatter (SSC) (Figure 1B). The percentage of HZ crystal⁺ neutrophils increased in a dose-dependent manner but independent of the exposure time (Figure 1C).

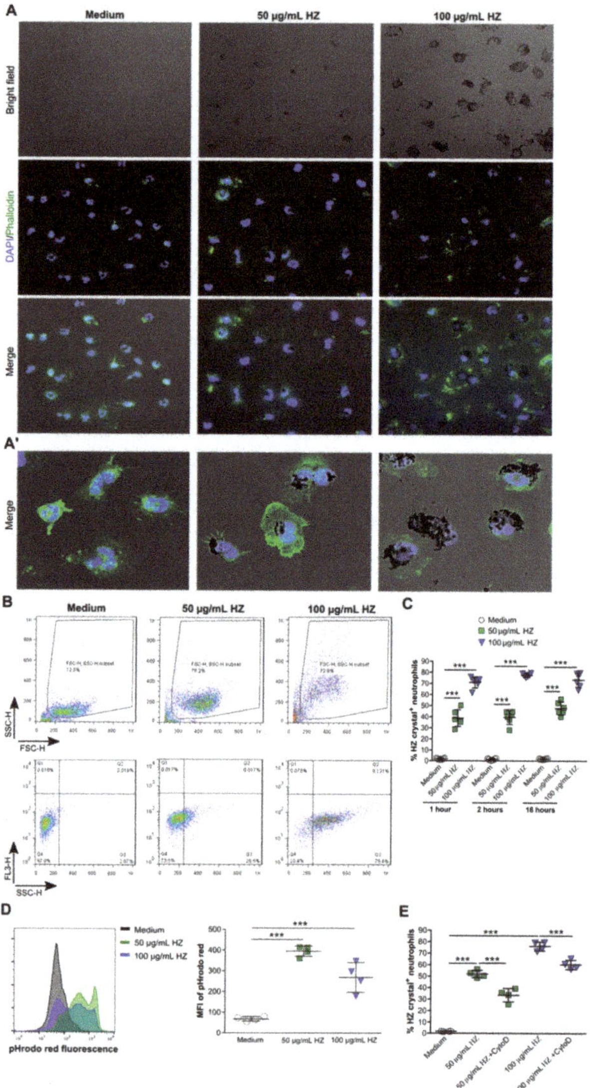

Figure 1. Neutrophils phagocytose large amounts of hemozoin (HZ) crystals. Human blood neutrophils were isolated from healthy volunteers and cultured in the presence or absence of hemozoin (HZ, 50

and 100 µg/mL) in Roswell Park Memorial Institute (RPMI) medium for up to 18 h, and fluorescence microscopy or flow cytometry were performed. (**A**,**A′**) Neutrophils were stained with phalloidin (green) and 4′,6-Diamidin-2-phenylindol (DAPI) (blue) for fluorescence microscopy (200× magnification (**A**)) and confocal microscopy (1000× magnification (**A′**)). (**B**) Representative images of the gating strategy to demonstrate the size of neutrophils (side scatter (SSC)-forward scatter (FSC)) and to quantify the percentage of neutrophils that had internalized HZ. (**C**) Percentage of HZ crystal$^+$ neutrophils after 1, 2, and 18 h (n = 5–6 duplicates from 2–3 donors, two-way ANOVA). (**D**) Neutrophils were stained with the pH-sensitive dye pHrodo red and cultured with or without HZ. Quantification of HZ uptake in neutrophils was indicated by an increased mean fluorescence intensity (MFI) of pHrodo red using flow cytometry (n = 4 duplicates from 2 donors). (**E**) Percentage of HZ crystal$^+$ neutrophils in the absence or presence of cytochalasin D (CytoD) (n = 4 duplicates from 2 donors, one-way ANOVA). Data are mean ± SD and representative of two independent experiments. *** $p < 0.001$; ns, not significant.

Next, to confirm the internalization of HZ, human neutrophils were cultured in the presence or absence of HZ in RPMI medium, and the mean fluorescence intensity (MFI) of the pH-sensitive dye pHrodo red was determined via flow cytometry. As shown in Figure 1D, the uptake of HZ was associated with an increase in the MFI of pHrodo red in HZ-treated neutrophils compared to medium control after 2 h. Blocking HZ uptake with the inhibitor of actin polymerization cytochalasin D significantly reduced the percentage of HZ crystal$^+$ neutrophils, although not completely, compared to untreated HZ crystal$^+$ neutrophils (Figure 1E). Taken together, our data showed that neutrophils internalized HZ crystals partially via phagocytosis and partially via other uptake mechanisms.

3.2. Hemozoin Uptake Caused Nuclei Enlargement and Vesicle Formation but not NET Release

To characterize the internalization process of HZ and the morphological abnormalities in more detail, we performed SEM and transmission electron microscopy (TEM) of human neutrophils in the presence or absence of HZ. Untreated neutrophils appeared round in shape with an even surface (Figure 2A, medium). After intracellular uptake of HZ, neutrophils increased in size and became activated, as illustrated by their rough membrane surface (Figure 2A′,A″). Neutrophils were also surrounded by clusters/aggregates of HZ crystals (white arrows) (Figure 2A′,A″). Under normal conditions (medium), neutrophils showed numerous dense granules and lysosomes in the cytoplasm (Figure 2B). The multi-lobed nucleus with the highly condensed heterochromatin (dark) was neatly marginalized to the edge of the nucleus, indicating intact cells (Figure 2B). However, internalization of HZ resulted in nuclei enlargement and loss of nucleus-associated heterochromatin, but the release of neutrophil extracellular traps (NETs) was not observed (Figure 2B′,B″). In addition, we observed that neutrophils ingested large HZ masses (Figure 2C, red arrows) into phagosomes (Figure 2C′,C″, as indicated by white arrow head). The uptake of HZ also resulted in nuclei enlargement with breakdown of the nuclear membrane (as indicated by #), the appearance of intracellular endosomes and lysosomes, and the release of extracellular vesicles (Figure 2D″, indicated by black arrows) as well as in the formation of vesicles/vacuoles to internalize smaller and single HZ crystals (Figure 2C″,D,D′, indicated by *). Thus, the intracellular uptake of HZ occurred via endocytosis into phagosomes and vesicles/vacuoles, which caused morphological changes in neutrophils without inducing cell membrane rupture or release of NETs.

3.3. Human Plasma Impaired Hemozoin Uptake in Neutrophils

Recent studies reported that HZ crystals can interact with blood molecules such as proteins, lipids, and DNA in malaria [16,17]. However, the effect of protein-coated HZ on the ability of neutrophils to internalize these crystals is currently not known. Indeed, ex vivo cell culture experiments with medium might produce artificial results because the uptake of HZ in malaria occurs at a plasma concentration of around 50%. To investigate this, we cultured neutrophils with or without increasing amounts of human plasma from healthy individuals in the presence or absence of HZ for 2 and 18 h. Flow cytometric analysis revealed that neutrophils cultured without plasma (w/o plasma) took up large amounts of HZ after 2 h, whereas in the presence of human plasma (10–50%) the ability of neutrophils to recognize and internalize HZ was significantly inhibited (Figure 3A), even upon exposure up to 18 h (Figure 3B). In contrast, human plasma had no effect on the capacity of neutrophils to take up silica particles of the same size (Figure 3C). Morphologically, the presence of human plasma did not change the appearance of neutrophils (Figures 2A and 3D–F). Those few neutrophils that had taken up HZ in the presence of plasma were activated, as indicated by their rough membrane surface (Figure 3D′,D″), and occasionally showed nuclei enlargement and loss of nuclear heterochromatin (Figure 3E′, indicated by #). Taken together, the data indicated that plasma altered the ability of neutrophils to recognize HZ as a danger signal, a vital mechanism during host defense.

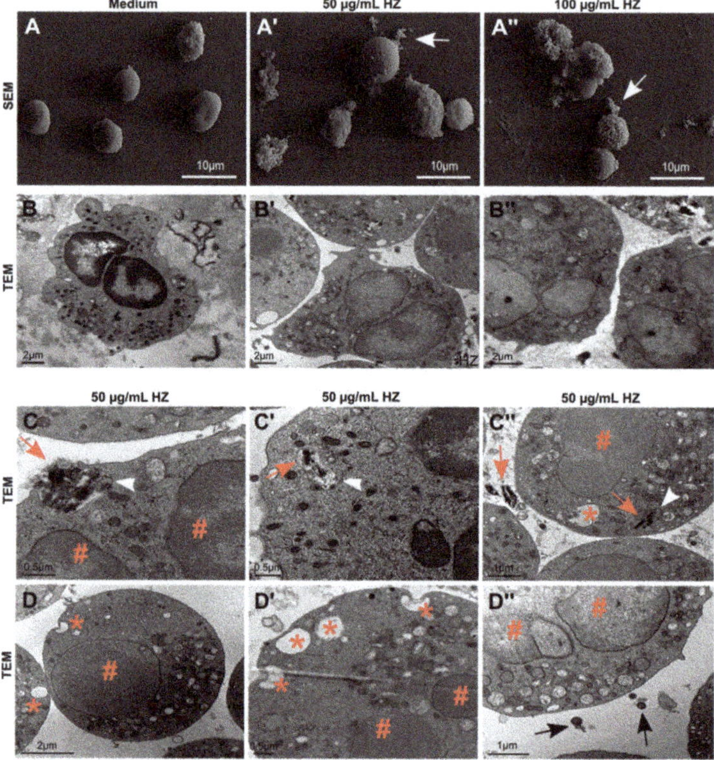

Figure 2. Hemozoin uptake induces nuclei enlargement, and intra- and extracellular vesicle formation in neutrophils but not neutrophil extracellular trap (NET) formation. Human neutrophils were isolated from healthy volunteers and cultured in the presence or absence of HZ (50 and 100 µg/mL) in RPMI medium for 2 h. (**A–C**) After stimulation, neutrophils were prepared for scanning and transmission electron microscopy (SEM and TEM, respectively). (**A**) SEM images of unstimulated neutrophils ((**A**) medium) and HZ-activated neutrophils, as indicated by a rough membrane surface and HZ clusters around neutrophils (white arrows) (**A′,A″**). (**B**) TEM images of unstimulated neutrophils (medium) showed dense nuclear hetero- and euchromatin, numerous granules, and few vesicles (**B**). Internalization of HZ led to loss of heterochromatin and nuclei enlargement (TEM, **B′,B″**). (**C,D**) TEM images of HZ-activated neutrophils showed large HZ aggregates (**C**, red arrows), HZ inside phagosomes (**C′** and **C″**, indicated by white arrow heads), granules/endosomes (**C″,D,D″**), formation of vesicles/vacuoles (**C″,D,D′**, indicated by *), loss of heterochromatin (**C,C″,D,D′,D″**, indicated by #), breakdown of the nuclear membrane (**C′**), and release of extracellular vesicles (**D″**, indicated by black arrows).

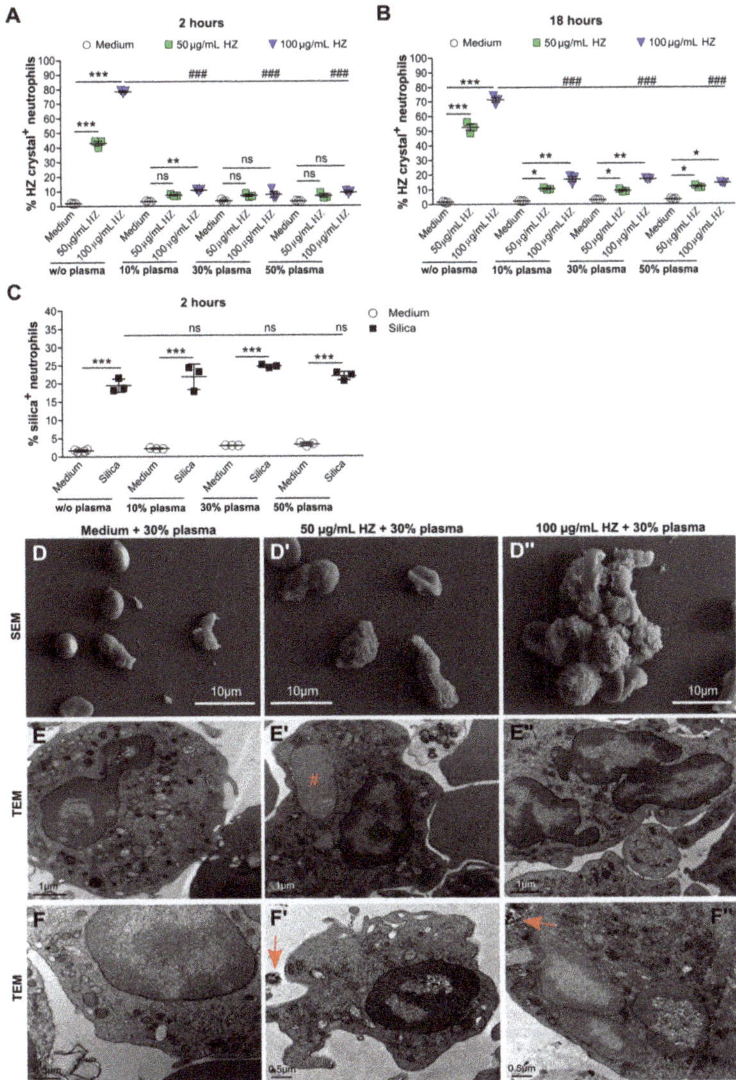

Figure 3. Human plasma impaired hemozoin but not silica uptake in neutrophils. Human neutrophils were isolated from healthy volunteers and cultured in the presence or absence of HZ (50 and 100 µg/mL) or with different amounts of human plasma for 2 and 18 h. (**A**,**B**) Percentage of HZ crystal$^+$ neutrophils was determined using flow cytometry after 2 h (**A**) and 18 h (**B**) ($n = 3$ donors). (**C**) Neutrophils stimulated with or without silica crystals and/or human plasma for 2 h. The percentage of neutrophils that had taken up silica was determined by flow cytometry ($n = 3$ donors). Data are mean ± SD and representative of two independent experiments. * $p < 0.05$; ** $p < 0.01$; *** $p < 0.001$; ns, not significant using two-way ANOVA. w/o indicates without. (**D**) Scanning electron microscopy (SEM) images of neutrophils treated with 30% plasma and/or HZ of 2 h. (**E**,**F**) Transmission electron microscopy (TEM) images of neutrophils treated with 30% serum and/or HZ of 2 h. TEM images showed HZ-activated neutrophils with normal morphology and occasionally loss of nuclear heterochromatin (**E′**, indicated by #), and extracellular and intracellular HZ (**F′**,**F″**, indicated by red arrows). ### $p < 0.001$.

3.4. Fibrinogen Altered the Uptake of Hemozoin by Human Neutrophils

In malaria, a variety of serum/plasma proteins bind to HZ crystals such as serum amyloid A, gelsolin, fibrinogen, albumin, and the lipopolysaccharide (LPS)-binding protein [16]. Among these, fibrinogen levels have also been shown to increase in children with malaria infection [21]. To test whether fibrinogen can influence the uptake of HZ in neutrophils, we pre-incubated HZ with or without fibrinogen prior to stimulation with neutrophils. Flow cytometric analysis revealed that fibrinogen significantly diminished the percentage of HZ crystal$^+$ neutrophils compared to HZ-treated neutrophils only under the plasma-free condition (Figure 4A). However, in the presence of 10% and 30% human plasma, fibrinogen had no additional effect on the uptake of HZ by after 2 h of stimulation (Figure 4B,C, respectively). Unlike fibrinogen, albumin and Ringer's solution (negative control) did not affect HZ uptake under the plasma-free condition (Figure 4D), suggesting that fibrinogen coating of HZ crystals inhibits the ability of neutrophils to internalize these crystals.

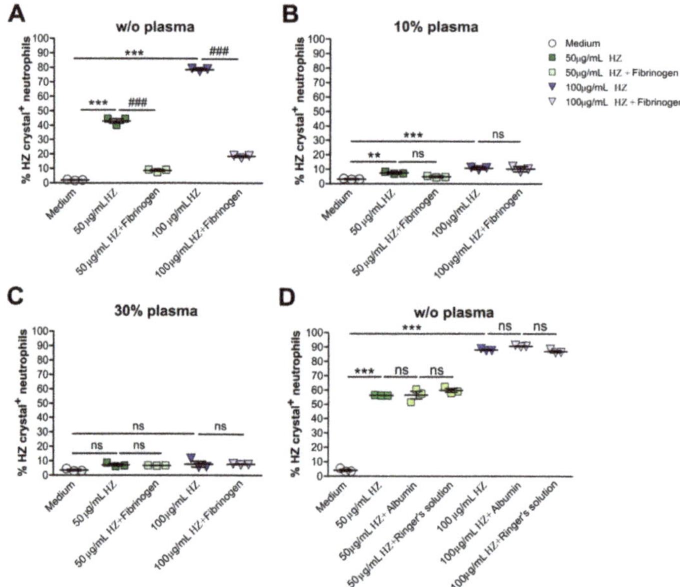

Figure 4. Fibrinogen impaired uptake of hemozoin by human neutrophils. Human neutrophils from healthy volunteers were cultured in the presence or absence of HZ (50 and 100 µg/mL) and/or with human plasma and/or fibrinogen for 2 h. (**A–C**) The percentage of HZ crystal$^+$ neutrophils incubated in the absence or presence of fibrinogen without (w/o) plasma (**A**) or with 10% (**B**) and 30% (**B**) human plasma determined by flow cytometry (n = 3 donors). (**D**) Neutrophils were cultured in the presence or absence of HZ with or without albumin or Ringer's solution in RPMI medium, and the percentage of HZ crystal$^+$ neutrophils determined by flow cytometry after 2 h (n = 3 donors). Data are mean ± SD and representative of two independent experiments. ** $p < 0.01$; *** $p < 0.001$; ns, not significant using one-way ANOVA. ### $p < 0.001$.

3.5. Removal of Platelets from Plasma Further Impaired HZ Uptake by Human Neutrophils

To investigate whether platelets play a role during neutrophil HZ uptake, we cultured human neutrophils with plasma or platelet-poor plasma in the presence of HZ for 2 h. Fluorescence microscopy revealed that neutrophils internalized very few HZ crystals in human platelet-poor plasma (Figure 5A). This observation was in line with a significant decrease in the percentage of HZ crystal$^+$ neutrophils in the presence of platelet-poor plasma compared with plasma only when cultured with 50 µg/mL HZ (Figure 5B) and 100 µg/mL HZ (Figure 5C). We also observed that the platelets in plasma accumulated around HZ and formed aggregates as illustrated by the positive actin staining for phalloidin and negative staining for the nuclear dye DAPI (Figure 5D). These data suggest that the uptake of HZ by neutrophils may depend on HZ-related platelet interaction.

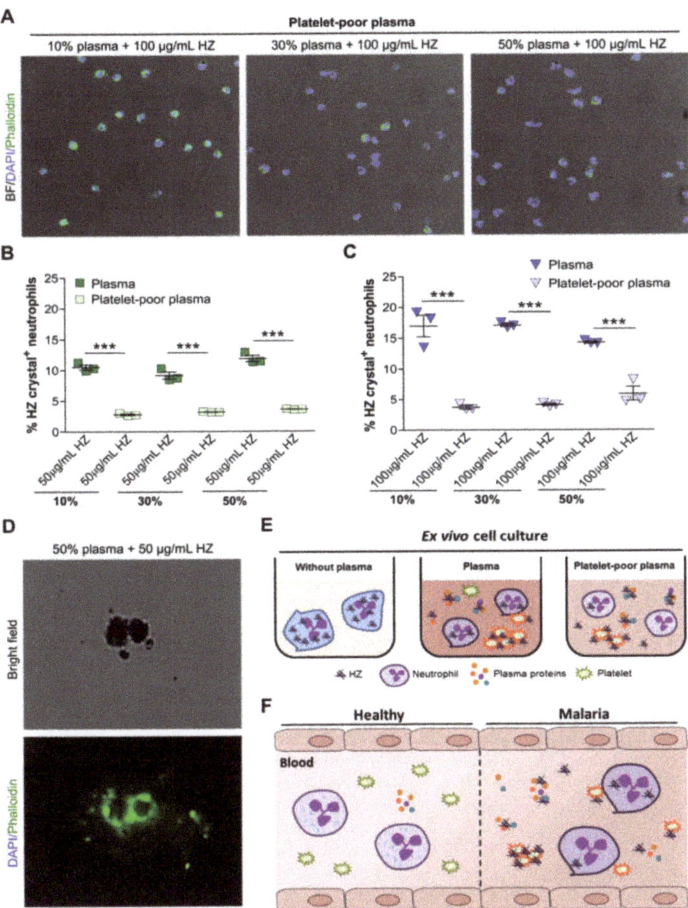

Figure 5. Platelet-poor plasma impaired hemozoin uptake by neutrophils. Human blood neutrophils were isolated from healthy volunteers and cultured with 10%, 30%, or 50% of platelet-poor plasma or plasma in the presence of HZ (50 and 100 µg/mL) for 2 h, and fluorescence microscopy or flow cytometry was performed. (**A**) Neutrophils cultured in platelet-poor plasma with HZ were stained with phalloidin (green) and DAPI (blue) for fluorescence microscopy. Images are shown as a merge of phalloidin and DAPI with bright field (BF) (200× magnification). (**B**,**C**) The percentage of neutrophils that had internalized HZ at concentrations of 50 µg/mL (**B**) and 100 µg/mL (**C**) in the presence of platelet-poor plasma or plasma were determined by flow cytometry (*n* = 3 donors). (**D**) Human plasma containing platelets was incubated with 50 µg/mL HZ and stained for phalloidin (green) for fluorescence microscopy (630× magnification). Data are mean ± SD and representative of two independent experiments. *** *p* < 0.001; ns, not significant using two-way ANOVA. (**E**) Schematic of ex vivo neutrophil culture experiments with plasma or platelet-poor plasma in the presence of HZ. (**F**) Schematic illustrating that during malaria HZ crystals bind to plasma proteins, which was associated with a diminished endocytotic capacity of neutrophils. Despite the impaired HZ uptake, those few neutrophils that did ingest HZ crystals relied on HZ-induced platelet activation.

4. Discussion

We hypothesized that human plasma would alter the ability of neutrophils to internalize malaria-related HZ crystals. Indeed, our ex vivo data revealed that the HZ internalization by neutrophils occurred via endocytosis into phagosomes as well as into vesicles/vacuoles (Figure 5E). Interestingly, plasma proteins including fibrinogen impaired this uptake process, whereas the presence of platelets enhanced it. These findings highlight the importance of factors regulating neutrophil endocytosis in vivo that are frequently ignored in ex vivo studies.

Neutrophils play an important role in the pathogenesis of malaria via processes including *Plasmodium* parasite killing and NET formation [11,12]. Recent reports have shown that heme, a known malaria danger-associated molecular pattern released during parasite egress, robustly induces NETs but not infected red blood cells, merozoites, and digestive vacuoles containing HZ, in tumor necrosis factor (TNF)-α-primed human neutrophils [14]. We found that human blood neutrophils internalized HZ in phagosomes and vesicles/vacuoles, which triggered morphological abnormalities without leading to cell membrane rupture and NET release. This suggests that although HZ does not directly induce NETs [14], they are known to significantly contribute to immune activation in other immune cells [5]. In contrast, very small nanoparticles (10 to 40 nm in size) and larger crystalline particles such as monosodium urate, calcium phosphate, cholesterol, and calcium oxalate crystals can induce mixed lineage kinase domain-like protein (MLKL)-driven neutrophil necroptosis and NET formation [19,22]. However, it is possible that neutrophils such as monocytes and macrophages remain viable after ingestion of HZ crystals, and that lysosome formation and acidification is normal [23], although HZ degradation might be impaired due to the inability of the lysosome to depolymerize HZ crystals. Thus, HZ can reside in these cells for long periods of time, but repeated phagocytosis or oxidative burst for further *Plasmodium* parasite killing is impaired [4,23–25], suggesting a state of sequestration of activated neutrophils [26]. Unresponsiveness of neutrophils in malaria accounts for increased susceptibility toward bacterial co-infections [27,28].

The process of endocytosis is characterized by polymerization of actin filaments and fusion of phagosomes with lysosomes to form phagolysosomes in macrophages [29] and human monocytes [30]. Unlike macrophages and monocytes, neutrophils do not form classical phagolysosomes and instead contain a large number of preformed granules that can rapidly fuse with phagosomes upon internalization of pathogens or larger amounts of particles [31]. Our data showed that human neutrophils ingested larger HZ crystal masses via direct uptake (phagocytosis) into phagolysosomes, whereas single and smaller HZ crystals might be internalized into vesicles/vacuoles via a different endocytotic uptake mechanism known as pinocytosis, due to the small size of HZ (0.1–1 μm). Previous studies have shown that pinocytosis does not require actin-dependent engulfment of small particles, for instance, zymosan, nanoparticles, or latex beads, by neutrophils [32], macrophages and endothelial cells [33], and non-phagocytic cells [34]. However, further studies are needed to confirm the clearance of HZ by neutrophils via pinocytosis.

The role of HZ-binding proteins in the recognition, immune modulation and physiological clearance of HZ in neutrophils remains to be elucidated. We report for the first time that human plasma from healthy individuals, specifically fibrinogen, impairs the ability of neutrophils to ingest HZ but not silica crystals ex vivo. This is in line with previous reports showing that blood proteins such as apolipoprotein E, serum amyloid A, LPS binding protein, complement factor H, albumin, and fibrinogen that were found to be elevated in malaria individuals are able to bind to HZ [16,17]. Hence, HZ-binding proteins alter the recognition of HZ as a danger signal for neutrophil clearance. The in vivo relevance of these findings remains to be proven, as the hematin-core crystal in HZ may remain shielded from serum proteins by the surrounding membranes/lipids [26,27].

It is known that circulating neutrophils and platelets interact during infection including malaria, inflammation, and thrombosis, and that they can modulate each other's functions [35,36]. In malaria patients, circulating platelets and platelet-bound neutrophils are reduced, hence these complexes are either lost, the neutrophils migrate to tissues, or they form NETs [13]. Our ex vivo data showed that the ability of neutrophils to clear HZ crystals even further decreases in platelet-poor plasma compared to normal human plasma. This may imply that neutrophils require platelets for HZ clearance. Previous reports have shown that activated platelets can initiate or amplify various neutrophil responses including phagocytosis, production of oxygen radicals, and NET formation. Such responses are initiated either by a direct contact or by the release of soluble mediators such as chemokine (C-C motif) ligand 5 (CCL5) and platelet factor 4 [37,38]. In addition, platelet interactions enhance the phagocytic capacity of neutrophils towards various bacteria in vitro [39–41]. Conversely, neutrophils can also release soluble mediators such as cathepsin G and elastase that augment platelet responses by activation of protease-activated receptors on platelets [42–44]. However, further studies are needed to investigate the crosstalk between HZ-mediated platelet activation and HZ crystal uptake by neutrophil.

Limitations of our study are that we lack access to plasma from malaria-infected patients to investigate the impact of malaria-related plasma proteins on the phagocytic capacity of neutrophils to ingest HZ. As mentioned above, many plasma proteins that can bind to HZ have been identified in malaria patients [16], and it is possible that besides fibrinogen, other plasma proteins may alter the uptake of HZ by neutrophils. Furthermore, the role of HZ in modulation of host innate and inflammatory responses has been investigated using different HZ preparation protocols. HZ can be synthesized from hematin (sHZ) or natural HZ (nHZ), or digestive vacuoles containing hemozoin can be purified from infected red blood cells in culture [27]. We used synthetic HZ and not nHZ or digestive vacuoles of *Plasmodia* for our ex vivo cell culture experiments. Although sHZ and nHZ crystals are similar in size, and capable of inducing the same level of inflammation, sHZ with a smaller or larger crystal size may differently affect the function of neutrophils.

5. Conclusions

In conclusion, we found that the engulfment of HZ crystals by neutrophils via endocytosis relies on crystal–platelet interaction, whereas plasma proteins such as fibrinogen inhibit HZ crystal uptake and clearance from the extracellular space. HZ ingestion does not trigger the release of NETs, as reported for many other crystalline microparticles (Figure 5F). These data raise the question of how malaria-related thrombozytopenia may affect HZ-driven manifestations and outcomes during malaria infection.

Supplementary Materials: The following are available online at http://www.mdpi.com/2073-4409/9/1/93/s1: Figure S1: Morphology of hemozoin crystals.

Author Contributions: S.S. designed the study concept and experiments; S.d.O.S.L., T.K., and S.S. conducted experiments and analyzed the data; S.d.O.S.L., D.L.B., and C.V.N. performed scanning and transmission electron microscopy of neutrophils; S.S., S.d.O.S.L., and H.-J.A. wrote the manuscript; all contributing authors reviewed the manuscript. All authors have read and agreed to the published version of the manuscript.

Funding: This work was supported by grants from the Deutsche Forschungsgemeinschaft (DFG) STE2437/2-1 to S.S.; AN372/14-3, 16-2, 24-1, and 27-1 to H.-J.A.; and Humboldt/CAPES to S.d.O.S.L.

Acknowledgments: We thank all healthy volunteers involved in this study.

Conflicts of Interest: The authors declare that they have no competing interests.

References

1. World Health Organization. World Malaria Report 2018. Available online: https://www.who.int/malaria/publications/world-malaria-report-2018/en/ (accessed on 28 November 2019).
2. Coronado, L.M.; Nadovich, C.T.; Spadafora, C. Malarial hemozoin: From target to tool. *Biochim. Biophys. Acta* **2014**, *1840*, 2032–2041. [CrossRef]
3. Polimeni, M.; Valente, E.; Ulliers, D.; Opdenakker, G.; Van den Steen, P.E.; Giribaldi, G.; Prato, M. Natural haemozoin induces expression and release of human monocyte tissue inhibitor of metalloproteinase-1. *PLoS ONE* **2013**, *8*, e71468. [CrossRef] [PubMed]
4. Shio, M.T.; Eisenbarth, S.C.; Savaria, M.; Vinet, A.F.; Bellemare, M.J.; Harder, K.W.; Sutterwala, F.S.; Bohle, D.S.; Descoteaux, A.; Flavell, R.A.; et al. Malarial hemozoin activates the NLRP3 inflammasome through Lyn and Syk kinases. *PLoS Pathog.* **2009**, *5*, e1000559. [CrossRef]

5. Gazzinelli, R.T.; Kalantari, P.; Fitzgerald, K.A.; Golenbock, D.T. Innate sensing of malaria parasites. *Nat. Rev. Immunol.* **2014**, *14*, 744–757. [CrossRef] [PubMed]

6. Oakley, M.S.; Gerald, N.; McCutchan, T.F.; Aravind, L.; Kumar, S. Clinical and molecular aspects of malaria fever. *Trends Parasitol.* **2011**, *27*, 442–449. [CrossRef]

7. Amulic, B.; Cazalet, C.; Hayes, G.L.; Metzler, K.D.; Zychlinsky, A. Neutrophil function, From mechanisms to disease. *Annu. Rev. Immunol.* **2012**, *30*, 459–489. [CrossRef]

8. Wickramasinghe, S.N.; Phillips, R.E.; Looareesuwan, S.; Warrell, D.A.; Hughes, M. The bone marrow in human cerebral malaria, Parasite sequestration within sinusoids. *Br. J. Haematol.* **1987**, *66*, 295–306. [CrossRef]

9. Leoratti, F.M.; Trevelin, S.C.; Cunha, F.Q.; Rocha, B.C.; Costa, P.A.; Gravina, H.D.; Tada, M.S.; Pereira, D.B.; Golenbock, D.T.; Antonelli, L.R.; et al. Neutrophil paralysis in Plasmodium vivax malaria. *PLoS Negl. Trop. Dis.* **2012**, *6*, e1710. [CrossRef]

10. Mohammed, A.O.; Elghazali, G.; Mohammed, H.B.; Elbashir, M.I.; Xu, S.; Berzins, K.; Venge, P. Human neutrophil lipocalin, A specific marker for neutrophil activation in severe Plasmodium falciparum malaria. *Acta Trop.* **2003**, *87*, 279–285. [CrossRef]

11. Boeltz, S.; Munoz, L.E.; Fuchs, T.A.; Herrmann, M. Neutrophil Extracellular Traps Open the Pandora's Box in Severe Malaria. *Front. Immunol.* **2017**, *8*, 874. [CrossRef]

12. Baker, V.S.; Imade, G.E.; Molta, N.B.; Tawde, P.; Pam, S.D.; Obadofin, M.O.; Sagay, S.A.; Egah, D.Z.; Iya, D.; Afolabi, B.B.; et al. Cytokine-associated neutrophil extracellular traps and antinuclear antibodies in Plasmodium falciparum infected children under six years of age. *Malar. J.* **2008**, *7*, 41. [CrossRef] [PubMed]

13. Kho, S.; Minigo, G.; Andries, B.; Leonardo, L.; Prayoga, P.; Poespoprodjo, J.R.; Kenangalem, E.; Price, R.N.; Woodberry, T.; Anstey, N.M.; et al. Circulating Neutrophil Extracellular Traps and Neutrophil Activation Are Increased in Proportion to Disease Severity in Human Malaria. *J. Infect. Dis.* **2019**, *219*, 1994–2004. [CrossRef] [PubMed]

14. Knackstedt, S.L.; Georgiadou, A.; Apel, F.; Abu-Abed, U.; Moxon, C.A.; Cunnington, A.J.; Raupach, B.; Cunningham, D.; Langhorne, J.; Kruger, R.; et al. Neutrophil extracellular traps drive inflammatory pathogenesis in malaria. *Sci. Immunol.* **2019**, *4*, eaaw0336. [CrossRef] [PubMed]

15. Lyke, K.E.; Diallo, D.A.; Dicko, A.; Kone, A.; Coulibaly, D.; Guindo, A.; Cissoko, Y.; Sangare, L.; Coulibaly, S.; Dakouo, B.; et al. Association of intraleukocytic Plasmodium falciparum malaria pigment with disease severity, clinical manifestations, and prognosis in severe malaria. *Am. J. Trop. Med. Hyg.* **2003**, *69*, 253–259. [CrossRef]

16. Kassa, F.A.; Shio, M.T.; Bellemare, M.J.; Faye, B.; Ndao, M.; Olivier, M. New inflammation-related biomarkers during malaria infection. *PLoS ONE* **2011**, *6*, e26495. [CrossRef]

17. Barrera, V.; Skorokhod, O.A.; Baci, D.; Gremo, G.; Arese, P.; Schwarzer, E. Host fibrinogen stably bound to hemozoin rapidly activates monocytes via TLR-4 and CD11b/CD18-integrin, A new paradigm of hemozoin action. *Blood* **2011**, *117*, 5674–5682. [CrossRef]

18. Nakazawa, D.; Kumar, S.V.; Marschner, J.; Desai, J.; Holderied, A.; Rath, L.; Kraft, F.; Lei, Y.; Fukasawa, Y.; Moeckel, G.W.; et al. Histones and Neutrophil Extracellular Traps Enhance Tubular Necrosis and Remote Organ Injury in Ischemic AKI. *J. Am. Soc. Nephrol.* **2017**, *28*, 1753–1768. [CrossRef]

19. Desai, J.; Foresto-Neto, O.; Honarpisheh, M.; Steiger, S.; Nakazawa, D.; Popper, B.; Buhl, E.M.; Boor, P.; Mulay, S.R.; Anders, H.J. Particles of different sizes and shapes induce neutrophil necroptosis followed by the release of neutrophil extracellular trap-like chromatin. *Sci. Rep.* **2017**, *7*, 15003. [CrossRef]

20. Honarpisheh, M.; Foresto-Neto, O.; Desai, J.; Steiger, S.; Gomez, L.A.; Popper, B.; Boor, P.; Anders, H.J.; Mulay, S.R. Phagocytosis of environmental or metabolic crystalline particles induces cytotoxicity by triggering necroptosis across a broad range of particle size and shape. *Sci. Rep.* **2017**, *7*, 15523. [CrossRef]

21. Omoigberale, A.I.; Abiodun, P.O.; Famodu, A.A. Fibrinolytic activity in children with Plasmodium falciparum malaria. *East Afr. Med. J.* **2005**, *82*, 103–105. [CrossRef]

22. Munoz, L.E.; Bilyy, R.; Biermann, M.H.; Kienhofer, D.; Maueroder, C.; Hahn, J.; Brauner, J.M.; Weidner, D.; Chen, J.; Scharin-Mehlmann, M.; et al. Nanoparticles size-dependently initiate self-limiting NETosis-driven inflammation. *Proc. Natl. Acad. Sci. USA* **2016**, *113*, E5856–E5865. [CrossRef]

23. Schwarzer, E.; Bellomo, G.; Giribaldi, G.; Ulliers, D.; Arese, P. Phagocytosis of malarial pigment haemozoin by human monocytes, A confocal microscopy study. *Parasitology* **2001**, *123*, 125–131. [CrossRef]

24. Schwarzer, E.; De Matteis, F.; Giribaldi, G.; Ulliers, D.; Valente, E.; Arese, P. Hemozoin stability and dormant induction of heme oxygenase in hemozoin-fed human monocytes. *Mol. Biochem. Parasitol.* **1999**, *100*, 61–72. [CrossRef]

25. Schwarzer, E.; Turrini, F.; Ulliers, D.; Giribaldi, G.; Ginsburg, H.; Arese, P. Impairment of macrophage functions after ingestion of Plasmodium falciparum-infected erythrocytes or isolated malarial pigment. *J. Exp. Med.* **1992**, *176*, 1033–1041. [CrossRef] [PubMed]

26. Dasari, P.; Reiss, K.; Lingelbach, K.; Baumeister, S.; Lucius, R.; Udomsangpetch, R.; Bhakdi, S.C.; Bhakdi, S. Digestive vacuoles of Plasmodium falciparum are selectively phagocytosed by and impair killing function of polymorphonuclear leukocytes. *Blood* **2011**, *118*, 4946–4956. [CrossRef] [PubMed]

27. Tyberghein, A.; Deroost, K.; Schwarzer, E.; Arese, P.; Van den Steen, P.E. Immunopathological effects of malaria pigment or hemozoin and other crystals. *Biofactors* **2014**, *40*, 59–78. [CrossRef] [PubMed]

28. Cunnington, A.J.; de Souza, J.B.; Walther, M.; Riley, E.M. Malaria impairs resistance to Salmonella through heme- and heme oxygenase-dependent dysfunctional granulocyte mobilization. *Nat. Med.* **2011**, *18*, 120–127. [CrossRef]

29. Vieira, O.V.; Botelho, R.J.; Grinstein, S. Phagosome maturation, Aging gracefully. *Biochem. J.* **2002**, *366*, 689–704. [CrossRef]

30. Olliaro, P.; Lombardi, L.; Frigerio, S.; Basilico, N.; Taramelli, D.; Monti, D. Phagocytosis of hemozoin (native and synthetic malaria pigment), and Plasmodium falciparum intraerythrocyte-stage parasites by human and mouse phagocytes. *Ultrastruct. Pathol.* **2000**, *24*, 9–13. [CrossRef]

31. Nordenfelt, P.; Tapper, H. Phagosome dynamics during phagocytosis by neutrophils. *J. Leukoc. Biol.* **2011**, *90*, 271–284. [CrossRef]

32. Botelho, R.J.; Tapper, H.; Furuya, W.; Mojdami, D.; Grinstein, S. Fc gamma R-mediated phagocytosis stimulates localized pinocytosis in human neutrophils. *J. Immunol.* **2002**, *169*, 4423–4429. [CrossRef] [PubMed]

33. Kuhn, D.A.; Vanhecke, D.; Michen, B.; Blank, F.; Gehr, P.; Petri-Fink, A.; Rothen-Rutishauser, B. Different endocytotic uptake mechanisms for nanoparticles in epithelial cells and macrophages. *Beilstein J. Nanotechnol.* **2014**, *5*, 1625–1636. [CrossRef] [PubMed]

34. Rejman, J.; Oberle, V.; Zuhorn, I.S.; Hoekstra, D. Size-dependent internalization of particles via the pathways of clathrin- and caveolae-mediated endocytosis. *Biochem. J.* **2004**, *377*, 159–169. [CrossRef] [PubMed]

35. Lisman, T. Platelet-neutrophil interactions as drivers of inflammatory and thrombotic disease. *Cell Tissue Res.* **2018**, *371*, 567–576. [CrossRef] [PubMed]

36. O'Sullivan, J.M.; O'Donnell, J.S. Platelets in malaria pathogenesis. *Blood* **2018**, *132*, 1222–1224. [CrossRef] [PubMed]

37. Von Hundelshausen, P.; Koenen, R.R.; Sack, M.; Mause, S.F.; Adriaens, W.; Proudfoot, A.E.; Hackeng, T.M.; Weber, C. Heterophilic interactions of platelet factor 4 and RANTES promote monocyte arrest on endothelium. *Blood* **2005**, *105*, 924–930. [CrossRef]

38. Pervushina, O.; Scheuerer, B.; Reiling, N.; Behnke, L.; Schroder, J.M.; Kasper, B.; Brandt, E.; Bulfone-Paus, S.; Petersen, F. Platelet factor 4/CXCL4 induces phagocytosis and the generation of reactive oxygen metabolites in mononuclear phagocytes independently of Gi protein activation or intracellular calcium transients. *J. Immunol.* **2004**, *173*, 2060–2067. [CrossRef]

39. Assinger, A.; Laky, M.; Schabbauer, G.; Hirschl, A.M.; Buchberger, E.; Binder, B.R.; Volf, I. Efficient phagocytosis of periodontopathogens by neutrophils requires plasma factors, platelets and TLR2. *J. Thromb. Haemost.* **2011**, *9*, 799–809. [CrossRef]

40. Peters, M.J.; Dixon, G.; Kotowicz, K.T.; Hatch, D.J.; Heyderman, R.S.; Klein, N.J. Circulating platelet-neutrophil complexes represent a subpopulation of activated neutrophils primed for adhesion, phagocytosis and intracellular killing. *Br. J. Haematol.* **1999**, *106*, 391–399. [CrossRef]

41. Hurley, S.M.; Kahn, F.; Nordenfelt, P.; Morgelin, M.; Sorensen, O.E.; Shannon, O. Platelet-Dependent Neutrophil Function Is Dysregulated by M Protein from Streptococcus pyogenes. *Infect. Immun.* **2015**, *83*, 3515–3525. [CrossRef]

42. Selak, M.A. Neutrophil elastase potentiates cathepsin G-induced platelet activation. *Thromb. Haemost.* **1992**, *68*, 570–576. [PubMed]

43. Sambrano, G.R.; Huang, W.; Faruqi, T.; Mahrus, S.; Craik, C.; Coughlin, S.R. Cathepsin G activates protease-activated receptor-4 in human platelets. *J. Biol. Chem.* **2000**, *275*, 6819–6823. [CrossRef] [PubMed]
44. Mihara, K.; Ramachandran, R.; Renaux, B.; Saifeddine, M.; Hollenberg, M.D. Neutrophil elastase and proteinase-3 trigger G protein-biased signaling through proteinase-activated receptor-1 (PAR1). *J. Biol. Chem.* **2013**, *288*, 32979–32990. [CrossRef] [PubMed]

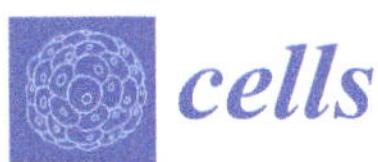 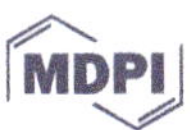

Review

Neutrophil Extracellular Traps: Current Perspectives in the Eye

Gibrán Alejandro Estúa-Acosta [1], Rocío Zamora-Ortiz [1], Beatriz Buentello-Volante [1], Mariana García-Mejía [1] and Yonathan Garfias [1,2,*]

[1] Research Unit, Cell and Tissue Biology, Institute of Ophthalmology Conde de Valenciana, Mexico City 06800, Mexico

[2] Department of Biochemistry, Faculty of Medicine, Universidad Nacional Autónoma de México, Mexico City 04510, Mexico

* Correspondence: yogarfias@insitutodeoftalmologia.org or ygarfias@bq.unam.mx; Tel.: +52-55-5442-1700 (ext. 3212)

Received: 6 August 2019; Accepted: 23 August 2019; Published: 27 August 2019

Abstract: Neutrophil extracellular traps (NETs) have been the subject of research in the field of innate immunity since their first description more than a decade ago. Neutrophils are the first cells recruited at sites of inflammation, where they perform their specific functions, including the release of NETs, which consist of web-like structures composed of granule proteins bound to decondensed chromatin fibres. This process has aroused interest, as it contributes to understanding how pathogenic microorganisms are contained, but they are also associated with pathophysiological processes of a wide range of diseases. Currently, there are growing reports of new molecules involved in the formation and release of NETs. However, whether the release of NETs contributes to eye diseases remains unclear. For this reason, the overall aim of this review is to gather current data of recent research in the ophthalmology field, where there is still much to discover.

Keywords: neutrophils extracellular traps; ophthalmology; diseases

---

1. Introduction

Neutrophils are the main effector cells of an acute inflammation. Their anti-inflammatory role is due to their specialised functions [1]. More than a decade ago, it was posited that, upon activation, neutrophils release extracellular structures composed of granular and nuclear constituents that neutralise bacteria. Since then, these fibrous networks have been called neutrophils extracellular traps (NETs) [2]. As this phenomenon was originally considered a particular form of cell death, different from necrosis or apoptosis, the process was labelled "NETosis" [3]. Recently, this concept has changed due to reports of two forms of NETosis: suicidal and vital [4]. The controversy continues as to whether a NETs release is a physiological host defence process or whether it is a consequence of cellular rupture [5]. It is important to be aware that robust effector functions may also lead to tissue damage [6]. The function of NETs is to offer a physical barrier that foils infectious spreading and raise the extracellular compartment of the concentration of antimicrobial substances [7]. Current research of NETs is expanding worldwide, and new research has uncovered new pathways in terms of understanding the mechanism for activating and releasing NETs. In the present review, we discuss the role of NETs in pathological responses, focusing specifically on eye diseases.

2. Structure of Neutrophil Extracellular Traps

Although the overall composition of NETs remains unknown, it has been described that the main components of NETs structures are nuclear DNA and histones. Also, proteins contained in different neutrophil granules like bactericidal enzymes, such as neutrophil elastase (NE), myeloperoxidase

(MPO), lactotransferrin (LTF), gelatinase, cathepsin G (CG), leukocyte proteinase 3 (PR3), calprotectin, cathelicidins, defensins, and actin, among many others, conform NETs [8].

NET scaffolds are composed of DNA fibres that are 15–17 nm in diameter and globular domains with diameters of 25–50 nm [9]. NETs can be studied using different techniques. In recent years, several strategies have been developed to identify NETs in vitro. Fluorescent microscopy is a versatile method that utilises different fluorescent-conjugated antibodies to specifically detect proteins, in combination with cell-membrane selective DNA-intercalating probes. Although there are some software programs that attempt to analyse NETs, but this technique is still observer-dependent, which is its main limitation. [10]. Another technique to study the release of NETs combines fluorescent microscopy and flow cytometry, also called multispectral imaging flow cytometry (MIFC) [11]. Scanning electron microscopy (SEM) has been useful to identify NETs. However, remnants of fibrin, fibronectin, and collagen can mimic NETs, revealing that SEM has limitations when NETs are analysed in tissue [12]. In order to quantify NETs, several methods have been described [11,13–16]. Each method offers alternatives for quantifying the release of NETs. So far, however, there is no single method for quantifying NETs.

3. Releasing of Neutrophil Extracellular Traps

The first description of NETs was performed with several stimuli, such as phorbol 12-myristate 13-acetate (PMA), bacterial lipopolysaccharide (LPS), and interleukin-8 (IL-8) [4,17]. Since then, a substantial number of inducers have been described, including harmful agents such as bacteria, fungi, protozoa and viruses, as well as their components [18]. In recent years, an increased number of activators have been proposed to induce the release of NETs, such as high-glucose medium, complement-derived peptides, autoantibodies, cigarette smoke, urate crystals, calcium ionophore, and activated platelets [4,19–21]. The mechanism by which neutrophils release NETs is not completely understood. It seems that the NETs releasing pathway depends on the stimuli. Recently, de Bont and colleagues reported that LPS, PMA, and the calcium ionophore A23187 promote NETs releasing through different pathways [22]. Another interesting study has mentioned that diverse stimuli for releasing NETs are heterogeneous in terms of both protein composition and post-translational modifications by means of proteomic approaches. This suggests that NETs induced in different conditions may have different biological effects [23].

4. Suicidal and Vital NETosis

Suicidal NETosis is the first and most studied model. Several stimuli can promote this process, but the best studied are those stimulated through PMA. In this context, it should be noted that this mechanism is dependent on reactive oxygen species (ROS) generation [4,5,24]. It persists for 2–4 h and consists of a specific neutrophil lysis, which begins with chromatin decondensation, followed by nuclear membrane disintegration and a mixture of DNA material and cytoplasmic components, including neutrophil granule contents. This leads to plasmatic membrane dissolution and cell death [24]. It has been reported that there are two different mechanisms of vital NETosis, depending on the origin of DNA release—nuclear or mitochondrial DNA. The former is a ROS-independent generation process; this mechanism has been described as occurring with staphylococcus aureus stimulation, and it has been observed that NETs release is through a vesicular-dependent manner and is very rapid (5–60 min) [25]. Meanwhile, in the latter process, NETs that are released contain only mitochondrial DNA [26]. In this non-cell death mechanism, the NETs release is preserved, as well as the phagocyte neutrophil capability. This seems to represent a response against microorganism aggression [6,26].

5. Neutrophil Extracellular Traps Pathways and Involved Molecules

The mechanism by which NETs are released is still controversial and is being studied by various research groups. Since their first description to date, we know that more than 30 components of the neutrophil granules are involved, and fibres are composed of DNA and histones. Thus, NETosis processes have been described as aforementioned. We also know that, on one hand, they contribute to inflammatory resolution processes, but on the other, they can contribute within the pathophysiological mechanism of diseases, although the exact molecular and biochemical mechanisms involved in NETs release are not completely understood.

The NETosis process has been described by several authors as dynamic, beginning with the disappearance of the nuclear structure and followed by a rupture of the nuclear envelope. Then, the components of the nucleus portion are commingled with the cytoplasm. Finally, the rupture of the neutrophil membrane occurs, although we know that the latter does not occur with certain stimuli. Independent of the stimulus, the NET release process is independent of transcription [27]. The release of NETs is evolutionarily conserved within the animal and plant kingdoms and has been described in different species [4].

It has been described that suicidal NETosis model depends on the protein kinase C activity (PCK) as the key modulator of this pathway, which is also NADPH oxidase 2 (Nox 2) dependent [5]. This pathway initiates with the recognition of any stimulus that activates receptors, which induces the activation of signal-related kinases, such as PKC, p38, PI3K, Src, Raf/MERK/Erk, Akt, and Ark [28–31]. All of them are well-known and important kinases for Nox2-dependent NETs formation [30,32]. Further downstream, the multimeric complex of NADPH oxidase assembles at the phagosomal membrane and generates ROS. With ROS generation, cytosolic calcium increases, acting as a cofactor for peptidyl arginase deaminase 4 (PAD4). PAD4 is an enzyme that endorses deamination of histones, and therefore, favours chromatin decondensation [24]. However, there is evidence suggesting that physiological stimuli induce PAD4-dependent ROS-independent NETosis [33].

At the same time, while neutrophil elastase (NE) and myeloperoxidase (MPO) translocate from cytoplasm to the nucleus [34,35], MPO binds to chromatin and synergises with NE decondensing chromatin [34]. Subsequently, Nox2 complex produces ROS that work as second messengers, promoting nuclear membrane disintegration. This oxidative activation is important because NE binds to F- actin filaments in the cytoplasm and must degrade them in order to enter the nucleus [35]. This process allows nuclear content mixtures into the cytoplasm, ultimately loosing the plasmatic membrane and then discharging the neutrophil contents as extracellular traps [6,24,36]. Interestingly, pharmacological inhibition of NADPH oxidase or ROS scavengers block NETs formation with certain stimuli [32]. Moreover, neutrophils from patients' chronic granulomatous disease, a primary immunodeficiency with mutations in NADPH oxidase subunits, lose their ability to release NETs in response to mitogens and some microbes, genetically confirming the relevance of ROS [37]. In contrast, there are some NETs stimuli, such as immune complexes, ionomycin and nicotine, that have been proposed to trigger NETosis independently of NADPH oxidase, depending instead on mitochondrial ROS [38].

Vital NETosis, in contrast to suicidal NETosis, is a live cell process at the time of releasing NETs. Neutrophils can release part of or the entire nucleus without breaching the cell membrane, resulting in an anuclear cytoplasm that is still able to move and phagocytose bacteria [4]. Thus, in this type of NETosis, neutrophils preserve some of their functions.

In this process, several molecules are involved, including MPO and NE. PAD4 is a nuclear enzyme that performs the citrullination of histones through the change of arginine for citrulline, making the overall charge of the histones less positive, particularly in histone H3 (H3Cit) [39]. This results in a lower affinity for the negatively charged DNA, thereby stimulating chromatin decondensation and eventually releasing NETs [22]. Although it has been described that PAD4 activation concludes in DNA decondensation, NE is sufficient for nuclei decondensation in vitro. However, the mechanism that disassembles the nuclear envelope in neutrophils is still unknown [34].

The mechanisms that regulate PAD4 activation in the NETs releasing process are not yet fully understood. There are still many controversies about the role of PAD4 activity in the release of NETs. For example, it has been described that when calcium ionophore is used, PAD4 is activated and a release of NETs occurs [22,38,40]. In contrast, neutrophil activation with PMA is a potent signal for releasing NETs in a PAD4-independent manner [41–43]. Moreover, it has recently been demonstrated that PAD4 activity is necessary to NET formation in a bacterial presence [44].

In this regard, Konig and Andrade have described two mechanisms that are different from NETosis: leukotoxic hypercitrullination (LTH) and defective mitophagy. Both have been erroneously classified as "NETosis" [40]. These authors showed evidence that PAD4 activation is independent of PMA. Actually, when PMA is used as an activator, all protein citrullination including H3Cit is abolished. Moreover, LTH is a NADPH oxidase-independent phenomenon and not necessarily bactericidal; in this process, NET-like structures (NLS) are released [40]. There are several features that distinguish LTH from NETosis—(1) NLS are triggered by prominent and sustained calcium influx and are inhibited by chelation of extracellular calcium [45], (2) NLS are generated independently of NADPH oxidase activity [45], (3) NLS require PAD4 activity and are suppressed by PAD inhibitors [41,46], (4) NLS undergo rapid formation (within minutes) [41], and (5) in LTH, protein citrullination is not limited to histones and transcription factors but encompasses proteins across all molecular weights [47]. On the other hand, defective mitophagy has not been associated with protein citrullination [40,48]. This has been explained as a compensatory mechanism for defect mithophagy. This mechanism is enhanced in neutrophils by inflammatory signals such LPS or C5a after priming with GM-CSF [26].

NETs and Disease

Despite NETs possessing antimicrobial activities and aiding in the resolution of inflammation [43], they also are pathologic in multiple diseases, such as autoimmune diseases [49], including arthritis [50,51], systemic lupus erythematosus [52–55], antiphospholipid antibody syndrome [56,57], small vessel vasculitis [58], and psoriasis [59–62]. In cancer, neutrophils affect health through multiple mechanisms, and evidence for the role of NETs have been found [63–69] and continue to emerge [38]. In the cardiovascular system, NETs have played a role in atherothrombosis and venous thrombosis [70–72]. Another important disease in which NETs have relevance in its pathophysiology is sepsis. In this process, it has been demonstrated that a release of NETs increases the risk of venous thromboembolism (VTE). It has also been shown that a high percentage of NETs correlates with a high risk to present sepsis [73]. Moreover, the presence of NETs has induced multiple organ damage in an experimental sepsis model [74]. In lung diseases, NETs have an important role in chronic inflammation, including cystic fibrosis [75,76] and chronic obstructive pulmonary disease (COPD) [21,77–79].

6. Eye Diseases

As we have discussed earlier, the release of NETs is an aspect of damage seen in a wide variety of diseases. For a long time, it was considered that the eye was an immune-privilege organ without any immune response. Nevertheless, this idea is not entirely true. Several works have described that ocular immune privilege provides the eye with immune protection against inflammation in order to minimise the risk to vision [80], and the focus was on the ocular privilege associated with Treg response. On the other hand, we know that different diseases have an immune response, and the eye has a series of mechanisms that defend against infections, but it is also true that there are pathologies that are not yet known to regulate this.

In recent years, there has been evidence of NETs and their implication within pathophysiology in ocular diseases.

7. Cornea and Ocular Surface

The cornea is the transparent and avascular dome-shaped tissue of the eye. It represents a physical immune barrier, and together with the tear film, provides the anterior ocular refractive surface. Its transparency is due to the composition and physiology of its cellular constituents [81].

Eye rheum is a medial angle accumulated discharge, independent of any disease. Its composition consists mainly of leukocytes, neutrophils, and their related proteins. Aggregated neutrophil extracellular traps (aggNETs) have also been measured in the eye rheum, and it has been concluded that their presence prevents the spreading of inflammation because they degrade inflammatory mediators [82,83]. However, it has been found that chronic accumulation of aggNETs contributes to inflammation and tissue damage.

7.1. Dry Eye Disease

Dry eye disease (DED) is defined as a multifactorial disease of the ocular surface, characterised by a loss of homeostasis of the tear film and accompanied by ocular symptoms, in which tear film instability and hyperosmolarity occurs. Ocular surface inflammation, damage and neurosensory abnormalities play etiological roles [84]. The dynamic turnover of the corneal epithelium is increased in DED. This is regulated by apoptosis, which stimulates the immune system, leading to the extracellular DNA (eDNA) release and NETosis. It has been suggested that, in healthy eyes, the eDNA is cleared by nucleases contained in tears, but in patients with DED (mainly in severe cases), it has been found to be nuclease deficient. This permits the tear gathering of eDNA and NETs to trigger and perpetrate inflammation of the ocular surface [85]. This theory was supported by Tibrewal and colleagues, who reported the presence of excessive amounts of eDNA in the tear fluid of patients with DED associated with a release of NETs, which was higher in patients with worse DED, which in turn is associated with hyperosmolar stress and the deprivation of nucleases [86]. Therefore, a high amount of NETs is expected to be found on the ocular surface in patients with DED. The outcomes of these studies were supported by Mun and colleagues, through a pilot clinical trial of recombinant human deoxyribonuclease I (0.1% DNase) eye drops in patients with DED. After comparing the use of DNase versus placebo eye drops in 41 patients four times a day for eight weeks, they demonstrated a significant reduction in symptomatic and clinical severity of DED. In relation to the mechanisms previously described, this result could possibly be explained due to degradation of the NETs [87].

Ocular sicca in chronic graft-versus-host disease (GVHD) has also been related to NETosis. GVHD is a complication that takes place in patients after hematopoietic stem cell transplantation, and ocular GVHD (oGVHD) is a particular clinical manifestation of chronic GVHD. Clinical signs and symptoms of oGVHD are related to eyelid disease and tear deficiency. However, it is not considered merely as a specific form of tear deficiency or dry eye. In fact, oGVHD has different pathophysiology and treatment than DED, but it is associated with a dysregulated immunity response. Through the analysis of ocular surface washing from patients with oGVHD, An and colleagues demonstrated an increase in associated NET-cytokines levels, such as MPO and IL-8, among others, which are well-known to be chronic inflammation contributors. Also, they showed therapeutic effects of sub-anticoagulant dose heparin (100 IU/mL) eye drops through the destabilisation and clearance of NETs from the ocular surface [88], demonstrating the essential role of NETs in oGVHD.

7.2. Infectious Keratitis

The leading cause of monocular blindness worldwide is corneal disease, and infectious keratitis is among the leading causes of corneal opacities. This pathology is more common among marginalised populations. The prognosis and clinical outcome of this ocular pathology is determined by the proper identification of the causative microorganism, as well as effective management.

In comparison with other tissues, the late immune response against infectious microbes could be significant because of corneal avascularity. The epidemiology of infectious keratitis is related to the population studied. While in developed countries it is associated with bacterial ulcers, mainly due to contact lens use, in developing countries, fungi are common causative agents [89]. Several keratitis cases in contact lens wearers are often caused by *Pseudomonas aeruginosa*, a Gramm negative bacterium with a harmful evolution that can cause permanent vision loss. The immune reaction against *Pseudomonas* is dominated by neutrophil response, but the infiltration pattern changes upon the *Pseudomonas* strain [90,91]. When Shan and colleagues tested the ability of *Pseudomonas* strains to release NETs and their vulnerability to be NET-captured, they found that even cytotoxic strains are better inductors of NETs and are less sensitive to be NET-captured [90]. Since the first description of NETs made by Brinkmann in 2004, the antimicrobial properties of NETs were described and explained through degradation of virulence factors and bacteria killing [2]. Current data has explained some NET evasion mechanisms in keratitis are caused by *Pseudomonas* strains. *Pseudomonas* employs virulence factors, like the type-3 secretion system (T3SS). T3SS also forms biofilms through Psl exopolysaccharide and favours bacterium NET escape. The inefficacy of neutrophils to penetrate *Pseudomonas* biofilm leads to the production and release of NETs as an attempt to avoid bacteria spreading [92]. The shedding of outer membrane vesicles (OMVs) contributes to avoid *Pseudomonas* linking to NETs; thus, the shedding of OMVs as a possible therapeutic target should be considered [93].

Mycotic keratitis is usually developed from corneal injury due to agricultural work or, less frequently, in contact lens users. Ulcers caused by fungi have worse outcomes than bacterial ulcers [93]. Although neutrophils can clear conidia fungi forms by phagocytosis, the hyphae of fungi are too large to be cleared by this mechanism, and NET release has been reported as a capture and kill neutrophil machinery in yeast and hyphal forms. Jin and colleagues studied the relationship between the quantification of NETs and the prognosis of fungal keratitis in vivo. They studied and measured DNA-releasing neutrophils in 14 patients with clinical and final diagnostic biopsy of fungal keratitis, in which the culture was positive for *Fusarium* sp., *Aspergylus* sp., *Candida*, and *Alternaria* sp. They demonstrated the existence of NETs in different stages from day 2 to day 22, suggesting their role in the entire stage of this infectious pathology, but they did not find any relationship between the number of NETs and the size of the ulcer. However, they did identify a close relationship between the patient response to therapy and the quantity of NETs [93].

8. Corneal Injuries and Repair

Due to its location, the cornea is susceptible to possible injuries like abrasions, burns, infections, and de-epithelisation. Depending on the damage, those stimuli can trigger the corneal wound healing process, impacting on the tissue transparency and, in some cases, producing permanent impairment of vision [94]. As previously studied, the exacerbated production of NETs offers the basis for the progress and preservation of inflammation. We have previously reported that NET release is presented in a rabbit corneal alkali burn, and intracameral injection of human amniotic mesenchymal stem cells (hAM-MSC) was able to significantly inhibit NET release. hAM-MSC were also able to reduce the number of inflammatory cells and infiltrated neutrophil, as well as neovascularisation and corneal opacity. These effects are attributable to their immunosuppressive molecules [95].

9. Uveitis

Uveitis refers to a group of eye diseases that are defined by intraocular inflammation, specifically affecting the uveal tract, which compromises the iris, ciliary body, and choroid [96]. It also includes other inflammation of adjacent intraocular structures, such as the retina, vitreous, and optic nerve and, depending on the severity, can generate imminently harmful ocular injuries [97]. Uveitis can be acute, chronic, or recurrent, infectious or non-infectious, granulomatous or non-granulomatous, and unilateral or bilateral [98,99].

The main non-infectious causes of uveitis are acute anterior uveitis, Behçet's disease (BD), Vogt-Koyanagi-Harada (VKH), and juvenile idiopathic arthritis (JIA), among others. Interestingly, it has been described that in non-infectious uveitis, the immune response is the main responsible cause [100].

The main infectious aetiologies of uveitis include pathogens like the herpes virus, *Toxoplasma gondii*, *Mycobacterium tuberculosis*, and *Treponema pallidum* [99], among others. To date, it is estimated that uveitis is responsible for about 10% of legal blindness in the United States per year. The socioeconomic impact of uveitis lies in the main affected age group being the young and middle working-age population; thus, the patients are usually economically active [101,102].

BD is a systemic vasculitis that affects arteries or veins [103]. Clinical features consist of recurrent oral and genital ulcers associated with inflammatory manifestations with skin, eyes, joints, gastrointestinal, and central nervous system involvement. It is histologically diagnosed by an intense neutrophilic infiltrate. There are reports that describe an inappropriate hyperactivity of neutrophils by cytokines and other molecules that produce increased volumes of superoxide anion via NADPH oxidase (Nox2) [103,104]. Clinical criteria for ocular BD diagnosis include anterior and posterior ocular segment involvement: uveitis, hypopyon iritis and retinitis. The wide range of ocular BD features include mild to severe clinical conditions. The most common anterior segment BD manifestation is bilateral non-granulomatous anterior uveitis, usually associated with transient hypopyon, that responds to topical steroid treatments. Posterior segment presentation includes retinitis, vitritis, and retinal vasculitis, which can provoke complications such as cystoid macular oedema and retinal ischaemia, with subsequent retinal neovascularization [105]. In a study conducted by Safi and colleagues, it was described that patients with BD had vasculitis as a result of a high release of NETs. It is also mentioned that 58% of patients had ocular manifestations, such as anterior uveitis, posterior uveitis, and panuveitis, among others [106], suggesting an active role of NETs release in BD aetiopathogenesis. In another study conducted by Perazzio and colleagues, they studied how the neutrophils from patients with severe BD showed up before and after PMA stimulation, with an increase in their oxidative burst activity via a CD40-dependent phosphoinositide 3-kinase/NF-κB pathway. This was compared with cells from patients with mild manifestations of BD [107]. This provided the basis for this team to study the effect of the soluble CD40 ligand (sCD40L), a member of the TNF family, in relation to the release of NETs. This soluble form of CD40 is related to the antigen-presenting cell process, T-cell activation, and platelet aggregation [107,108]. Current data has shown a rise of sCD40L serum levels in BD patients. Recently, Perazzio and colleagues demonstrated a significant increase of NET release and reactive oxygen species production after neutrophil stimulation with sCD40L and a decrease by blocking this molecule [107]. This indicates an active function of this molecule as a possible target for the treatment for BD or other related NET releasing pathologies.

Although increased NET release has been studied in systemic lupus erythematosus and rheumatoid arthritis, there are no current studies of NET release and its association with ocular manifestations of these diseases [50,53]. We consider BD as ocular symptoms that are required criteria for the diagnoses.

10. Vitreoretinal Pathologies

Diabetic retinopathy (DR) is one of the main causes of avoidable bilateral blindness worldwide [109–111]. It has been considered as a microvascular complication related to diabetes mellitus, and its diagnosis and classification is based on visible vascular lesions on the retina. There are two main stages—non-proliferative DR (NPDR) and proliferative diabetic retinopathy (PDR). In the first stage of PDR, microaneurysms, retinal haemorrhages, and vascular tortuosity are present in the ophthalmoscopical examination, while in the second stage, frank neovascularization is found [111]. An important additional categorisation in DR is diabetic macular oedema (DME), which is a fluid accumulation into the neural retina that leads to abnormal retinal thickening and often cystoid oedema of the macula [111]. It is one of the major complications of DR [112]. The hallmark of DR pathophysiology lies in the compromised integrity of blood–retinal barrier (BRB). It has been described that long-term hyperglycaemia promotes an increase in vascular capillary permeability, letting neutrophils pass through it, infiltrating choroid and retina and therefore enabling retinopathy progression, which is caused by this chronic inflammation condition [113,114].

Within the pathophysiology of DR there are reports of pro-inflammatory molecules, as well as growth factors involved in the exacerbation of the disease. Several inflammatory cytokines, such as IL-1ß, IL-6, IL-8, tumour necrosis factor-alpha (TNF-α), and monocyte chemoattractant protein-1 (MCP-1), have been reported as elevated in vitreous samples from NPDR patients [115]. In contrast, another study of patients with PDR described elevated levels of pro inflammatory cytokines, IL-1ß, IL-6, IL8, and CCL2. However, they reported that IL-10 was similar to that obtained in the controls [116].

Some important factors such as endothelin 1 (EDN1, also called ET-1), vascular endothelial growth factor (VEGF), and TNF-α have been involved in the inflammatory reactivity and neovascularisation of PDR. By another hand, in patients with DME, it has been found that the levels of angiopoietin-2 (ANg2), an important modulator of angiogenesis of VEGF, is elevated in comparison to controls [111].

In recent years, the use of therapy based on intravitreal injection of anti-vascular endothelial growth factor (anti-VEGF) drugs has become the first line of treatment for PDR [112]. In order to describe another therapy, experiments in vitro have demonstrated that corticosteroids also modulate vascular permeability by suppressing the production of VEGF mRNA, VEGF-mediated protein expression, and VEGF receptor in human cell cultures, macrophages, and endothelial cells [112].

As aforementioned, DME is the major complication in PDR; thus, treatment alternatives have been investigated. Intravitreal steroid administration has shown to be an alternative to anti-VEGF drugs in treatment of naïve eyes affected by DME. This reduced the frequency of anti-VEGF intravitreal injections in patients with coronary diseases, for whom anti-VEGF agents are contraindicated [112,117].

Certain studies associated NET release as a factor involved in the pathogenesis of DR. Wang and colleagues showed that neutrophils from diabetic patients, especially in PDR, are able to promote spontaneous release of NETs and that neutrophils of healthy controls are able to release NETs when they are stimulated by high glucose levels. They also studied the association between high glucose-induced NETosis and NADPH oxidase-derived ROS pathways [113].

Although it has been studied and reported that high glucose medium can increase NET release in vivo and in vitro [118], it has even been reported that levels of NET markers are independent factors for diabetic retinopathy [119]; yet, the molecular mechanisms that stimulate its release has not been clearly elucidated.

The existence of NETosis has been reported in ocular inflammation induced by proinflammatory cytokines in a mouse model and in samples obtained via standard pars plana vitrectomy of diabetic patients with PDR. In the same study, they confirmed the presence of NETs, and these authors proved in their mouse model that NETs can be degraded with DNase I, which has been reported to help in clinical NETs association when used as eye drops [86].

Barliya and colleagues have demonstrated the existence of NET release in a mouse model and human samples. They injected two well-known inflammatory cytokines, IL-8 and TNF-α, into murine eyes as NET inductors. NETosis was measured by considering specific marker staining for MPO, NE, and H3Cit. They found aggregate neutrophils in anterior and posterior chambers with NET staining markers. Their results confirmed eDNA through the inhibition of H3Cit staining when DNAase treatment was applied. In the same study, the authors analysed vitreous human samples of diabetic patients with proliferative retinopathy that underwent vitrectomy and correlated NET release with the severity of the disease. As expected, they reported that those patients with worse clinical features showed a higher release of NETs [120].

11. Age Macular Degeneration

Age macular degeneration (AMD) is an acquired central retina degeneration and the leading cause of irreversible visual impairment in elderly people. Within its aetiology, environmental factors are well-described as triggers for the disease in both of its forms: dry or atrophic and exudative or neovascular "wet" AMD. The latter is less frequent but the most serious because it causes severe visual loss [121].

The pathogenesis of neovascular AMD is multifactorial; however, it is well-known that the hallmark of macular oedema is the breakdown of the blood retinal barrier (BRB), which leads to vascular leakage. This condition is common in retinal diseases, such as diabetic retinopathy, cystoid macular oedema, ischaemic retinal vein occlusion and some forms of posterior uveitis [122]. The breakdown of the BRB facilitates immune cell infiltration, as previous reports show [123]. Although the molecular mechanisms are not well-understood, it has been reported in histopathological studies of AMD eyes that the presence of "drusen", lipoproteinaceous undigested products of retinal pigment epithelium (RPE) exist between the RPE and Bruch's membrane, as well as basal laminar deposits, which are remarkably related to choroidal neovascularisation [124]. Histological reports of these infiltrates have proven the existence of complement molecules like C3, C5b-9, and the membrane attack complex (MAC), as well as macrophages that, due to TNF stimulation, initiate VEGF production by RPE [121,125]. The retina is susceptible to these factors and produces inflammatory cytokines such as VEGF and tissue factors that induce fibrin growth, which act as a platform for Choroidal Neovascularisation (CNV) development [121].

Furthermore, it is known that VEGF not only contributes to vascular dysfunctions, but acts as a pro-inflammatory molecule, as long as it endorses the expression of inflammatory cytokines like IL-8 [126], a biomarker of NET release, and promotes ROS production derived from NADPH oxidase in turn [115]. VEGF is also a regulator of angiogenesis and a main contributor of macular oedema development either in AMD or DR. While the molecular pathogenesis of these pathologies is different, they have a background of inflammatory microenvironment in common [111,127].

Although there is no current data of NETosis related to AMD, as previously mentioned, there is a study on a diabetic rat model where the existence of NETs was demonstrated in eye tissues, specifically vitreous body and retina. Their presence was justified by peripheral neutrophils that had infiltrated when BRB broke. In the same study, authors reported a reduction in NETs release after anti-VEGF therapy [113]. As shown, the research field on AMD is promising.

12. Future Perspectives

The overall aim of this review has been to condense current data of NETs related to healthy eyes and ocular diseases. As demonstrated, the better the understanding of molecular processes during inflammation, the better the assessment of intervention pathways to control it.

Future work concerns taking a deeper approach of NET release mechanisms and molecules involved, in order to obtain new proposals that help with the diagnosis, prognosis and management of ocular pathologies.

A better understanding of NETosis triggers during diseases may aid in discovering new therapeutic potential interventions based on ocular molecular components. Therapeutic interventions centred on clearing NETs as well as inhibiting their signalling molecules could yield innovative targets to work with.

Molecule systems involved in NET release production should be a focus of future research. Assessment of those molecular changes implicated in the NET release process will provide new insights into the pathogenesis and therefore the potential management of a wide range of diseases.

A schematic summary is presented in Figure 1.

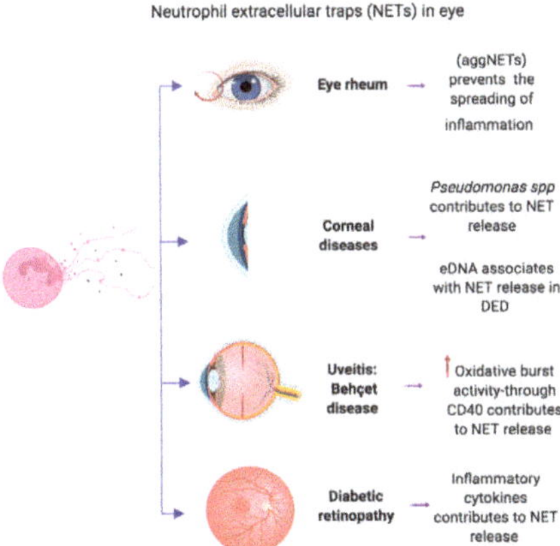

Figure 1. Neutrophil extracellular traps in eye. Neutrophil extracellular traps (NETs) are involved in several diseases in eye. NETs are associated with the pathophysiological mechanism, contributing to the exacerbation of the disease in some cases, such as diabetic retinopathy, in corneal diseases for instance, dry eye disease (DED), another disease is uveitis. However, a benefit of the NETs in eye, we can see it in the eye rheum, in which the NETs prevent the spread of inflammation. AggNETS: Aggregated neutrophil extracellular traps; eDNA: extracellular DNA; DED: Dry eye disease. Created with: biorender.com.

Funding: This study was supported by grants from Consejo Nacional de Ciencia y Tecnología (CONACyT): Problemas Nacionales 0311; Fondo Sectorial en Salud 273349. UNAM-PAPIIT-DGAPA: IN215617.

Acknowledgments: Gibrán Alejandro Estúa Acosta is a doctoral student from Programa de Doctorado en Ciencias Biomédicas, Universidad Nacional Autónoma de México (UNAM) and was supported by CONACyT CVU: 661449.

Conflicts of Interest: The authors declare no conflict of interest.

References

1. Kolaczkowska, E.; Kubes, P. Neutrophil recruitment and function in health and inflammation. *Nat. Rev. Immunol.* **2013**, *13*, 159–175. [CrossRef]
2. Brinkmann, V. Neutrophil Extracellular Traps Kill Bacteria. *Science* **2004**, *303*, 1532–1535. [CrossRef]
3. Fuchs, T.A.; Abed, U.; Goosmann, C.; Hurwitz, R.; Schulze, I.; Wahn, V.; Weinrauch, Y.; Brinkmann, V.; Zychlinsky, A. Novel cell death program leads to neutrophil extracellular traps. *J. Cell Boil.* **2007**, *176*, 231–241. [CrossRef] [PubMed]
4. Brinkmann, V. Neutrophil Extracellular Traps in the Second Decade. *J. Innate Immun.* **2018**, *10*, 414–421. [CrossRef] [PubMed]
5. Yipp, B.G.; Kubes, P. NETosis: How vital is it? *Blood* **2013**, *122*, 2784–2794. [CrossRef] [PubMed]
6. Wang, J. Neutrophils in tissue injury and repair. *Cell Tissue Res.* **2018**, *371*, 531–539. [CrossRef] [PubMed]
7. Kruger, P.; Saffarzadeh, M.; Weber, A.N.R.; Rieber, N.; Radsak, M.; Von Bernuth, H.; Benarafa, C.; Roos, D.; Skokowa, J.; Hartl, D. Neutrophils: Between Host Defence, Immune Modulation, and Tissue Injury. *PLOS Pathog.* **2015**, *11*, e1004651. [CrossRef] [PubMed]
8. Urban, C.F.; Ermert, D.; Schmid, M.; Abu-Abed, U.; Goosmann, C.; Nacken, W.; Brinkmann, V.; Jungblut, P.R.; Zychlinsky, A. Neutrophil extracellular traps contain calprotectin, a cytosolic protein complex involved in host defense against Candida albicans. *PLOS Pathog.* **2009**, *5*, e1000639. [CrossRef]
9. Jabłońska, E.; Garley, M.; Iwaniuk, A.; Wrona, W.R.; Dąbrowska, D. New Aspects of the Biology of Neutrophil Extracellular Traps. *Scand. J. Immunol.* **2016**, *84*, 317–322.
10. Van Der Linden, M.; Westerlaken, G.H.A.; Van Der Vlist, M.; Van Montfrans, J.; Meyaard, L. Differential Signalling and Kinetics of Neutrophil Extracellular Trap Release Revealed by Quantitative Live Imaging. *Sci. Rep.* **2017**, *7*, 6529. [CrossRef]
11. Zhao, W.; Fogg, D.K.; Kaplan, M.J. A novel image-based quantitative method for the characterization of NETosis. *J. Immunol. Methods* **2015**, *423*, 104–110. [CrossRef]
12. Krautgartner, W.D.; Klappacher, M.; Hannig, M.; Obermayer, A.; Hartl, D.; Marcos, V.; Vitkov, L. Fibrin Mimics Neutrophil Extracellular Traps in SEM. *Ultrastruct. Pathol.* **2010**, *34*, 226–231. [CrossRef]
13. Brinkmann, V.; Goosmann, C.; Kühn, L.I.; Zychlinsky, A. Automatic quantification of in vitro NET formation. *Front. Immunol.* **2012**, *3*, 413. [CrossRef]
14. de Buhr, N.; von Köckritz-Blickwede, M. How Neutrophil Extracellular Traps Become Visible. *J. Immunol. Res.* **2016**, *2016*, 4604713. [CrossRef]
15. Mohanty, T.; Sørensen, O.E.; Nordenfelt, P. NETQUANT: Automated Quantification of Neutrophil Extracellular Traps. *Front. Immunol.* **2018**, *8*, 1999. [CrossRef]
16. Arends, E.J.; Van Dam, L.S.; Kraaij, T.; Kamerling, S.W.; Rabelink, T.J.; Van Kooten, C.; Teng, Y.O. A High-throughput Assay to Assess and Quantify Neutrophil Extracellular Trap Formation. *J. Vis. Exp.* **2019**, e59150. [CrossRef]
17. Takei, H.; Araki, A.; Watanabe, H.; Ichinose, A.; Sendo, F. Rapid killing of human neutrophils by the potent activator phorbol 12-myristate 13-acetate (PMA) accompanied by changes different from typical apoptosis or necrosis. *J. Leukoc. Boil.* **1996**, *59*, 229–240. [CrossRef]
18. Branzk, N.; Lubojemska, A.; Hardison, S.E.; Wang, Q.; Gutierrez, M.G.; Brown, G.D.; Papayannopoulos, V. Neutrophils sense microbial size and selectively release neutrophil extracellular traps in response to large pathogens. *Nat. Immunol.* **2014**, *15*, 1017–1025. [CrossRef]
19. Hoppenbrouwers, T.; Autar, A.S.A.; Sultan, A.R.; Abraham, T.E.; van Cappellen, W.A.; Houtsmuller, A.B.; van Wamel, W.J.B.; van Beusekom, H.M.M.; van Neck, J.W.; de Maat, M.P.M. In vitro induction of NETosis: Comprehensive live imaging comparison and systematic review. *PLOS ONE* **2017**, *12*, e0176472. [CrossRef]

20. Mitroulis, I.; Kambas, K.; Chrysanthopoulou, A.; Skendros, P.; Apostolidou, E.; Kourtzelis, I.; Drosos, G.I.; Boumpas, D.T.; Ritis, K. Neutrophil Extracellular Trap Formation Is Associated with IL-1β and Autophagy-Related Signaling in Gout. *PLOS ONE* **2011**, *6*, e29318. [CrossRef]

21. Qiu, S.-L.; Deng, J.-M.; Liu, G.-N.; Zhang, H.; Tang, Q.-Y.; Bai, J.; He, Z.-Y.; Li, M.-H.; Zhong, X.-N. Neutrophil extracellular traps induced by cigarette smoke activate plasmacytoid dendritic cells. *Thorax* **2017**, *72*, 1084–1093. [CrossRef]

22. De Bont, C.M.; Koopman, W.J.; Boelens, W.C.; Pruijn, G.J. Stimulus-dependent chromatin dynamics, citrullination, calcium signalling and ROS production during NET formation. *Biochim. et Biophys. Acta (BBA)-Bioenerg.* **2018**, *1865*, 1621–1629. [CrossRef]

23. Petretto, A.; Bruschi, M.; Pratesi, F.; Croia, C.; Candiano, G.; Ghiggeri, G.; Migliorini, P. Neutrophil extracellular traps (NET) induced by different stimuli: A comparative proteomic analysis. *PLOS ONE* **2019**, *14*, e0218946. [CrossRef]

24. Delgado-Rizo, V.; Martínez-Guzmán, M.A.; Iñiguez-Gutierrez, L.; García-Orozco, A.; Alvarado-Navarro, A.; Fafutis-Morris, M. Neutrophil Extracellular Traps and Its Implications in Inflammation: An Overview. *Front. Immunol.* **2017**, *8*, 81. [CrossRef]

25. Pilsczek, F.H.; Salina, D.; Poon, K.K.H.; Fahey, C.; Yipp, B.G.; Sibley, C.D.; Robbins, S.M.; Green, F.H.Y.; Surette, M.G.; Sugai, M.; et al. A Novel Mechanism of Rapid Nuclear Neutrophil Extracellular Trap Formation in Response to Staphylococcus aureus. *J. Immunol.* **2010**, *185*, 7413–7425. [CrossRef]

26. Yousefi, S.; Mihalache, C.; Kozlowski, E.; Schmid, I.; Simon, H.-U. Viable neutrophils release mitochondrial DNA to form neutrophil extracellular traps. *Cell Death Differ.* **2009**, *16*, 1438–1444. [CrossRef]

27. Sollberger, G.; Amulic, B.; Zychlinsky, A. Neutrophil Extracellular Trap Formation Is Independent of De Novo Gene Expression. *PLOS ONE* **2016**, *11*, e0157454. [CrossRef]

28. Saitoh, T.; Komano, J.; Saitoh, Y.; Misawa, T.; Takahama, M.; Kozaki, T.; Uehata, T.; Iwasaki, H.; Omori, H.; Yamaoka, S.; et al. Neutrophil Extracellular Traps Mediate a Host Defense Response to Human Immunodeficiency Virus-1. *Cell Host Microbe* **2012**, *12*, 109–116. [CrossRef]

29. DeSouza-Vieira, T.; Guimarães-Costa, A.; Rochael, N.C.; Lira, M.N.; Nascimento, M.T.; Lima-Gomez, P.S.; Mariante, R.M.; Persechini, P.M.; Saraiva, E.M. Neutrophil extracellular traps release induced by Leishmania: Role of PI3Kγ, ERK, PI3Kσ, PKC, and [Ca2+]. *J. Leukoc. Biol.* **2016**, *100*, 801–810. [CrossRef]

30. Douda, D.N.; Yip, L.; Khan, M.A.; Grasemann, H.; Palaniyar, N. Akt is essential to induce NADPH-dependent NETosis and to switch the neutrophil death to apoptosis. *Blood* **2014**, *123*, 597–600. [CrossRef]

31. Remijsen, Q.; Vanden Berghe, T.; Wirawan, E.; Asselbergh, B.; Parthoens, E.; De Rycke, R.; Noppen, S.; Delforge, M.; Willems, J.; Vandenabeele, P. Neutrophil extracellular trap cell death requires both autophagy and superoxide generation. *Cell Res.* **2011**, *21*, 290–304. [CrossRef]

32. Hakkim, A.; Fuchs, T.A.; Martinez, N.E.; Hess, S.; Prinz, H.; Zychlinsky, A.; Waldmann, H. Activation of the Raf-MEK-ERK pathway is required for neutrophil extracellular trap formation. *Nat. Chem. Biol.* **2011**, *7*, 75–77. [CrossRef]

33. Tatsiy, O.; McDonald, P.P. Physiological Stimuli Induce PAD4-Dependent, ROS-Independent NETosis, With Early and Late Events Controlled by Discrete Signaling Pathways. *Front. Immunol.* **2018**, *9*, 9. [CrossRef]

34. Papayannopoulos, V.; Metzler, K.D.; Hakkim, A.; Zychlinsky, A. Neutrophil elastase and myeloperoxidase regulate the formation of neutrophil extracellular traps. *J. Cell Boil.* **2010**, *191*, 677–691. [CrossRef]

35. Metzler, K.D.; Goosmann, C.; Lubojemska, A.; Zychlinsky, A.; Papayannopoulos, V. A Myeloperoxidase-Containing Complex Regulates Neutrophil Elastase Release and Actin Dynamics during NETosis. *Cell Rep.* **2014**, *8*, 883–896. [CrossRef]

36. Khan, M.A.; Palaniyar, N. Transcriptional firing helps to drive NETosis. *Sci. Rep.* **2017**, *7*, 41749. [CrossRef]

37. Bianchi, M.; Hakkim, A.; Brinkmann, V.; Siler, U.; Seger, R.A.; Zychlinsky, A.; Reichenbach, J. Restoration of NET formation by gene therapy in CGD controls aspergillosis. *Blood* **2009**, *114*, 2619–2622. [CrossRef]

38. Papayannopoulos, V. Neutrophil extracellular traps in immunity and disease. *Nat. Rev. Immunol.* **2018**, *18*, 134–147. [CrossRef]

39. Nomura, K.; Miyashita, T.; Yamamoto, Y.; Munesue, S.; Harashima, A.; Takayama, H.; Fushida, S.; Ohta, T. Citrullinated Histone H3: Early Biomarker of Neutrophil Extracellular Traps in Septic Liver Damage. *J. Surg. Res.* **2019**, *234*, 132–138. [CrossRef]

40. Konig, M.F.; Andrade, F. A Critical Reappraisal of Neutrophil Extracellular Traps and NETosis Mimics Based on Differential Requirements for Protein Citrullination. *Front. Immunol.* **2016**, *7*, 209. [CrossRef]

41. Wang, Y.; Li, M.; Stadler, S.; Correll, S.; Li, P.; Wang, D.; Hayama, R.; Leonelli, L.; Han, H.; Grigoryev, S.A.; et al. Histone hypercitrullination mediates chromatin decondensation and neutrophil extracellular trap formation. *J. Cell Boil.* **2009**, *184*, 205–213. [CrossRef]

42. Neeli, I.; Radic, M. Opposition between PKC isoforms regulates histone deimination and neutrophil extracellular chromatin release. *Front. Immunol.* **2013**, *4*, 38. [CrossRef]

43. Holmes, C.L.; Shim, D.; Kernien, J.; Johnson, C.J.; Nett, J.E.; Shelef, M.A. Insight into Neutrophil Extracellular Traps through Systematic Evaluation of Citrullination and Peptidylarginine Deiminases. *J. Immunol. Res.* **2019**, *2019*, 1–11. [CrossRef]

44. Saha, P.; Yeoh, B.S.; Xiao, X.; Golonka, R.M.; Singh, V.; Wang, Y.; Vijay-Kumar, M. PAD4-dependent NETs generation are indispensable for intestinal clearance of Citrobacter rodentium. *Mucosal Immunol.* **2019**, *12*, 761–771. [CrossRef]

45. Parker, H.; Dragunow, M.; Hampton, M.B.; Kettle, A.J.; Winterbourn, C.C. Requirements for NADPH oxidase and myeloperoxidase in neutrophil extracellular trap formation differ depending on the stimulus. *J. Leukoc. Boil.* **2012**, *92*, 841–849. [CrossRef]

46. Lewis, H.D.; Liddle, J.; Coote, J.E.; Atkinson, S.J.; Barker, M.D.; Benjamin, D.B.; Bicker, K.L.; Bingham, R.P.; Campbell, M.; Chen, Y.H.; et al. Inhibition of PAD4 activity is sufficient to disrupt mouse and human NET formation. *Nat. Methods* **2015**, *11*, 189–191. [CrossRef]

47. Darrah, E.; Rosen, A.; Giles, J.T.; Andrade, F. Peptidylarginine deiminase 2, 3 and 4 have distinct specificities against cellular substrates: Novel insights into autoantigen selection in rheumatoid arthritis. *Ann. Rheum. Dis.* **2012**, *71*, 92–98. [CrossRef]

48. Caielli, S.; Athale, S.; Domic, B.; Murat, E.; Chandra, M.; Banchereau, R.; Baisch, J.; Phelps, K.; Clayton, S.; Gong, M.; et al. Oxidized mitochondrial nucleoids released by neutrophils drive type I interferon production in human lupus. *J. Exp. Med.* **2016**, *213*, 697–713. [CrossRef]

49. Lee, K.H.; Kronbichler, A.; Park, D.D.-Y.; Park, Y.; Moon, H.; Kim, H.; Choi, J.H.; Choi, Y.; Shim, S.; Lyu, I.S.; et al. Neutrophil extracellular traps (NETs) in autoimmune diseases: A comprehensive review. *Autoimmun. Rev.* **2017**, *16*, 1160–1173. [CrossRef]

50. Chowdhury, C.S.; Giaglis, S.; A Walker, U.; Buser, A.; Hahn, S.; Hasler, P. Enhanced neutrophil extracellular trap generation in rheumatoid arthritis: Analysis of underlying signal transduction pathways and potential diagnostic utility. *Arthritis Res. Ther.* **2014**, *16*, R122. [CrossRef]

51. Yu, H.-C.; Lu, M.-C. The roles of anti-citrullinated protein antibodies in the immunopathogenesis of rheumatoid arthritis. *Tzu Chi Med J.* **2019**, *31*, 5–10.

52. Kahlenberg, J.M.; Carmona-Rivera, C.; Smith, C.K.; Kaplan, M.J. Neutrophil extracellular trap-associated protein activation of the NLRP3 inflammasome is enhanced in lupus macrophages. *J. Immunol.* **2013**, *190*, 1217–1226. [CrossRef]

53. Hakkim, A.; Fürnrohr, B.G.; Amann, K.; Laube, B.; Abu Abed, U.; Brinkmann, V.; Herrmann, M.; Voll, R.E.; Zychlinsky, A. Impairment of neutrophil extracellular trap degradation is associated with lupus nephritis. *Proc. Natl. Acad. Sci. USA* **2010**, *107*, 9813–9818. [CrossRef]

54. Khandpur, R.; Carmona-Rivera, C.; Vivekanandan-Giri, A.; Gizinski, A.; Yalavarthi, S.; Knight, J.S.; Friday, S.; Li, S.; Patel, R.M.; Subramanian, V.; et al. NETs are a source of citrullinated autoantigens and stimulate inflammatory responses in rheumatoid arthritis. *Sci. Transl. Med.* **2013**, *5*, 178ra40. [CrossRef]

55. Van Dam, L.S.; Kraaij, T.; A Kamerling, S.W.; Bakker, J.A.; Scherer, U.H.; Rabelink, T.J.; Van Kooten, C.; Teng, Y.O. Neutrophil extracellular trap formation is intrinsically distinct in ANCA -associated vasculitis and systemic lupus erythematosus. *Arthritis Rheumatol.* **2019**. [CrossRef]

56. Meng, H.; Yalavarthi, S.; Kanthi, Y.; Mazza, L.F.; Elfline, M.A.; Luke, C.E.; Pinsky, D.J.; Henke, P.K.; Knight, J.S. In vivo role of neutrophil extracellular traps in antiphospholipid antibody-mediated venous thrombosis. *Arthritis Rheumatol.* **2017**, *69*, 655–667. [CrossRef]

57. Yalavarthi, S.; Gould, T.J.; Rao, A.N.; Mazza, L.F.; Morris, A.E.; Núñez-Álvarez, C.; Hernández-Ramírez, D.; Bockenstedt, P.L.; Liaw, P.C.; Cabral, A.R.; et al. Release of neutrophil extracellular traps by neutrophils stimulated with antiphospholipid antibodies: A newly identified mechanism of thrombosis in the antiphospholipid syndrome. *Arthritis Rheumatol.* **2015**, *67*, 2990–3003. [CrossRef]

58. Kessenbrock, K.; Krumbholz, M.; Schönermarck, U.; Back, W.; Gross, W.L.; Werb, Z.; Gröne, H.-J.; Brinkmann, V.; E Jenne, D. Netting neutrophils in autoimmune small-vessel vasculitis. *Nat. Med.* **2009**, *15*, 623–625. [CrossRef]

59. Hu, S.C.-S.; Yu, H.-S.; Yen, F.-L.; Lin, C.-L.; Chen, G.-S.; Lan, C.-C.E. Neutrophil extracellular trap formation is increased in psoriasis and induces human β-defensin-2 production in epidermal keratinocytes. *Sci. Rep.* **2016**, *6*, 31119. [CrossRef]

60. Zabieglo, K.; Majewski, P.; Majchrzak-Gorecka, M.; Wlodarczyk, A.; Grygier, B.; Zegar, A.; Kapinska-Mrowiecka, M.; Naskalska, A.; Pyrc, K.; Dubin, A.; et al. The inhibitory effect of secretory leukocyte protease inhibitor (SLPI) on formation of neutrophil extracellular traps. *J. Leukoc. Boil.* **2015**, *98*, 99–106. [CrossRef]

61. Hoffmann, J.H.; Enk, A.H. Neutrophil extracellular traps in dermatology: Caught in the NET. *J. Dermatol. Sci.* **2016**, *84*, 3–10. [CrossRef]

62. Shao, S.; Fang, H.; Dang, E.; Xue, K.; Zhang, J.; Li, B.; Qiao, H.; Cao, T.; Zhuang, Y.; Shen, S.; et al. Neutrophil Extracellular Traps Promote Inflammatory Responses in Psoriasis via Activating Epidermal TLR4/IL-36R Crosstalk. *Front. Immunol.* **2019**, *10*. [CrossRef]

63. Demers, M.; Krause, D.S.; Schatzberg, D.; Martinod, K.; Voorhees, J.R.; Fuchs, T.A.; Scadden, D.T.; Wagner, D.D. Cancers predispose neutrophils to release extracellular DNA traps that contribute to cancer-associated thrombosis. *Proc. Natl. Acad. Sci. USA* **2012**, *109*, 13076–13081. [CrossRef]

64. Cedervall, J.; Zhang, Y.; Huang, H.; Zhang, L.; Femel, J.; Dimberg, A.; Olsson, A.-K. Neutrophil Extracellular Traps Accumulate in Peripheral Blood Vessels and Compromise Organ Function in Tumor-Bearing Animals. *Cancer Res.* **2015**, *75*, 2653–2662. [CrossRef]

65. Demers, M.; Wong, S.L.; Martinod, K.; Gallant, M.; Cabral, J.E.; Wang, Y.; Wagner, D.D. Priming of neutrophils toward NETosis promotes tumor growth. *OncoImmunology* **2016**, *5*, e1134073. [CrossRef]

66. Park, J.; Wysocki, R.W.; Amoozgar, Z.; Maiorino, L.; Fein, M.R.; Jorns, J.; Schott, A.F.; Kinugasa-Katayama, Y.; Lee, Y.; Won, N.H.; et al. Cancer cells induce metastasis-supporting neutrophil extracellular DNA traps. *Sci. Transl. Med.* **2016**, *8*, 361ra138. [CrossRef]

67. Berger-Achituv, S.; Brinkmann, V.; Abu-Abed, U.; Kühn, L.I.; Ben-Ezra, J.; Elhasid, R.; Zychlinsky, A. A proposed role for neutrophil extracellular traps in cancer immunoediting. *Front. Immunol.* **2013**, *4*, 48. [CrossRef]

68. Coffelt, S.B.; Wellenstein, M.D.; De Visser, K.E. Neutrophils in cancer: Neutral no more. *Nat. Rev. Cancer* **2016**, *16*, 431–446. [CrossRef]

69. Nicolás-Ávila, J.Á.; Adrover, J.M.; Hidalgo, A. Neutrophils in Homeostasis, Immunity, and Cancer. *Immunity* **2017**, *46*, 15–28.

70. Fuchs, T.A.; Brill, A.; Duerschmied, D.; Schatzberg, D.; Monestier, M.; Myers, D.D.; Wrobleski, S.K.; Wakefield, T.W.; Hartwig, J.H.; Wagner, D.D. Extracellular DNA traps promote thrombosis. *Proc. Natl. Acad. Sci. USA* **2010**, *107*, 15880–15885. [CrossRef]

71. Napirei, M.; Ludwig, S.; Mezrhab, J.; Klöckl, T.; Mannherz, H.G. Murine serum nucleases - contrasting effects of plasmin and heparin on the activities of DNase1 and DNase1-like 3 (DNase1l3). *FEBS J.* **2009**, *276*, 1059–1073. [CrossRef]

72. Von Brühl, M.-L.; Stark, K.; Steinhart, A.; Chandraratne, S.; Konrad, I.; Lorenz, M.; Khandoga, A.; Tirniceriu, A.; Coletti, R.; Köllnberger, M.; et al. Monocytes, neutrophils, and platelets cooperate to initiate and propagate venous thrombosis in mice in vivo. *J. Exp. Med.* **2012**, *209*, 819–835. [CrossRef]

73. Kumar, S.; Gupta, E.; Kaushik, S.; Srivastava, V.K.; Saxena, J.; Mehta, S.; Jyoti, A. Quantification of NETs formation in neutrophil and its correlation with the severity of sepsis and organ dysfunction. *Clin. Chim. Acta* **2019**, *495*, 606–610. [CrossRef]

74. Czaikoski, P.G.; Mota, J.M.; Nascimento, D.C.; Sônego, F.; Castanheira, F.V.; Melo, P.H.; Scortegagna, G.T.; Silva, R.L.; Barroso-Sousa, R.; Souto, F.O.; et al. Neutrophil Extracellular Traps Induce Organ Damage during Experimental and Clinical Sepsis. *PLoS ONE* **2016**, *11*, e0148142. [CrossRef]

75. Dwyer, M.; Shan, Q.; D'Ortona, S.; Maurer, R.; Mitchell, R.; Olesen, H.; Thiel, S.; Huebner, J.; Gadjeva, M. Cystic fibrosis sputum DNA has NETosis characteristics and neutrophil extracellular trap release is regulated by macrophage migration-inhibitory factor. *J. Innate Immun.* **2014**, *6*, 765–779. [CrossRef]

76. Marcos, V.; Zhou-Suckow, Z.; Önder Yildirim, A.; Bohla, A.; Hector, A.; Vitkov, L.; Krautgartner, W.D.; Stoiber, W.; Griese, M.; Eickelberg, O.; et al. Free DNA in cystic fibrosis airway fluids correlates with airflow obstruction. *Mediators Inflamm.* **2015**, *2015*, 408935. [CrossRef]

77. Grabcanovic-Musija, F.; Obermayer, A.; Stoiber, W.; Krautgartner, W.-D.; Steinbacher, P.; Winterberg, N.; Bathke, A.C.; Klappacher, M.; Studnicka, M. Neutrophil extracellular trap (NET) formation characterises stable and exacerbated COPD and correlates with airflow limitation. *Respir. Res.* **2015**, *16*, 347. [CrossRef]

78. Obermayer, A.; Stoiber, W.; Krautgartner, W.-D.; Klappacher, M.; Kofler, B.; Steinbacher, P.; Vitkov, L.; Grabcanovic-Musija, F.; Studnicka, M. New Aspects on the Structure of Neutrophil Extracellular Traps from Chronic Obstructive Pulmonary Disease and In Vitro Generation. *PLOS ONE* **2014**, *9*, e97784. [CrossRef]

79. Hosseinzadeh, A.; Thompson, P.R.; Segal, B.H.; Urban, C.F. Nicotine induces neutrophil extracellular traps. *J. Leukoc. Boil.* **2016**, *100*, 1105–1112. [CrossRef]

80. Keino, H.; Horie, S.; Sugita, S. Immune Privilege and Eye-Derived T-Regulatory Cells. *J. Immunol. Res.* **2018**, *2018*, 1–12. [CrossRef]

81. Delmonte, D.W.; Kim, T. Anatomy and physiology of the cornea. *J. Cataract. Refract. Surg.* **2011**, *37*, 588–598. [CrossRef] [PubMed]

82. Mahajan, A.; Grüneboom, A.; Petru, L.; Podolska, M.J.; Kling, L.; Maueröder, C.; Dahms, F.; Christiansen, S.; Günter, L.; Krenn, V.; et al. Frontline Science: Aggregated neutrophil extracellular traps prevent inflammation on the neutrophil-rich ocular surface. *J. Leukoc. Boil.* **2019**, *105*, 1087–1098. [CrossRef] [PubMed]

83. Thanabalasuriar, A.; Kubes, P. Rise and shine: Open your eyes to produce anti-inflammatory NETs. *J. Leukoc. Boil.* **2019**, *105*, 1083–1084. [CrossRef] [PubMed]

84. Craig, J.P.; Nichols, K.K.; Akpek, E.K.; Caffery, B.; Dua, H.S.; Joo, C.-K.; Liu, Z.; Nelson, J.D.; Nichols, J.J.; Tsubota, K.; et al. TFOS DEWS II Definition and Classification Report. *Ocul. Surf.* **2017**, *15*, 276–283. [CrossRef] [PubMed]

85. Sonawane, S.; Khanolkar, V.; Namavari, A.; Chaudhary, S.; Gandhi, S.; Tibrewal, S.; Jassim, S.H.; Shaheen, B.; Hallak, J.; Horner, J.H.; et al. Ocular Surface Extracellular DNA and Nuclease Activity Imbalance: A New Paradigm for Inflammation in Dry Eye Disease. *Investig. Opthalmology Vis. Sci.* **2012**, *53*, 8253–8263. [CrossRef] [PubMed]

86. Tibrewal, S.; Ivanir, Y.; Sarkar, J.; Nayeb-Hashemi, N.; Bouchard, C.S.; Kim, E.; Jain, S. Hyperosmolar Stress Induces Neutrophil Extracellular Trap Formation: Implications for Dry Eye Disease. *Investig. Opthalmology Vis. Sci.* **2014**, *55*, 7961–7969. [CrossRef] [PubMed]

87. Mun, C.; Gulati, S.; Tibrewal, S.; Chen, Y.-F.; An, S.; Surenkhuu, B.; Raju, I.; Buwick, M.; Ahn, A.; Kwon, J.-E.; et al. A Phase I/II Placebo-Controlled Randomized Pilot Clinical Trial of Recombinant Deoxyribonuclease (DNase) Eye Drops Use in Patients With Dry Eye Disease. *Transl. Vis. Sci. Technol.* **2019**, *8*, 10. [CrossRef] [PubMed]

88. An, S.; Raju, I.; Surenkhuu, B.; Kwon, J.-E.; Gulati, S.; Karaman, M.; Pradeep, A.; Sinha, S.; Mun, C.; Jain, S. Neutrophil extracellular traps (NETs) contribute to pathological changes of ocular graft-vs.-host disease (oGVHD) dry eye: Implications for novel biomarkers and therapeutic strategies. *Ocul. Surf.* **2019**. [CrossRef] [PubMed]

89. Austin, A.; Lietman, T.; Rose-Nussbaumer, J. Update on the Management of Infectious Keratitis. *Ophthalmology* **2017**, *124*, 1678–1689. [CrossRef] [PubMed]

90. Shan, Q.; Dwyer, M.; Rahman, S.; Gadjeva, M. Distinct Susceptibilities of Corneal Pseudomonas aeruginosa Clinical Isolates to Neutrophil Extracellular Trap-Mediated Immunity. *Infect. Immun.* **2014**, *82*, 4135–4143. [CrossRef] [PubMed]

91. Cole, N.; Willcox, M.D.P.; Fleiszig, S.M.J.; Stapleton, F.; Bao, B.; Tout, S.; Husband, A. Different strains of Pseudomonas aeruginosa isolated from ocular infections or inflammation display distinct corneal pathologies in an animal model. *Curr. Eye Res.* **1998**, *17*, 730–735. [CrossRef] [PubMed]

92. Thanabalasuriar, A.; Scott, B.N.V.; Peiseler, M.; Willson, M.E.; Zeng, Z.; Warrener, P.; Keller, A.E.; Surewaard, B.G.J.; Dozier, E.A.; Korhonen, J.T.; et al. Neutrophil Extracellular Traps Confine Pseudomonas aeruginosa Ocular Biofilms and Restrict Brain Invasion. *Cell Host Microbe* **2019**, *25*, 526–536.e4. [CrossRef] [PubMed]

93. Jin, X.; Zhao, Y.; Zhang, F.; Wan, T.; Fan, F.; Xie, X.; Lin, Z. Neutrophil extracellular traps involvement in corneal fungal infection. *Mol. Vis.* **2016**, *22*, 944–952. [PubMed]

94. Ljubimov, A.V.; Saghizadeh, M. Progress in corneal wound healing. *Prog. Retin. Eye Res.* **2015**, *49*, 17–45. [CrossRef] [PubMed]

95. Navas, A.; Magaña-Guerrero, F.S.; Domínguez-López, A.; Chávez-García, C.; Partido, G.; Graue-Hernández, E.O.; Sánchez-García, F.J.; Garfias, Y. Anti-Inflammatory and Anti-Fibrotic Effects of

Human Amniotic Membrane Mesenchymal Stem Cells and Their Potential in Corneal Repair. *STEM CELLS Transl. Med.* **2018**, *7*, 906–917. [CrossRef] [PubMed]

96. Bertrand, P.J.; Jamilloux, Y.; Ecochard, R.; Richard-Colmant, G.; Gerfaud-Valentin, M.; Guillaud, M.; Denis, P.; Kodjikian, L.; Sève, P. Uveitis: Autoimmunity . . . and beyond. *Autoimmun. Rev.* **2019**, *18*, 102351. [CrossRef]

97. Krishna, U.; Ajanaku, D.; Denniston, A.K.; Gkika, T. Uveitis: A sight-threatening disease which can impact all systems. *Postgrad. Med. J.* **2017**, *93*, 766–773. [CrossRef]

98. Kim, J.S.; Knickelbein, J.E.; Nussenblatt, R.B.; Sen, H.N. Clinical Trials in Noninfectious Uveitis. *Int. Ophthalmol. Clin.* **2015**, *55*, 79–110. [CrossRef]

99. Tsirouki, T.; Dastiridou, A.; Symeonidis, C.; Tounakaki, O.; Brazitikou, I.; Kalogeropoulos, C.; Androudi, S. A Focus on the Epidemiology of Uveitis. *Ocul. Immunol. Inflamm.* **2018**, *26*, 2–16. [CrossRef]

100. Rothova, A.; Hajjaj, A.; de Hoog, J.; Thiadens, A.A.H.J.; Dalm, V.A.S.H. Uveitis causes according to immune status of patients. *Acta Ophthalmol.* **2019**, *97*, 53–59. [CrossRef]

101. Suttorp-Schulten, M.S.; Rothova, A. The possible impact of uveitis in blindness: A literature survey. *Br. J. Ophthalmol.* **1996**, *80*, 844–848. [CrossRef]

102. Sève, P.; Cacoub, P.; Bodaghi, B.; Trad, S.; Sellam, J.; Bellocq, D.; Bielefeld, P.; Sène, D.; Kaplanski, G.; Monnet, D.; et al. Uveitis: Diagnostic work-up. A literature review and recommendations from an expert committee. *Autoimmun. Rev.* **2017**, *16*, 1254–1264. [CrossRef] [PubMed]

103. Emmi, G.; Becatti, M.; Bettiol, A.; Hatemi, G.; Prisco, D.; Fiorillo, C. Behçet's Syndrome as a Model of Thrombo-Inflammation: The Role of Neutrophils. *Front. Immunol.* **2019**, *10*, 1085. [CrossRef] [PubMed]

104. Jennette, J.C. Overview of the 2012 Revised International Chapel Hill Consensus Conference Nomenclature of Vasculitides. *Clin. Exp. Nephrol.* **2013**, *17*, 603–606. [CrossRef] [PubMed]

105. International Team for the Revision of the International Criteria for Behçet's Disease (ITR-ICBD). The International Criteria for Behçet's Disease (ICBD): A collaborative study of 27 countries on the sensitivity and specificity of the new criteria. *J. Eur. Acad. Dermatol. Venereol.* **2014**, *28*, 338–347. [CrossRef] [PubMed]

106. Safi, R.; Kallas, R.; Bardawil, T.; Mehanna, C.J.; Abbas, O.; Hamam, R.; Uthman, I.; Kibbi, A.-G.; Nassar, D. Neutrophils contribute to vasculitis by increased release of neutrophil extracellular traps in Behçet's disease. *J. Dermatol. Sci.* **2018**, *92*, 143–150. [CrossRef] [PubMed]

107. Perazzio, S.F.; Soeiro-Pereira, P.V.; Dos Santos, V.C.; De Brito, M.V.; Salu, B.; Oliva, M.L.V.; Stevens, A.M.; De Souza, A.W.S.; Ochs, H.D.; Torgerson, T.R.; et al. Soluble CD40L is associated with increased oxidative burst and neutrophil extracellular trap release in Behçet's disease. *Arthritis Res. Ther.* **2017**, *19*, 235. [CrossRef] [PubMed]

108. Hassan, G.S.; Merhi, Y.; Mourad, W. CD40 Ligand: A neo-inflammatory molecule in vascular diseases. *Immunobiology* **2012**, *217*, 521–532. [CrossRef]

109. Congdon, N.G.; Friedman, D.S.; Lietman, T. Important Causes of Visual Impairment in the World Today. *JAMA* **2003**, *290*, 2057. [CrossRef]

110. Klein, B.E.K. Overview of Epidemiologic Studies of Diabetic Retinopathy. *Ophthalmic Epidemiol.* **2007**, *14*, 179–183. [CrossRef]

111. Rübsam, A.; Parikh, S.; Fort, P.E. Role of Inflammation in Diabetic Retinopathy. *Int. J. Mol. Sci.* **2018**, *19*, 942. [CrossRef] [PubMed]

112. Semeraro, F.; Morescalchi, F.; Cancarini, A.; Russo, A.; Rezzola, S.; Costagliola, C. Diabetic retinopathy, a vascular and inflammatory disease: Therapeutic implications. *Diabetes Metab.* Available online: https://doi.org/10.1016/j.diabet.2019.04.002 (accessed on 18 April 2019). [CrossRef] [PubMed]

113. Wang, L.; Zhou, X.; Yin, Y.; Mai, Y.; Wang, D.; Zhang, X. Hyperglycemia Induces Neutrophil Extracellular Traps Formation Through an NADPH Oxidase-Dependent Pathway in Diabetic Retinopathy. *Front. Immunol.* **2018**, *9*, 3076. [CrossRef] [PubMed]

114. Wellen, K.E.; Hotamisligil, G.S. Inflammation, stress, and diabetes. *J. Clin. Investig.* **2005**, *115*, 1111–1119. [CrossRef] [PubMed]

115. Boss, J.D.; Singh, P.K.; Pandya, H.K.; Tosi, J.; Kim, C.; Tewari, A.; Juzych, M.S.; Abrams, G.W.; Kumar, A. Assessment of Neurotrophins and Inflammatory Mediators in Vitreous of Patients With Diabetic Retinopathy. *Investig. Opthalmology Vis. Sci.* **2017**, *58*, 5594–5603. [CrossRef] [PubMed]

116. Zhou, J.; Wang, S.; Xia, X. Role of Intravitreal Inflammatory Cytokines and Angiogenic Factors in Proliferative Diabetic Retinopathy. *Curr. Eye Res.* **2012**, *37*, 416–420. [CrossRef] [PubMed]

117. Lattanzio, R.; Cicinelli, M.V.; Bandello, F.; Zarbin, M.; Zucchiatti, I. Intravitreal Steroids in Diabetic Macular Edema. *Vital Dye. Vitreoretinal Surg.* **2017**, *60*, 78–90.

118. Park, J.-H.; Kim, J.-E.; Gu, J.-Y.; Yoo, H.J.; Nam-Goong, I.S. Evaluation of Circulating Markers of Neutrophil Extracellular Trap (NET) Formation as Risk Factors for Diabetic Retinopathy in a Case-Control Association Study. *Exp. Clin. Endocrinol. Diabetes* **2016**, *124*, 557–561. [CrossRef]

119. Carestia, A.; Frechtel, G.; Cerrone, G.; Linari, M.A.; Gonzalez, C.D.; Casais, P.; Schattner, M. NETosis before and after Hyperglycemic Control in Type 2 Diabetes Mellitus Patients. *PLOS ONE* **2016**, *11*, e0168647. [CrossRef]

120. Barliya, T.; Dardik, R.; Nisgav, Y.; Dachbash, M.; Gaton, D.; Kenet, G.; Ehrlich, R.; Weinberger, D.; Livnat, T. Possible involvement of NETosis in inflammatory processes in the eye: Evidence from a small cohort of patients. *Mol. Vis.* **2017**, *23*, 922–932.

121. Kumar-Singh, R. The role of complement membrane attack complex in dry and wet AMD - From hypothesis to clinical trials. *Exp. Eye Res.* **2019**, *184*, 266–277. [CrossRef] [PubMed]

122. Klaassen, I.; Van Noorden, C.J.; Schlingemann, R.O. Molecular basis of the inner blood-retinal barrier and its breakdown in diabetic macular edema and other pathological conditions. *Prog. Retin. Eye Res.* **2013**, *34*, 19–48. [CrossRef] [PubMed]

123. Soto, I.; Krebs, M.P.; Reagan, A.M.; Howell, G.R. Vascular Inflammation Risk Factors in Retinal Disease. *Annu. Rev. Vis. Sci.* **2019**, *5*. [CrossRef] [PubMed]

124. Kliffen, M.; Van Der Schaft, T.L.; Mooy, C.M.; De Jong, P.T. Morphologic changes in age-related maculopathy. *Microsc. Res. Tech.* **1997**, *36*, 106–122. [CrossRef]

125. El-Mollayess, G.M.; Noureddine, B.N.; Bashshur, Z.F. Bevacizumab and Neovascular Age Related Macular Degeneration: Pathogenesis and Treatment. *Semin. Ophthalmol.* **2011**, *26*, 69–76. [CrossRef] [PubMed]

126. Lee, T.-H.; Avraham, H.; Lee, S.-H.; Avraham, S. Vascular Endothelial Growth Factor Modulates Neutrophil Transendothelial Migration via Up-regulation of Interleukin-8 in Human Brain Microvascular Endothelial Cells. *J. Boil. Chem.* **2002**, *277*, 10445–10451. [CrossRef] [PubMed]

127. Rezar-Dreindl, S.; Eibenberger, K.; Pollreisz, A.; Bühl, W.; Georgopoulos, M.; Krall, C.; Weigert, G.; Schmidt-Erfurth, U.; Sacu, S. The Intraocular Cytokine Profile and Therapeutic Response in Persistent Neovascular Age-Related Macular Degeneration. *Investig. Opthalmology Vis. Sci.* **2016**, *57*, 4144. [CrossRef]

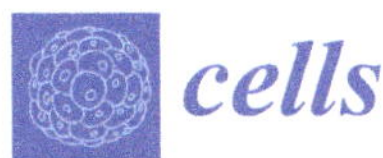 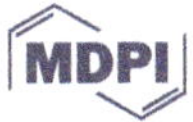

Review

Neutrophil Extracellular Traps in Periodontitis

Antonio Magán-Fernández [1], Sarmad Muayad Rasheed Al-Bakri [1], Francisco O'Valle [2,3], Cristina Benavides-Reyes [4,*], Francisco Abadía-Molina [5,6,†] and Francisco Mesa [1,†]

[1] Periodontology Department, School of Dentistry, University of Granada, 18071 Granada, Spain; amaganf@ugr.es (A.M.-F.); sarmad89@correo.ugr.es (S.M.R.A.-B.); fmesa@ugr.es (F.M.)

[2] Pathology Department, School of Medicine (IBIMER, CIBM), University of Granada, 18071 Granada, Spain; fovalle@ugr.es

[3] Biosanitary Research Institute (IBS-GRANADA), University of Granada, 18012 Granada, Spain

[4] Department of Operative Dentistry, School of Dentistry, University of Granada, 18071 Granada, Spain

[5] Department of Cell Biology, University of Granada, 18071 Granada, Spain; fmolina@ugr.es

[6] INYTA, Institute of Nutrition and Food Technology "José Mataix", University of Granada, Armilla, 18100 Granada, Spain

*   Correspondence: crisbr@ugr.es; Tel.: +34-9-5824-0654

†   These authors contributed equally to this work.

Received: 3 January 2020; Accepted: 17 June 2020; Published: 19 June 2020

Abstract: Neutrophils are key cells of the immune system and have a decisive role in fighting foreign pathogens in infectious diseases. Neutrophil extracellular traps (NETs) consist of a mesh of DNA enclosing antimicrobial peptides and histones that are released into extracellular space following neutrophil response to a wide range of stimuli, such as pathogens, host-derived mediators and drugs. Neutrophils can remain functional after NET formation and are important for periodontal homeostasis. Periodontitis is an inflammatory multifactorial disease caused by a dysbiosis state between the gingival microbiome and the immune response of the host. The pathogenesis of periodontitis includes an immune-inflammatory component in which impaired NET formation and/or elimination can be involved, contributing to an exacerbated inflammatory reaction and to the destruction of gingival tissue. In this review, we summarize the current knowledge about the role of NETs in the pathogenesis of periodontitis.

Keywords: innate immunity; periodontitis; neutrophil functions; neutrophil extracellular traps

---

1. Periodontitis

Periodontitis is a chronic inflammatory disease that affects the tooth-supporting tissues and exhibits a wide range of clinical, microbiological and immunological manifestations. It is associated with, and caused by, a multifaceted dynamic interaction among specific infectious agents, host immune responses, hazardous environmental exposure and genetic propensity [1]. The process of developing the disease starts with the accumulation of a complex bacterial biofilm. The composition of this biofilm has been estimated in approximately 700 species [2]. This biofilm creates a coat for the dental root and its structure is capable of protecting against antimicrobial substances. In healthy subjects, there is a homeostasis between the periodontium and the host response. However, when the plaque biofilm persists in a susceptible host it generates an inflammatory reaction that causes a dysbiosis, where periodontal pathogens thrive [3]. This leads to a chronic inflammatory state, which consequentially causes the destruction of the connective tissue. The process can progress to destroying surrounding support tissues—gingiva, cementum, periodontal ligament and alveolar bone—and eventually end in the loss of the affected teeth [4].

As a result of gingivitis, the bacteria penetrate the sulcus between the gum and the tooth, and then attack the gum attachment to progress deeper along the root. During this migration, toxins produced by bacteria and consequent inflammatory reactions will irreversibly destroy the attachment and the tooth-supporting tissues. This leads to the formation of periodontal pockets, which are located between the deep periodontal tissues and the tooth and are considered to be the main clinical feature of periodontitis [5].

The frequency and severity of periodontitis increases with age, with incidence peaking around the age of 60 [6]. Periodontitis is considered the main cause of tooth loss in people older than 40, having a higher prevalence than caries [7]. A high prevalence of periodontitis has been reported, with more than 47% of adults (more than 60 million) in the USA affected, and the prevalence continues to grow every year [8,9].

Periodontal inflammation is characterized by a chronic inflammatory infiltrate of varying intensity. This infiltrate is mainly composed of lymphocytes, plasma cells and macrophages distributed in patches on the lamina propria, frequently surrounding vascular structures [10]. Neutrophils are abundant in the periodontal inflammatory-immune response infiltrate and are considered a first-line cell defense mechanism against bacterial invasion [11]. However, in a susceptible host in which neutrophils do not properly contribute to the restraint of the invading bacteria, the homeostasis between the biofilm and the host response is altered, leading to an increase in tissue destruction [12,13]. Due to this immune-inflammatory component, periodontitis has been related to several systemic diseases, including rheumatoid arthritis (RA) [14]. Previous studies have indicated that neutrophils derived from patients with periodontitis are hyperactive and have an increased activity and production of reactive oxygen species (ROS) in response to a microbial invasion [15].

2. Periodontal Neutrophils

Neutrophils are the most abundant cell type of the granulocyte family (95%) and represent 50% to 70% of the blood leukocytes [11], approximately $(1–2) \times 10^{11}$ neutrophils are produced daily and released from the bone marrow into the bloodstream [16]. Peripheral blood neutrophils are eventually recruited from the bloodstream into the site of the infection. Naturally present in the oral cavity, neutrophils attach to the endothelial cells through the interaction with selectin and integrin receptors; by extravasation they abandon the bloodstream and migrate from the periodontal sulcus into the oral cavity. In case of infection, neutrophils are the first of the immune cells to arrive at the site through periodontal tissues and into gingival crevices as part of normal immune control. Although neutrophils are one of the predominant immune cells present in the oral cavity, T cells in periodontal tissue constitute the prevalent immune cell type [17]. Additionally, oral neutrophils have been found to show different chemotactic and antimicrobial functions than circulating neutrophils [18,19].

Mutations in genes affecting neutrophil differentiation and egression from the bone marrow have been related to periodontitis. Severe periodontitis has been described in patients with Severe Congenital Neutropenia due to mutations in the neutrophil elastase (NE) ELA2/ELANE or the HAX1 gene (hematopoietic cell-specific Lyn substrate) 1-associated gene X1 [20]. Patients with warts, hypogammaglobulinemia, immunodeficiency and myelokathexis (WHIM) syndrome have been reported to present with severe periodontitis [21,22]. WHIM is an autosomal dominant immunodeficiency caused by mutations in the CXCR4 chemokine receptor leading to defects in neutrophil exiting from the bone marrow.

Different neutrophil defects have been described affecting all stages of neutrophil recruitment and extravasation to periodontal tissue: tethering, rolling, adhesion and endothelial transmigration [23,24]. Most notably, leukocyte adhesion deficiency-I (LAD-I) immunodeficiency, which alters neutrophil extravasation into tissues, presents with periodontitis [25]. LAD-I results from mutation in the CD18 gene [26] preventing normal integrin dimerization and leukocyte adhesion and extravasation. Endothelial cell-derived developmental endothelial locus-1 (DEL-1) inhibits neutrophil adhesion to the endothelial cells [27] thereby restraining neutrophil transmigration; consequently, both DEL-1 upregulation and deficiency have been related to periodontitis [28].

Periodontitis is associated with reduced neutrophil chemotaxis. Dysfunctional neutrophil chemotaxis may predispose patients with periodontitis to disease by increasing tissue transit times, thereby exacerbating neutrophil-mediated collateral host tissue damage [29]. The absence of tissue neutrophils due to defective recruitment and extravasation [23] can also lead to persistent periodontal inflammation and bone loss [30,31]. Both an excessive presence or absence of neutrophils in the tissue can lead to periodontitis, indicating how important neutrophil balance is in periodontal homeostasis. A comprehensive understanding of defective neutrophil behavior in periodontitis would help in the development of new therapeutic approaches.

3. Neutrophil Extracellular Traps (NETs)

3.1. NET Formation

Neutrophils contribute to host defense at sites of tissue injury by patroling through the circulatory system [32]. The function of eliminating invading pathogens in periodontal tissues is mediated through ROS production, phagocytosis, extracellular and intracellular degranulation [11] and most recently neutrophil extracellular trap (NET) production. Brinkmann first described NETs as bactericidal traps, disarming and promoting the elimination of extracellular bacteria [33]. The formation of NETs involves the extrusion of nuclear chromatin into the extracellular space through the rupture of the nuclear and plasma membranes, and this extruded chromatin is embedded with cytoplasmic granule-derived proteins [34]. The term NETosis has been used in the past years to describe the combination of NET formation and neutrophil death [35]. However, concerns have been raised and the use of this term has been discouraged in some reports, and other terms such as "NET formation" or "NETotic cell death" have been proposed [36,37]. NETs are web-like structures of decondensed nuclear chromatin fibers combined with various antimicrobial compounds, including histones and antimicrobial peptides (AMPs) from azurophilic granules, specific granules and tertiary granules (gelatinase) released out of the neutrophil after activation. These AMPs were found to be effective not only against bacterial species but also against viruses, fungi and other microorganisms [38,39].

Many stimuli have been revealed to induce NET formation, such as viruses, fungi, parasites and host-derived components, such as cytokines and activated platelets [40]. Three main forms of NET formation have been identified. The classical form of NET formation is defined as a programmed cell death, different from necrosis and apoptosis, characterized by disruption of the nuclear membrane that lasts from two to four hours, which gives neutrophils the ability to fight pathogens beyond their lifespan. NET formation starts with the recognition of several stimuli (e.g., bacteria, fungi, viruses) through neutrophil receptors (such as toll-like receptors (TLRs), IgG-Fc receptors and cytokine receptors) [41]. Then, the mobilization of stored calcium ions from the endoplasmic reticulum would also be crucial for the process, the calcium being necessary for the citrullination of the histones and for the activation of protein-arginine deiminase 4 (PAD4) and the release of ROS [42]. The histone deamination by PAD4 is known as a major event in the decondensation of chromatin and the release of NET. ROS play an essential part in promoting the breakdown of the nuclear membrane. NE and deferoxamine are involved in the further decondensation of the nuclear chromatin phenomenon [43]. In addition, NE and myeloperoxidase are dismissed from azurophilic granules and then translocate into the nucleus. Then the nuclear chromatin is extruded into the extracellular space; suicidal NETosis can be recognized microscopically by the presence of disrupted neutrophils in the tissue (Figure 1). NET extrusion from cell death would cause damage of periodontal tissues through an autoimmune phenomenon [44]. However, in 2012, Pilsczek et al. offered another mechanism and stated that the neutrophils formed NETs during highly developed infection with *Staphylococcus aureus* (*S. aureus*), but the neutrophils are still viable, and have the normal function of vital neutrophils in terms of phagocytosis and other purposes. NET formation involves the use of vesicles that carry the chromatin without extracellular release of DNA [45]. This phenomenon is very rapid; it takes place between 5 and 60 min after stimulation and does not involve NADPH oxidase. In this second form, called vital NET formation, neutrophils create NETs but there is no breakdown of the plasma or nuclear membranes [46]. More recently, NET formation from mitochondrial DNA in viable neutrophils has been described [47]; mitochondrial DNA is released instead of nuclear DNA. Mitochondrial NET formation is not related to cell death but is dependent on ROS formation [47]. Mitochondrial NETs are identified in neutrophils within 15 min when stimulated with C5a or lipopolysaccharide (LPS). These findings are not in line with those of Brinkmann et al., who stated that NET formation leads inexorably to the death of the neutrophil [48]; moreover, it is not clear whether the mitochondrial DNA content would be enough for the amount of DNA detected in the traps [40]. The mechanisms that result in the formation of NETs through the release of mitochondrial DNA or through viable cells are still unknown. Interestingly, mitochondrial NETs may be a faster antimicrobial mechanism, which allows cells to remain viable and to prevent the extrusion of phagocytosed bacteria [49], an event that to our knowledge has not yet been studied in relation with periodontitis.

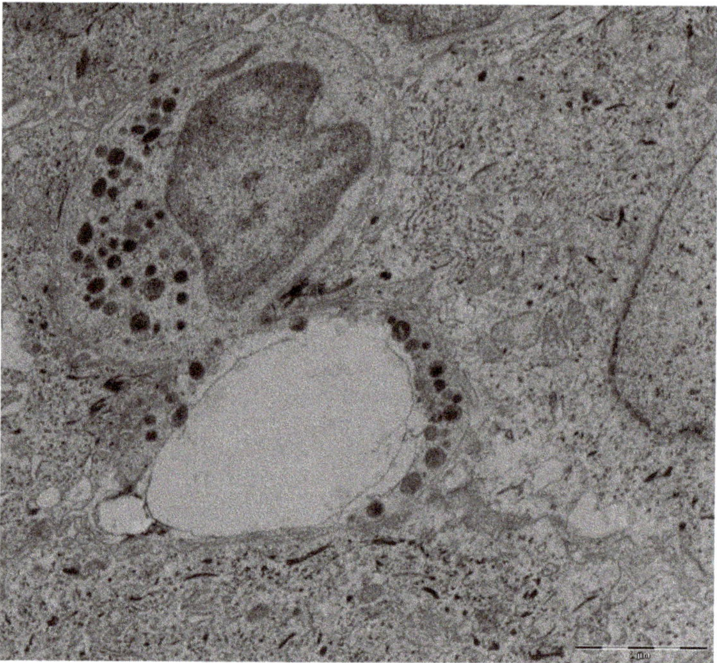

Figure 1. Transmission electron microscopy micrograph from a gingival tissue sample with periodontitis. An emptied disrupted neutrophil alongside an intact one are shown. Scale bar, 2 μm.

3.2. Microbicidal Effects of NETs

Since 2004, many studies have highlighted the ability of NETs to participate in destroying infectious agents, such as bacteria, parasites, fungi and more recently viruses. Bacteria are powerful stimuli that activate the release of NETs [50]. NETs can trap microorganisms and slow their spread from the initial site of infection, probably through the electrostatic interactions between cationic components of NETs and the anionic surface of the pathogen [48]. NETs can also inactivate the virulence factors of pathogenic microorganisms; whose function is to modify and destroy the host cells. This had already been confirmed in the first evidence on NETs, where extracellular NE as a component of NETs actively targeted bacterial virulence factors of *Shigella* spp., such as the adhesin IcsA protein and the invasion plasmid antigen B. The antimicrobial activity of NETs depends on the structure of the NETs, as it provides a high local concentration of proteins with anti-infectious activity in the direct proximity of the trapped pathogen [33]. These proteins' proteases include enzymes such as antimicrobial peptides and lysozyme. Histones, the most abundant proteins of NETs, also possess a strong ability to kill microorganisms. NETs are involved in the elimination of Gram-positive and Gram-negative bacteria. Among Gram-positive bacteria, *S. aureus* can be destroyed by a mechanism dependent on peroxidase activity of the NET's MPO [51]. NETs can also kill Gram-negative bacteria, including *Shigella flexneri*, *Escherichia coli* and *Salmonella typhimurium* [34].

3.3. Microorganisms' Strategies to Escape the Action of NETs

Identifying strategies to escape NETs in various microorganisms highlights the long coexistence of neutrophils and infectious agents in evolution, as well as the importance of this mechanism for combating infections [50]. Among these strategies, some bacteria produce DNases and other extracellular nucleases in order to destroy the DNA backbone of NETs and therefore evade this mechanism. This has been demonstrated with *S. aureus* [52] and *Streptococcus pneumonia* (*S. Pneumonia*) [53]. DNase production has been reported by a wide range of periodontal bacterial species and this expression appeared to be a trait in species that have been classically considered as periodontal pathogens, such as species from red (*Porphyromonas gingivalis* (*P. gingivalis*) and *Tannerella forsythia* (*T. forsythia*)), orange (*Fusobacterium nucleatum* (*F. nucleatum*), *Prevotella intermedia* (*P. intermedia*) and *Prevotella nigrescens* (*P. nigrescens*)) and yellow (*Streptococcus gordonii* (*S. gordonii*)) microbial complexes. As *P. gingivalis* is one of the most important periodontal pathogens, the DNase expression of six different strains was analyzed, showing all of them had different degrees of DNase activity [54]. *P. gingivalis* is a potent inducer of NET formation that is mediated by gingipains, but its proteolytical activity has shown to inactivate the bactericidal components of NETs through the activation of protease-activated receptor-2 [55]. Several mutant and wild-type strains of *P. gingivalis* have been analyzed and their results showed that mutant strains induced a characteristic NET formation [56]. *P. intermedia* has also shown a strong nuclease activity when compared with other periodontal bacterial species, suggesting that this species could have a major role in the biofilm ability to evade the action of NETs. In the same study, another major periodontal pathogen such as *Aggregatibacter actinomycetemcomitans* (*A. actinomycetemcomitans*) showed no DNase activity [57].

3.4. Removal of NETs

Many investigations about the removal of NETs have been published recently. While the investigations appreciated that the removal of NETs is essential for tissue homeostasis, the processes involved and time required in removing NETs are not well understood. In 2010, it was reported that NETs produced in vitro were stable for over 90 h. DNase 1 is one of the mechanisms responsible for NET degradation, and the presence of DNase 1 inhibitors or anti-NET antibodies that also blocked the access of the enzyme would be responsible for the removal of impaired NETs in cases of autoimmune diseases such as systemic lupus erythematosus [58]. NETs are degraded by macrophages through lysosomic action. However, the whole specific nuclease pathway involved in this process remains difficult to find. A key to this process is that the mechanism of NET removal is similar to that of apoptosis, whereby macrophages do not release pro-inflammatory cytokines [59]. Recently it has been reported that NET degradation is increased in treated periodontitis patients, what indicates that NET degradation contributes to a decreased pro-inflammatory state [60,61].

4. NETs and Periodontitis

4.1. NETs in Periodontitis Studies

In Table 1, we summarize the articles to date that have studied the role of NETs in periodontitis.

Table 1. Summary table of the studies assessing the role of neutrophil extracellular traps (NETs) in periodontitis and the induction of NET formation by periodontal bacteria.

Studies on the Expression of NETs in Periodontitis Patients					
Author	Year	Participants	Types of samples	NET marker	Results
Zhang et al. [62]	2020	27 periodontitis, 17 gingivitis and 20 controls	Peripheral blood neutrophils	IL-8 and TNF-alpha as NETs inducers	Periodontitis showed lower expression of IL-8 compared to controls
Moonen et al. A [61]	2019	1st part:38 periodontitis and 38 controls 2nd part: 91 periodontitis before and after treatment	Peripheral blood neutrophils	SYTOX Green	No differences in NET degradation between healthy subjects and periodontitis. Periodontal therapy increased NET degradation
Magán-Fernández et al. [63]	2019	6 Chronic periodontitis, 5 gingivitis and 2 controls	Gingival tissue biopsies	CitH3 and MPO	Higher H3 in gingivitis and MPO higher in periodontitis
Levy et al. [64]	2019	3 Localized aggressive periodontitis and 3 controls and HL60 neutrophils	Peripheral blood neutrophils and HL60 neutrophils incubated with nupharidine	SYTOX Green	NET formation was higher in the neutrophils exposed to Nupharidine
Kaneko et al. [65]	2018	40 Rheumatoid arthritis and periodontitis, 30 periodontitis and 43 controls	Serum samples	NET-associated MPO-DNA complexes by ELISA	NETs increased in the RA + periodontitis group. NETs were associated with moderate to severe periodontitis. Periodontal treatment reduced NETs
White et al. [60]	2016	Chronic periodontitis and controls (40 pairs)	Peripheral blood neutrophils stimulated with PMA or HOCl	SYTOX Green	NET formation decreased and NET removal was restored following periodontal treatment
Fine et al. [66]	2016	17 Chronic periodontitis and 11 controls	Blood and oral neutrophils	CitH3, MPO, CD18	Proinflammatory oral neutrophils from periodontitis showed high levels of NET formation compared to controls
Hirschfeld et al. [67]	2015	14 Experimental gingivitis and 6 controls	Supragingival plaque, peripheral blood neutrophils	CitH3, Histone H1, CD-177, MPO, NE, Cathepsin-G.	NETs were found within the oral biofilm. Bacterial isolates tested induced NET formation.
Vitkov et al. [68]	2010	26 Periodontitis	GCF (18); Purulent crevicular exudate (8)	Scanning electron microscopy (SEM); CitH3 and DNA	All neutrophils in the samples were citrullinated. 78% of them showed dispersed NETs
Vitkov et al. [69]	2009	22 Chronic Periodontitis	Purulent crevicular exudate (22); Gingival biopsies (12)	Exudates: NE and DNA; Biopsies: Transmission electron microscopy (TEM) and SEM (with and without DNase).	NETs were found on all the exudate samples. DNase caused the disappearance of NETs

Table 1. *Cont.*

In Vitro Studies on NET Formation Induced by Periodontal Bacteria					
Author	Year	Participants	Types of samples	NET marker	Results
Bryzek et al. [55]	2019	Human donors	Peripheral blood neutrophils stimulated with different *P. gingivalis* strains, antigens and gingipains	NE, Hoechst 33342, ADNbc PicoGreen® and DNase I	Gingipains from *P. gingivalis* induce NETs formation and prevent *P. gingivalis* entrapment and killing
Alyami et al. [70]	2019	In vitro PMN layers	Human primary neutrophils infected with *Aggregatibacter actinomycetemcomitans, P. gingivalis and F. nucleatum*	SYTOX Orange, NE, CitH3, DAPI	*F. nucleatum* induced rapid and robust NET formation trough NOD1 and NOD 2 receptors
Hirschfeld et al. [71]	2017	10 Healthy donors	Peripheral blood neutrophils. Stimulation with 19 periodontal bacteria	FITC NET-DNA, NE, and MPO	Certain species stimulated higher NET formation.
Doke et al. [57]	2017	Healthy donors	PMA-stimulated peripheral blood neutrophils. Nucleases from several periodontal bacteria.	SYTOX Orange, NE and DAPI	*Prevotella intermedia* demonstrated the highest NET degradation of all the Gram—periodontal bacteria
Roberts et al. [72]	2016	5 Papillon–Lefévre syndrome (PLS) patients and 5 controls	Peripheral blood neutrophils stimulated with periodontal bacteria	SYTOX Green, NE, NET-bound MPO, NET-bound CG	Neutrophils from PLS patients have a reduced capacity for NET formation and a compromised antimicrobial activity
Palmer et al. [73]	2016	Healthy donors	Peripheral blood neutrophils incubated with oral bacteria in different complement blocking conditions	NET-DNA fluorometry	Complement and IgG enhance NET formation by several periodontal bacteria
Hirschfeld et al. [74]	2016	Healthy donors	Peripheral blood neutrophils with A.a., A.a. leucotoxin	Micrococcal nuclease	The leucotoxic strain of A.a. and high concentrations of A.a. leucotoxin induced NET formation
Jayaprakash et al. [56]	2015	Healthy donors	In vitro PMA-generated NETs;	FITC-labeled *P. gingivalis*, F-actin, DNA	*P. gingivalis* strains K1A and E8 induced NET formation
Palmer et al. [54]	2012	Healthy donors	In vitro PMA-generated NETs	DNase activity of periodontal bacterial species. SYTOX Green	DNase producing species caused the degradation of NETs

Table 1. *Cont.*

Other Studies Regarding NET Formation in Oral Neutrophils				
Moonen et al. [18]	2019	9 Healthy donors	PMA-stimulated venous blood neutrophils and oral neutrophils	SYTOX Green	Oral neutrophils showed greater NET formation than circulating neutrophils in both stimulated and non-stimulated groups

With regard to previous results published by our group, we were able to characterize NETs in tissue samples with periodontitis and gingivitis using immunofluorescence, immunohistochemistry and electron microscopy analysis (Figure 2). The comparison of periodontitis and gingivitis showed that NET composition changed, and the general expression of citrullinated histone H3 was found to be higher in gingivitis. These findings suggested that the potential role of NETs in periodontitis may be associated with early and more acute phases of the inflammatory process [63].

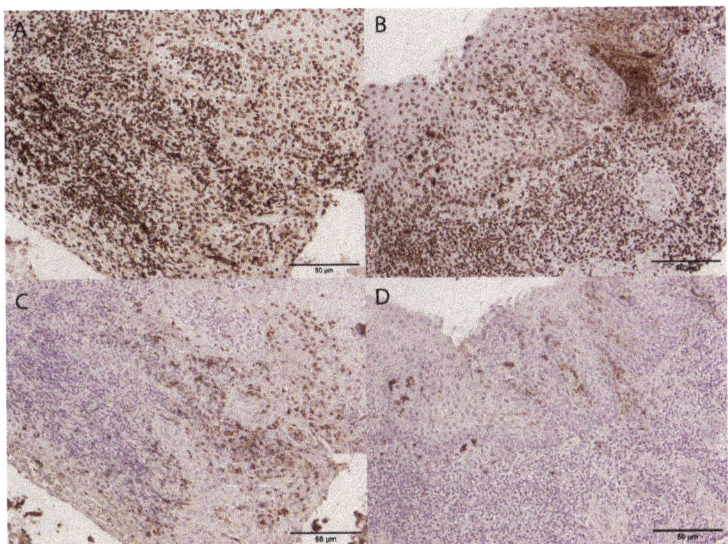

Figure 2. Micrographs from gingivitis (**A,C**) and periodontitis (**B,D**) gingival tissue samples. Immunostaining of citrullinated histone H3 (**A,B**) and MPO (**C,D**) are shown. Although citrullinated histone H3 expression did not differ between gingivitis and periodontitis (**A,B**), a higher MPO expression in gingivitis compared to periodontitis was found. This suggested that NET formation might be more associated with gingivitis. Scale bar, 50 μm.

Previous investigations (see Table 1) showed that periodontitis led to an increased formation of ROS and NETs. In addition, interferon alpha (IFN-α) was found in significant amounts in periodontitis patients. This mediator is very important for stimulating NET formation and the periodontal pocket provides ideal O_2 levels and pH for ROS formation [75]. Thus, for all the previous reasons this provides a friendly environment for ROS formation. Investigations suggest that the loss of bone and progression of disease depend on the nature of the inflammatory response of the patient and the type of pathogen.

4.2. Microbial Agents Alter NET Formation

Lipopolysaccharide is a key component of Gram-negative bacterial cell walls, where it maintains the structural integrity, stability and negative charge of the bacteria. LPS does not have the capacity to directly induce neutrophils to release NETs; however, there is a growing belief that LPS can activate platelets, which subsequently initiate NET release. It has recently been discovered that TLR4 is present on platelets, which is indicative of platelets having the capacity to recognize and respond to LPS from Gram-negative bacteria [76]. Early studies identified *P. gingivalis*, *Agregatibacter actinomycetemcomitans* and *Tannerella forsythia* as causative agents in periodontal disease and found them to be involved in NET-related processes [77]. NET formation is dependent on the activation of protease-activated receptor 2 (PAR2) by *P. gingivalis*-derived proteases. *P. gingivalis* is found in the oral cavity, where it is implicated in periodontal disease. Furthermore, a novel role has also been demonstrated for proteases as bacterial virulence factors antagonizing the antibacterial activity of NETs [55]. Additionally, the suggested generation of NETs in the periodontium leads to increased inflammation and can be considered another virulence strategy used by *P. gingivalis*. The presentation of intracellular self-antigens modified by gingipains may have immunological consequences, as the excessive presentation of cryptic antigens creates a developed part of systemic diseases associated with periodontitis [78]. Hirschfeld et al. indicated that some bacteria (*Propionibacterium acnes*, *Veillonella parvula* and *Streptococcus gordonii*) led to an enhancement of NET-derived DNA production, via NADPH oxidase-independent mechanisms [71]. It was previously mentioned in this review that NET formation depends strongly on the formation of ROS for its release. Periodontal bacteria produce DNases that reduce NET release levels, and pathogen colonization might increase in the periodontal tissue. Most aggressive pathogens release DNase, disseminating NET contents that lead to the liberation of their antimicrobial components in the surrounding tissue, resulting in a harmful effect on periodontal tissue [54].

As neutrophils are the major and first immune cell to reach the infected area, they are involved in the initial steps of the inflammatory response. Therefore, neutrophils are a determinant component of the immune response in periodontal status [15]. It is reasonable to assume that NET production or effectiveness in periodontitis may be reduced, a reduction in the effectiveness of the NET function would allow easier bacterial infiltration of periodontal tissues, leading to more inflammatory response in the infected area and resulting in tissue destruction. The digestion of NETs via DNase leads to the liberation of NET-associated antimicrobial peptides, which in turn leads to more tissue destruction [44].

4.3. Defective Neutrophils and Impaired NET Formation in Periodontitis

Previous evidence has already shown that neutrophils show hyperactivity to bacterial species found in subgingival plaque and an upregulated ROS release [15,79]. Neutrophils in healthy periodontal tissue are moved towards dental biofilms, in which they are stimulated by oral bacteria and their components to form NETs. The migrated oral neutrophil is a viable cell with a hyperactive phenotype, as evidenced by the increased adhesion and internalization of microbes and 13 times more NET formation capacity than the circulating neutrophils [18]. In 2017, Hirschfeld et al. suggested that the variability in neutrophils, such as deficiencies in the number or abnormal function of neutrophils toward various bacteria, might contribute to the pathogenesis of periodontal disease [71]. Periodontitis patients presented with over four times higher oral neutrophil counts compared to healthy periodontal tissue, which was a predictor for protease activity. More oral neutrophils were apoptotic in periodontitis patients than in healthy ones [80,81]. The neutrophil-mediated antimicrobial action fails to stop the bacteria in cases of periodontitis, leading to tissue damage and destruction of both bacterial and immune origin. NET formation is also considered a potential factor changing the influence of the individual course of periodontitis [82]. Periodontitis in Papillon–Lefèvre (PLS) syndrome arises from the failure to eliminate periodontal pathogens because of cathepsin C deficiency [83]. PLS neutrophils reduced the capacity for NET production, characterized by the absence of the NET-related proteins such as chorionic gonadotropin, MPO and NE. ROS formation was higher in PLS [72]. The failure of activities of neutrophil antimicrobial proteins might maintain the stimulus for the wrongful recruiting of highly responsive neutrophils in periodontal tissues, providing a reasonable explanation for the acute inflammation and bone loss that characterize PLS periodontitis patients [84,85]. Interestingly, individuals with PLS do not suffer any systemic infections—rarely are there any skin abscesses. Therefore, the defects of neutrophils appear to be localized in areas of the human body more susceptible to a direct and chronic bacterial challenge, such as the oral cavity [86].

This hyper-reactivity may come from the excessive NET formation in response to periodontal pathogens and/or local mediators [66]. The implication of the neutrophils and their enzymes is supported by the fact that high levels of NETs remain in the tissue for an extended period. In addition, this supports the hypothesis that NET formation is dependent on ROS formation, which has been shown to be higher in periodontitis [15]. The neutrophil function in periodontitis may be a key determinant of the patient's periodontal health status.

In addition, increased neutrophil ROS formation is associated with elevated IFNα levels in periodontitis, indicating that this class of signaling proteins is also important in NET formation [75,87]. High levels of NETs within periodontal tissue could stimulate an autoimmune response, resulting in augmented neutrophil levels and causing more tissue destruction [73]. This hypothesis of NETs' hyperactivity in periodontitis is supported by Vitkov et al. They investigated NETs in exudate samples from the gingiva of periodontitis patients and compared the results with previous examinations of abscesses. In addition, they found that the samples collected had high levels of NETs and that in seven samples 22 trapped bacteria were associated with the NETs. In addition, based on the use of electron microscopy and analysis of gingival biopsies, patients with chronic periodontitis showed the presence of NETs [69]. In a recent study from the same authors, they hypothesize that there is a dissemination phenomenon of bacterial species, LPS and antigens citrullinated by NETs from the infected periodontal tissue. This dissemination could contribute to exacerbated autoimmune diseases such as RA via the activation of TLR receptors [78]. Therefore, both mechanisms of NET formation may be responsible for tissue destruction [88]. The impaired degradation of NETs and the escape of pathogens from the effect of NETs by virulence factors leads to a response from neutrophils, upregulating the release of NETs, resulting in the immobilization and localization of neutrophils instead of trapping bacteria, which leads to tissue destruction [34] (Figure 3).

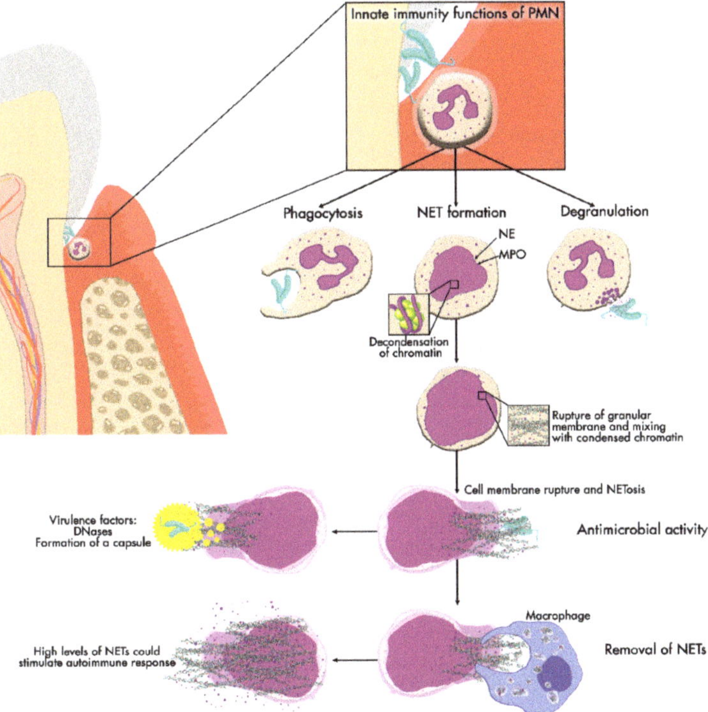

Figure 3. NET release. NET formation may be one of the main neutrophil functions in periodontal tissue. NET production starts with chromatin decondensation, which is then embedded with cytoplasmic antimicrobial peptide granules. NETs are then released into the extracellular space after cell membrane rupture to exert their antimicrobial effect and later removed from the tissue. If NET removal fails, persistent high levels of NETs could cause damage to periodontal tissues.

5. Role of NETs in Systemic Diseases

The formation of NETs could promote thrombosis via histones [61]. NETs in combination with platelets may damage the blood vessels during sepsis, destroying endothelial cells and causing vascular occlusions [76,89]. On the other hand, it has been reported that NETs might promote the implantation of metastases through the uptake of circulating malignant cells [90]. Garley et al. indicated in 2018 that the neutrophils of patients with oral inflammation with stage I/II cancer produce increased formation of NETs compared to the neutrophils of healthy humans. However, the amount of NETs in stage III/IV cancer patients was lower than the amount of NETs in inflammation and early-stage cancer patients [91].

NETs have been described as a source of auto-antigens in various autoimmune diseases, such as vasculitis, lupus, psoriasis and RA [92]. NETs exhibit proteins normally restricted to the interior of the granules, nucleus or cytoplasm. This exposure would result in immunization against self-antigens and create autoimmune disorders. For example, in anti-neutrophil cytoplasmic antibody-associated vasculitis, proteinase 3 and MPO are self-antigens targeted by auto-antibodies, and these two enzymes are associated with NETs [93]. NETs have also been shown to have adverse effects in pre-eclampsia, where placenta-derived cytokine-activated neutrophils activated NET extrusion. NETs were found in the intervillous space of placental tissue samples [94]. In atherosclerosis, dendritic cell activation by NETs is similar to that which occurs in lupus, and these dendritic cells are one of the cell populations found in atheromatous plaques [95].

The Relationship between Rheumatoid Arthritis, Periodontitis and NETs

Periodontitis and RA are considered to be two chronic inflammatory diseases with a common pathogenesis. RA is an autoimmune inflammatory disease defined by the destruction and inflammation of joints and internal organs in which citrullination is a central feature leading to the generation of auto-antibodies to citrullinated protein antigens. In periodontitis, citrullination either by NET formation or *P. gingivalis*-derived peptydil arginine deiminase activity has been suggested [96], although citrullination independent of oral bacteria has also been reported [97]. Evidence has suggested that citrullinated antigens in RA are mostly derived from NETs [98]. Patients with periodontitis may have RA and vice versa [99]. A recent publication has suggested that periodontal indices such as gingival index, probing pocket depth (PPD) and bleeding on probing (BOP) have positive relationships with RA. Anti-*P. gingivalis* antibody levels were associated with BOP, PPD and GI and the severity of periodontitis; thus, increasing the values of periodontitis indices could be a sign of advanced disease development in RA patients [100]. In addition, a high level of anti-*P. gingivalis* antibody could be regarded as a warning sign in RA patients suffering from periodontitis [101]. Non-surgical periodontal treatment has shown to improve symptoms in both diseases [102–104]. Previous studies demonstrated that NETs were increased in the synovial fluid, rheumatoid nodules, peripheral blood and skin of RA patients [92]. Increased NET formation in the oral cavity of periodontitis patients perhaps plays a part in the initiation of RA [105]. *P. gingivalis* is the most important pathogen responsible for periodontitis. Further, it was shown that *P. gingivalis* could induce NET generation [55]. Interestingly, a study has demonstrated that patients with periodontitis and RA showed significantly higher serum levels of NETs than the control group. Furthermore, a periodontal cure remarkably decreased the serum levels of NETs in patients with RA and periodontitis [65]. However, more studies are required with a greater number of cases and a longer evolution time in order to understand the relation between the two diseases.

6. Conclusions and Future Research Lines

NETs trap and/or kill a wide variety of microorganisms, bacteria, fungi and parasites through their antimicrobial agents, such as MPO, NE and proteinase. NET formation has been associated with different diseases, such as inflammatory diseases including periodontitis and autoimmune diseases such as RA. Excess formation of NETs can be harmful to periodontal tissue if they are not correctly removed; consequently, increased NET degradation has been reported following periodontal treatment. As stated by a recently published consensus document, several areas regarding the study of NETs are still controversial. Specifically, the origin of the DNA found in NETs should be identified in order to find a clear way to distinguish NET formation from other forms of programmed cell death, and to identify all the pathways that regulate NET formation, since it is very unlikely that it is mediated by a single pathway. There is also a great need for standardization of the methodologies used for the identification of NETs [37]. Finally, NETs are currently considered potential therapeutic targets. Treatment with Nupharidine, an agent purified from the plant *Nuphar lutea*, has been shown to increase NET extrusions by neutrophil-like cells by 106%. However, the authors claim that whether the increase in NET extrusion by this compound has a detrimental or protective effect on the periodontal tissues requires further in vivo research [64]. Therefore, NETs can be considered as potential therapeutic targets for periodontitis as well as for other diseases of autoimmune origin. Certainly, the role of NETs in periodontitis needs to be further studied to enable a full understanding of their role in the pathogenicity of the disease.

Funding: This research has received no external funding.

Conflicts of Interest: The authors declare no conflict of interest.

References

1. Lamont, R.J.; Koo, H.; Hajishengallis, G. The oral microbiota: Dynamic communities and host interactions. *Nat. Rev. Microbiol.* **2018**, *16*, 745–759. [CrossRef] [PubMed]
2. Darveau, R.P. Periodontitis: A polymicrobial disruption of host homeostasis. *Nat. Rev. Microbiol.* **2010**, *8*, 481–490. [CrossRef] [PubMed]
3. Nibali, L.; Henderson, B.; Sadiq, S.T.; Donos, N. Genetic dysbiosis: The role of microbial insults in chronic inflammatory diseases. *J. Oral. Microbiol.* **2014**, *6*, 22962. [CrossRef]
4. Nauseef, W.M. Proteases, neutrophils, and periodontitis: The net effect. *J. Clin. Investig.* **2014**, *124*, 4237–4239. [CrossRef] [PubMed]
5. Bascones-Martinez, A.; Munoz-Corcuera, M.; Noronha, S.; Mota, P.; Bascones-Ilundain, C.; Campo-Trapero, J. Host defence mechanisms against bacterial aggression in periodontal disease: Basic mechanisms. *Med. Oral Patol. Oral Cir. Bucal.* **2009**, *14*, e680–e685. [CrossRef]
6. Kassebaum, N.J.; Bernabe, E.; Dahiya, M.; Bhandari, B.; Murray, C.J.; Marcenes, W. Global burden of severe periodontitis in 1990–2010: A systematic review and meta-regression. *J. Dent. Res.* **2014**, *93*, 1045–1053. [CrossRef]
7. Frencken, J.E.; Sharma, P.; Stenhouse, L.; Green, D.; Laverty, D.; Dietrich, T. Global epidemiology of dental caries and severe periodontitis—A comprehensive review. *J. Clin. Periodontol.* **2017**, *44*, S94–S105. [CrossRef]
8. Marcenes, W.; Kassebaum, N.J.; Bernabe, E.; Flaxman, A.; Naghavi, M.; Lopez, A.; Murray, C.J. Global burden of oral conditions in 1990–2010: A systematic analysis. *J. Dent. Res.* **2013**, *92*, 592–597. [CrossRef]
9. Eke, P.I.; Dye, B.A.; Wei, L.; Slade, G.D.; Thornton-Evans, G.O.; Borgnakke, W.S.; Taylor, G.W.; Page, R.C.; Beck, J.D.; Genco, R.J. Update on prevalence of periodontitis in adults in the united states: Nhanes 2009 to 2012. *J. Periodontol.* **2015**, *86*, 611–622. [CrossRef] [PubMed]
10. Mesa, F.; Liebana, J.; Galindo-Moreno, P.; J. O'Valle, F. Oral pathogens, immunity, and periodontal diseases. *Curr. Immunol. Rev.* **2011**, *7*, 83–91. [CrossRef]
11. Jaillon, S.; Galdiero, M.R.; Del Prete, D.; Cassatella, M.A.; Garlanda, C.; Mantovani, A. Neutrophils in innate and adaptive immunity. *Semin. Immunopathol.* **2013**, *35*, 377–394. [CrossRef] [PubMed]
12. Scott, D.A.; Krauss, J. Neutrophils in periodontal inflammation. *Front. Oral Biol.* **2012**, *15*, 56–83. [PubMed]
13. Cortes-Vieyra, R.; Rosales, C.; Uribe-Querol, E. Neutrophil functions in periodontal homeostasis. *J. Immunol. Res.* **2016**, *2016*, 1396106. [CrossRef]
14. De Smit, M.; Westra, J.; Vissink, A.; Doornbos-van der Meer, B.; Brouwer, E.; van Winkelhoff, A.J. Periodontitis in established rheumatoid arthritis patients: A cross-sectional clinical, microbiological and serological study. *Arthritis Res. Ther.* **2012**, *14*, R222. [CrossRef] [PubMed]

15. Matthews, J.B.; Wright, H.J.; Roberts, A.; Ling-Mountford, N.; Cooper, P.R.; Chapple, I.L. Neutrophil hyper-responsiveness in periodontitis. *J. Dent. Res.* **2007**, *86*, 718–722. [CrossRef]

16. Eash, K.J.; Greenbaum, A.M.; Gopalan, P.K.; Link, D.C. Cxcr2 and cxcr4 antagonistically regulate neutrophil trafficking from murine bone marrow. *J. Clin. Investig.* **2010**, *120*, 2423–2431. [CrossRef] [PubMed]

17. Thorbert-Mros, S.; Larsson, L.; Berglundh, T. Cellular composition of long-standing gingivitis and periodontitis lesions. *J. Periodontal. Res.* **2015**, *50*, 535–543. [CrossRef]

18. Moonen, C.G.J.; Hirschfeld, J.; Cheng, L.; Chapple, I.L.C.; Loos, B.G.; Nicu, E.A. Oral neutrophils characterized: Chemotactic, phagocytic, and neutrophil extracellular trap (net) formation properties. *Front. Immunol.* **2019**, *10*, 635. [CrossRef]

19. Hirschfeld, J. Neutrophil subsets in periodontal health and disease: A mini review. *Front. Immunol.* **2019**, *10*, 3001. [CrossRef]

20. Zeidler, C.; Germeshausen, M.; Klein, C.; Welte, K. Clinical implications of ela2-, hax1-, and g-csf-receptor (csf3r) mutations in severe congenital neutropenia. *Br. J. Haematol.* **2009**, *144*, 459–467. [CrossRef]

21. Mc Guire, P.J.; Cunningham-Rundles, C.; Ochs, H.; Diaz, G.A. Oligoclonality, impaired class switch and b-cell memory responses in whim syndrome. *Clin. Immunol.* **2010**, *135*, 412–421. [CrossRef] [PubMed]

22. Hajishengallis, E.; Hajishengallis, G. Neutrophil homeostasis and periodontal health in children and adults. *J. Dent. Res.* **2014**, *93*, 231–237. [CrossRef] [PubMed]

23. Silva, L.M.; Brenchley, L.; Moutsopoulos, N.M. Primary immunodeficiencies reveal the essential role of tissue neutrophils in periodontitis. *Immunol. Rev.* **2019**, *287*, 226–235. [CrossRef] [PubMed]

24. Hajishengallis, G. New developments in neutrophil biology and periodontitis. *Periodontology 2000* **2020**, *82*, 78–92. [CrossRef]

25. Almarza Novoa, E.; Kasbekar, S.; Thrasher, A.J.; Kohn, D.B.; Sevilla, J.; Nguyen, T.; Schwartz, J.D.; Bueren, J.A. Leukocyte adhesion deficiency-i: A comprehensive review of all published cases. *J. Allergy Clin. Immunol. Pract.* **2018**, *6*, 1418–1420. [CrossRef] [PubMed]

26. Hanna, S.; Etzioni, A. Leukocyte adhesion deficiencies. *Ann. N. Y. Acad. Sci.* **2012**, *1250*, 50–55. [CrossRef] [PubMed]

27. Choi, E.Y.; Chavakis, E.; Czabanka, M.A.; Langer, H.F.; Fraemohs, L.; Economopoulou, M.; Kundu, R.K.; Orlandi, A.; Zheng, Y.Y.; Prieto, D.A.; et al. Del-1, an endogenous leukocyte-endothelial adhesion inhibitor, limits inflammatory cell recruitment. *Science* **2008**, *322*, 1101–1104. [CrossRef]

28. Kourtzelis, I.; Li, X.; Mitroulis, I.; Grosser, D.; Kajikawa, T.; Wang, B.; Grzybek, M.; von Renesse, J.; Czogalla, A.; Troullinaki, M.; et al. Del-1 promotes macrophage efferocytosis and clearance of inflammation. *Nat. Immunol.* **2019**, *20*, 40–49. [CrossRef]

29. Roberts, H.M.; Ling, M.R.; Insall, R.; Kalna, G.; Spengler, J.; Grant, M.M.; Chapple, I.L. Impaired neutrophil directional chemotactic accuracy in chronic periodontitis patients. *J. Clin. Periodontol.* **2015**, *42*, 1–11. [CrossRef] [PubMed]

30. Moutsopoulos, N.M.; Konkel, J.; Sarmadi, M.; Eskan, M.A.; Wild, T.; Dutzan, N.; Abusleme, L.; Zenobia, C.; Hosur, K.B.; Abe, T.; et al. Defective neutrophil recruitment in leukocyte adhesion deficiency type i disease causes local il-17-driven inflammatory bone loss. *Sci. Transl. Med.* **2014**, *6*, 229–240. [CrossRef]

31. Moutsopoulos, N.M.; Zerbe, C.S.; Wild, T.; Dutzan, N.; Brenchley, L.; DiPasquale, G.; Uzel, G.; Axelrod, K.C.; Lisco, A.; Notarangelo, L.D.; et al. Interleukin-12 and interleukin-23 blockade in leukocyte adhesion deficiency type 1. *N. Engl. J. Med.* **2017**, *376*, 1141–1146. [CrossRef] [PubMed]

32. Nakazawa, D.; Kumar, S.; Desai, J.; Anders, H.J. Neutrophil extracellular traps in tissue pathology. *Histol. Histopathol.* **2017**, *32*, 203–213. [PubMed]

33. Brinkmann, V.; Reichard, U.; Goosmann, C.; Fauler, B.; Uhlemann, Y.; Weiss, D.S.; Weinrauch, Y.; Zychlinsky, A. Neutrophil extracellular traps kill bacteria. *Science* **2004**, *303*, 1532–1535. [CrossRef] [PubMed]

34. Delgado-Rizo, V.; Martinez-Guzman, M.A.; Iniguez-Gutierrez, L.; Garcia-Orozco, A.; Alvarado-Navarro, A.; Fafutis-Morris, M. Neutrophil extracellular traps and its implications in inflammation: An overview. *Front. Immunol.* **2017**, *8*, 81. [CrossRef] [PubMed]

35. Desai, J.; Kumar, S.V.; Mulay, S.R.; Konrad, L.; Romoli, S.; Schauer, C.; Herrmann, M.; Bilyy, R.; Muller, S.; Popper, B.; et al. Pma and crystal-induced neutrophil extracellular trap formation involves ripk1-ripk3-mlkl signaling. *Eur. J. Immunol.* **2016**, *46*, 223–229. [CrossRef]

36. Galluzzi, L.; Vitale, I.; Aaronson, S.A.; Abrams, J.M.; Adam, D.; Agostinis, P.; Alnemri, E.S.; Altucci, L.; Amelio, I.; Andrews, D.W.; et al. Molecular mechanisms of cell death: Recommendations of the nomenclature committee on cell death 2018. *Cell Death Differ.* **2018**, *25*, 486–541. [CrossRef]

37. Boeltz, S.; Amini, P.; Anders, H.J.; Andrade, F.; Bilyy, R.; Chatfield, S.; Cichon, I.; Clancy, D.M.; Desai, J.; Dumych, T.; et al. To net or not to net:Current opinions and state of the science regarding the formation of neutrophil extracellular traps. *Cell Death Differ.* **2019**, *26*, 395–408. [CrossRef]

38. Sierra, J.M.; Fuste, E.; Rabanal, F.; Vinuesa, T.; Vinas, M. An overview of antimicrobial peptides and the latest advances in their development. *Expert Opin. Biol. Ther.* **2017**, *17*, 663–676. [CrossRef]

39. Kang, H.K.; Kim, C.; Seo, C.H.; Park, Y. The therapeutic applications of antimicrobial peptides (amps): A patent review. *J. Microbiol.* **2017**, *55*, 1–12. [CrossRef]

40. Brinkmann, V. Neutrophil extracellular traps in the second decade. *J. Innate Immun.* **2018**, *10*, 414–421. [CrossRef]

41. Fuchs, T.A.; Abed, U.; Goosmann, C.; Hurwitz, R.; Schulze, I.; Wahn, V.; Weinrauch, Y.; Brinkmann, V.; Zychlinsky, A. Novel cell death program leads to neutrophil extracellular traps. *J. Cell Biol.* **2007**, *176*, 231–241. [CrossRef]

42. Gupta, A.K.; Giaglis, S.; Hasler, P.; Hahn, S. Efficient neutrophil extracellular trap induction requires mobilization of both intracellular and extracellular calcium pools and is modulated by cyclosporine a. *PLoS ONE* **2014**, *9*, e97088. [CrossRef] [PubMed]

43. Papayannopoulos, V.; Metzler, K.D.; Hakkim, A.; Zychlinsky, A. Neutrophil elastase and myeloperoxidase regulate the formation of neutrophil extracellular traps. *J. Cell Biol.* **2010**, *191*, 677–691. [CrossRef] [PubMed]

44. Cooper, P.R.; Palmer, L.J.; Chapple, I.L. Neutrophil extracellular traps as a new paradigm in innate immunity: Friend or foe? *Periodontology 2000* **2013**, *63*, 165–197. [CrossRef]

45. Pilsczek, F.H.; Salina, D.; Poon, K.K.; Fahey, C.; Yipp, B.G.; Sibley, C.D.; Robbins, S.M.; Green, F.H.; Surette, M.G.; Sugai, M.; et al. A novel mechanism of rapid nuclear neutrophil extracellular trap formation in response to staphylococcus aureus. *J. Immunol.* **2010**, *185*, 7413–7425. [CrossRef] [PubMed]

46. Li, P.; Li, M.; Lindberg, M.R.; Kennett, M.J.; Xiong, N.; Wang, Y. Pad4 is essential for antibacterial innate immunity mediated by neutrophil extracellular traps. *J. Exp. Med.* **2010**, *207*, 1853–1862. [CrossRef]

47. Yousefi, S.; Mihalache, C.; Kozlowski, E.; Schmid, I.; Simon, H.U. Viable neutrophils release mitochondrial DNA to form neutrophil extracellular traps. *Cell Death Differ.* **2009**, *16*, 1438–1444. [CrossRef]

48. Brinkmann, V.; Zychlinsky, A. Beneficial suicide: Why neutrophils die to make nets. *Nat. Rev. Microbiol.* **2007**, *5*, 577–582. [CrossRef]

49. Jorch, S.K.; Kubes, P. An emerging role for neutrophil extracellular traps in noninfectious disease. *Nat. Med.* **2017**, *23*, 279–287. [CrossRef]

50. Arazna, M.; Pruchniak, M.P.; Demkow, U. Neutrophil extracellular traps in bacterial infections: Strategies for escaping from killing. *Respir. Physiol. Neurobiol.* **2013**, *187*, 74–77. [CrossRef] [PubMed]

51. Parker, H.; Albrett, A.M.; Kettle, A.J.; Winterbourn, C.C. Myeloperoxidase associated with neutrophil extracellular traps is active and mediates bacterial killing in the presence of hydrogen peroxide. *J. Leukoc. Biol.* **2012**, *91*, 369–376. [CrossRef]

52. Berends, E.T.; Horswill, A.R.; Haste, N.M.; Monestier, M.; Nizet, V.; von Kockritz-Blickwede, M. Nuclease expression by staphylococcus aureus facilitates escape from neutrophil extracellular traps. *J. Innate Immun.* **2010**, *2*, 576–586. [CrossRef] [PubMed]

53. Beiter, K.; Wartha, F.; Albiger, B.; Normark, S.; Zychlinsky, A.; Henriques-Normark, B. An endonuclease allows streptococcus pneumoniae to escape from neutrophil extracellular traps. *Curr. Biol.* **2006**, *16*, 401–407. [CrossRef] [PubMed]

54. Palmer, L.J.; Chapple, I.L.; Wright, H.J.; Roberts, A.; Cooper, P.R. Extracellular deoxyribonuclease production by periodontal bacteria. *J. Periodontal. Res.* **2012**, *47*, 439–445. [CrossRef]

55. Bryzek, D.; Ciaston, I.; Dobosz, E.; Gasiorek, A.; Makarska, A.; Sarna, M.; Eick, S.; Puklo, M.; Lech, M.; Potempa, B.; et al. Triggering netosis via protease-activated receptor (par)-2 signaling as a mechanism of hijacking neutrophils function for pathogen benefits. *PLoS Pathog.* **2019**, *15*, e1007773. [CrossRef]

56. Jayaprakash, K.; Demirel, I.; Khalaf, H.; Bengtsson, T. The role of phagocytosis, oxidative burst and neutrophil extracellular traps in the interaction between neutrophils and the periodontal pathogen porphyromonas gingivalis. *Mol. Oral Microbiol.* **2015**, *30*, 361–375. [CrossRef]

57. Doke, M.; Fukamachi, H.; Morisaki, H.; Arimoto, T.; Kataoka, H.; Kuwata, H. Nucleases from prevotella intermedia can degrade neutrophil extracellular traps. *Mol. Oral Microbiol.* **2017**, *32*, 288–300. [CrossRef] [PubMed]

58. Hakkim, A.; Furnrohr, B.G.; Amann, K.; Laube, B.; Abed, U.A.; Brinkmann, V.; Herrmann, M.; Voll, R.E.; Zychlinsky, A. Impairment of neutrophil extracellular trap degradation is associated with lupus nephritis. *Proc. Natl. Acad. Sci. USA* **2010**, *107*, 9813–9818. [CrossRef] [PubMed]

59. Farrera, C.; Fadeel, B. Macrophage clearance of neutrophil extracellular traps is a silent process. *J. Immunol.* **2013**, *191*, 2647–2656. [CrossRef] [PubMed]

60. White, P.; Sakellari, D.; Roberts, H.; Risafi, I.; Ling, M.; Cooper, P.; Milward, M.; Chapple, I. Peripheral blood neutrophil extracellular trap production and degradation in chronic periodontitis. *J. Clin. Periodontol.* **2016**, *43*, 1041–1049. [CrossRef]

61. Moonen, C.G.; Buurma, K.G.; Faruque, M.R.; Balta, M.G.; Liefferink, E.; Bizzarro, S.; Nicu, E.A.; Loos, B.G. Periodontal therapy increases neutrophil extracellular trap degradation. *Innate Immun.* **2019**. [CrossRef] [PubMed]

62. Zhang, F.; Yang, X.M.; Jia, S.Y. Characteristics of neutrophil extracellular traps in patients with periodontitis and gingivitis. *Braz. Oral Res.* **2020**, *34*, e015. [CrossRef] [PubMed]

63. Magan-Fernandez, A.; O'Valle, F.; Abadia-Molina, F.; Munoz, R.; Puga-Guil, P.; Mesa, F. Characterization and comparison of neutrophil extracellular traps in gingival samples of periodontitis and gingivitis: A pilot study. *J. Periodontal Res.* **2019**, *54*, 218–224. [CrossRef] [PubMed]

64. Levy, D.H.; Chapple, I.L.C.; Shapira, L.; Golan-Goldhirsh, A.; Gopas, J.; Polak, D. Nupharidine enhances aggregatibacter actinomycetemcomitans clearance by priming neutrophils and augmenting their effector functions. *J. Clin. Periodontol.* **2019**, *46*, 62–71. [CrossRef]

65. Kaneko, C.; Kobayashi, T.; Ito, S.; Sugita, N.; Murasawa, A.; Nakazono, K.; Yoshie, H. Circulating levels of carbamylated protein and neutrophil extracellular traps are associated with periodontitis severity in patients with rheumatoid arthritis: A pilot case-control study. *PLoS ONE* **2018**, *13*, e0192365. [CrossRef]

66. Fine, N.; Hassanpour, S.; Borenstein, A.; Sima, C.; Oveisi, M.; Scholey, J.; Cherney, D.; Glogauer, M. Distinct oral neutrophil subsets define health and periodontal disease states. *J. Dent. Res.* **2016**, *95*, 931–938. [CrossRef]

67. Hirschfeld, J.; Dommisch, H.; Skora, P.; Horvath, G.; Latz, E.; Hoerauf, A.; Waller, T.; Kawai, T.; Jepsen, S.; Deschner, J.; et al. Neutrophil extracellular trap formation in supragingival biofilms. *Int. J. Med. Microbiol.* **2015**, *305*, 453–463. [CrossRef]

68. Vitkov, L.; Klappacher, M.; Hannig, M.; Krautgartner, W.D. Neutrophil fate in gingival crevicular fluid. *Ultrastruct. Pathol.* **2010**, *34*, 25–30. [CrossRef]

69. Vitkov, L.; Klappacher, M.; Hannig, M.; Krautgartner, W.D. Extracellular neutrophil traps in periodontitis. *J. Periodontal. Res.* **2009**, *44*, 664–672. [CrossRef]

70. Alyami, H.M.; Finoti, L.S.; Teixeira, H.S.; Aljefri, A.; Kinane, D.F.; Benakanakere, M.R. Role of nod1/nod2 receptors in fusobacterium nucleatum mediated netosis. *Microb. Pathog.* **2019**, *131*, 53–64. [CrossRef]

71. Hirschfeld, J.; White, P.C.; Milward, M.R.; Cooper, P.R.; Chapple, I.L.C. Modulation of neutrophil extracellular trap and reactive oxygen species release by periodontal bacteria. *Infect. Immun.* **2017**, *85*. [CrossRef] [PubMed]

72. Roberts, H.; White, P.; Dias, I.; McKaig, S.; Veeramachaneni, R.; Thakker, N.; Grant, M.; Chapple, I. Characterization of neutrophil function in papillon-lefevre syndrome. *J. Leukoc. Biol.* **2016**, *100*, 433–444. [CrossRef] [PubMed]

73. Palmer, L.J.; Damgaard, C.; Holmstrup, P.; Nielsen, C.H. Influence of complement on neutrophil extracellular trap release induced by bacteria. *J. Periodontal Res.* **2016**, *51*, 70–76. [CrossRef]

74. Hirschfeld, J.; Roberts, H.M.; Chapple, I.L.; Parcina, M.; Jepsen, S.; Johansson, A.; Claesson, R. Effects of aggregatibacter actinomycetemcomitans leukotoxin on neutrophil migration and extracellular trap formation. *J. Oral Microbiol.* **2016**, *8*, 33070. [CrossRef]

75. Wright, H.J.; Matthews, J.B.; Chapple, I.L.; Ling-Mountford, N.; Cooper, P.R. Periodontitis associates with a type 1 ifn signature in peripheral blood neutrophils. *J. Immunol.* **2008**, *181*, 5775–5784. [CrossRef]

76. Clark, S.R.; Ma, A.C.; Tavener, S.A.; McDonald, B.; Goodarzi, Z.; Kelly, M.M.; Patel, K.D.; Chakrabarti, S.; McAvoy, E.; Sinclair, G.D.; et al. Platelet tlr4 activates neutrophil extracellular traps to ensnare bacteria in septic blood. *Nat. Med.* **2007**, *13*, 463–469. [CrossRef]

77. White, P.; Cooper, P.; Milward, M.; Chapple, I. Differential activation of neutrophil extracellular traps by specific periodontal bacteria. *Free Radic. Biol. Med.* **2014**, *75*, S53. [CrossRef] [PubMed]

78. Vitkov, L.; Hannig, M.; Minnich, B.; Herrmann, M. Periodontal sources of citrullinated antigens and tlr agonists related to ra. *Autoimmunity* **2018**, *51*, 304–309. [CrossRef] [PubMed]

79. Matthews, J.B.; Wright, H.J.; Roberts, A.; Cooper, P.R.; Chapple, I.L. Hyperactivity and reactivity of peripheral blood neutrophils in chronic periodontitis. *Clin. Exp. Immunol.* **2007**, *147*, 255–264. [CrossRef]

80. Nicu, E.A.; Rijkschroeff, P.; Wartewig, E.; Nazmi, K.; Loos, B.G. Characterization of oral polymorphonuclear neutrophils in periodontitis patients: A case-control study. *BMC Oral Health* **2018**, *18*, 149. [CrossRef]

81. Borenstein, A.; Fine, N.; Hassanpour, S.; Sun, C.; Oveisi, M.; Tenenbaum, H.C.; Glogauer, M. Morphological characterization of para- and proinflammatory neutrophil phenotypes using transmission electron microscopy. *J. Periodontal Res.* **2018**, *53*, 972–982. [CrossRef]

82. Cekici, A.; Kantarci, A.; Hasturk, H.; Van Dyke, T.E. Inflammatory and immune pathways in the pathogenesis of periodontal disease. *Periodontology 2000* **2014**, *64*, 57–80. [CrossRef] [PubMed]

83. Bullon, P.; Castejon-Vega, B.; Roman-Malo, L.; Jimenez-Guerrero, M.P.; Cotan, D.; Forbes-Hernandez, T.Y.; Varela-Lopez, A.; Perez-Pulido, A.J.; Giampieri, F.; Quiles, J.L.; et al. Autophagic dysfunction in patients with papillon-lefevre syndrome is restored by recombinant cathepsin c treatment. *J. Allergy Clin. Immunol.* **2018**, *142*, 1131–1143. [CrossRef] [PubMed]

84. Jepsen, S.; Caton, J.G.; Albandar, J.M.; Bissada, N.F.; Bouchard, P.; Cortellini, P.; Demirel, K.; de Sanctis, M.; Ercoli, C.; Fan, J.; et al. Periodontal manifestations of systemic diseases and developmental and acquired conditions: Consensus report of workgroup 3 of the 2017 world workshop on the classification of periodontal and peri-implant diseases and conditions. *J. Periodontol.* **2018**, *89*, S237–S248. [CrossRef]

85. Hahn, J.; Schauer, C.; Czegley, C.; Kling, L.; Petru, L.; Schmid, B.; Weidner, D.; Reinwald, C.; Biermann, M.H.C.; Blunder, S.; et al. Aggregated neutrophil extracellular traps resolve inflammation by proteolysis of cytokines and chemokines and protection from antiproteases. *FASEB J.* **2019**, *33*, 1401–1414. [CrossRef]

86. Byrd, A.S.; O'Brien, X.M.; Johnson, C.M.; Lavigne, L.M.; Reichner, J.S. An extracellular matrix-based mechanism of rapid neutrophil extracellular trap formation in response to candida albicans. *J. Immunol.* **2013**, *190*, 4136–4148. [CrossRef] [PubMed]

87. Martinelli, S.; Urosevic, M.; Daryadel, A.; Oberholzer, P.A.; Baumann, C.; Fey, M.F.; Dummer, R.; Simon, H.U.; Yousefi, S. Induction of genes mediating interferon-dependent extracellular trap formation during neutrophil differentiation. *J. Biol. Chem.* **2004**, *279*, 44123–44132. [CrossRef]

88. Kaplan, M.J.; Radic, M. Neutrophil extracellular traps: Double-edged swords of innate immunity. *J. Immunol.* **2012**, *189*, 2689–2695. [CrossRef]

89. McDonald, B.; Davis, R.P.; Kim, S.J.; Tse, M.; Esmon, C.T.; Kolaczkowska, E.; Jenne, C.N. Platelets and neutrophil extracellular traps collaborate to promote intravascular coagulation during sepsis in mice. *Blood* **2017**, *129*, 1357–1367. [CrossRef]

90. Cools-Lartigue, J.; Spicer, J.; McDonald, B.; Gowing, S.; Chow, S.; Giannias, B.; Bourdeau, F.; Kubes, P.; Ferri, L. Neutrophil extracellular traps sequester circulating tumor cells and promote metastasis. *J. Clin. Investig.* **2013**, *123*, 3446–3458. [CrossRef]

91. Garley, M.; Dziemianczyk-Pakiela, D.; Grubczak, K.; Surazynski, A.; Dabrowska, D.; Ratajczak-Wrona, W.; Sawicka-Powierza, J.; Borys, J.; Moniuszko, M.; Palka, J.A.; et al. Differences and similarities in the phenomenon of nets formation in oral inflammation and in oral squamous cell carcinoma. *J. Cancer* **2018**, *9*, 1958–1965. [CrossRef] [PubMed]

92. Khandpur, R.; Carmona-Rivera, C.; Vivekanandan-Giri, A.; Gizinski, A.; Yalavarthi, S.; Knight, J.S.; Friday, S.; Li, S.; Patel, R.M.; Subramanian, V.; et al. Nets are a source of citrullinated autoantigens and stimulate inflammatory responses in rheumatoid arthritis. *Sci. Transl. Med.* **2013**, *5*, 178ra140. [CrossRef]

93. Panda, R.; Krieger, T.; Hopf, L.; Renne, T.; Haag, F.; Rober, N.; Conrad, K.; Csernok, E.; Fuchs, T.A. Neutrophil extracellular traps contain selected antigens of anti-neutrophil cytoplasmic antibodies. *Front. Immunol.* **2017**, *8*, 439. [CrossRef]

94. Gupta, A.; Hasler, P.; Gebhardt, S.; Holzgreve, W.; Hahn, S. Occurrence of neutrophil extracellular DNA traps (nets) in pre-eclampsia: A link with elevated levels of cell-free DNA? *Ann. NY Acad. Sci.* **2006**, *1075*, 118–122. [CrossRef] [PubMed]

95. Drechsler, M.; Doring, Y.; Megens, R.T.; Soehnlein, O. Neutrophilic granulocytes—Promiscuous accelerators of atherosclerosis. *Thromb. Haemost.* **2011**, *106*, 839–848. [PubMed]

96. Olsen, I.; Singhrao, S.K.; Potempa, J. Citrullination as a plausible link to periodontitis, rheumatoid arthritis, atherosclerosis and alzheimer's disease. *J. Oral Microbiol.* **2018**, *10*, 1487742. [CrossRef] [PubMed]

97. Engstrom, M.; Eriksson, K.; Lee, L.; Hermansson, M.; Johansson, A.; Nicholas, A.P.; Gerasimcik, N.; Lundberg, K.; Klareskog, L.; Catrina, A.I.; et al. Increased citrullination and expression of peptidylarginine deiminases independently of p. Gingivalis and a. Actinomycetemcomitans in gingival tissue of patients with periodontitis. *J. Trans. Med.* **2018**, *16*, 214. [CrossRef]

98. Corsiero, E.; Pratesi, F.; Prediletto, E.; Bombardieri, M.; Migliorini, P. Netosis as source of autoantigens in rheumatoid arthritis. *Front. Immunol.* **2016**, *7*, 485. [CrossRef]

99. Zhao, X.; Liu, Z.; Shu, D.; Xiong, Y.; He, M.; Xu, S.; Si, S.; Guo, B. Association of periodontitis with rheumatoid arthritis and the effect of non-surgical periodontal treatment on disease activity in patients with rheumatoid arthritis. *Med. Sci. Monit. Int. Med. J. Exp. Clin. Res.* **2018**, *24*, 5802–5810. [CrossRef]

100. Kim, J.H.; Choi, I.A.; Lee, J.Y.; Kim, K.H.; Kim, S.; Koo, K.T.; Kim, T.I.; Seol, Y.J.; Ku, Y.; Rhyu, I.C.; et al. Periodontal pathogens and the association between periodontitis and rheumatoid arthritis in korean adults. *J. Periodontal Implant. Sci.* **2018**, *48*, 347–359. [CrossRef]

101. Lee, J.Y.; Choi, I.A.; Kim, J.H.; Kim, K.H.; Lee, E.Y.; Lee, E.B.; Lee, Y.M.; Song, Y.W. Association between anti-porphyromonas gingivalis or anti-alpha-enolase antibody and severity of periodontitis or rheumatoid arthritis (ra) disease activity in ra. *BMC Musculoskelet. Disord.* **2015**, *16*, 190. [CrossRef] [PubMed]

102. Bizzarro, S.; Van der Velden, U.; Loos, B.G. Local disinfection with sodium hypochlorite as adjunct to basic periodontal therapy: A randomized controlled trial. *J. Clin. Periodontol.* **2016**, *43*, 778–788. [CrossRef] [PubMed]

103. Bizzarro, S.; van der Velden, U.; Teeuw, W.J.; Gerdes, V.E.A.; Loos, B.G. Effect of periodontal therapy with systemic antimicrobials on parameters of metabolic syndrome: A randomized clinical trial. *J. Clin. Periodontol.* **2017**, *44*, 833–841. [CrossRef] [PubMed]

104. Bialowas, K.; Radwan-Oczko, M.; Dus-Ilnicka, I.; Korman, L.; Swierkot, J. Periodontal disease and influence of periodontal treatment on disease activity in patients with rheumatoid arthritis and spondyloarthritis. *Rheumatol. Int.* **2020**, *40*, 455–463. [CrossRef]

105. He, Y.; Yang, F.Y.; Sun, E.W. Neutrophil extracellular traps in autoimmune diseases. *Chin. Med. J. Engl.* **2018**, *131*, 1513–1519. [CrossRef]

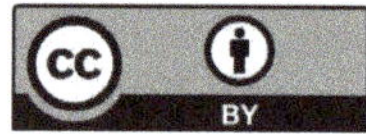

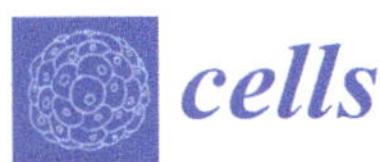 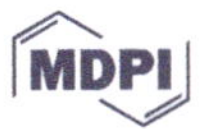

Article

Farnesol, a Quorum-Sensing Molecule of *Candida albicans* Triggers the Release of Neutrophil Extracellular Traps

Marcin Zawrotniak, Karolina Wojtalik and Maria Rapala-Kozik *

Department of Comparative Biochemistry and Bioanalytics, Faculty of Biochemistry, Biophysics and Biotechnology, Jagiellonian University in Krakow, 7 Gronostajowa st., 30387 Krakow, Poland; marcin.zawrotniak@uj.edu.pl (M.Z.); karolinawojtalik13@gmail.com (K.W.)
* Correspondence: maria.rapala-kozik@uj.edu.pl; Tel.: +48-1266-46526

Received: 30 October 2019; Accepted: 9 December 2019; Published: 11 December 2019

Abstract: The efficient growth of pathogenic bacteria and fungi in the host organism is possible due to the formation of microbial biofilms that cover the host tissues. Biofilms provide optimal local environmental conditions for fungal cell growth and increased their protection against the immune system. A common biofilm-forming fungus—*Candida albicans*—uses the quorum sensing (QS) mechanism in the cell-to-cell communication, which determines the biofilm development and, in consequence, host colonization. In the presented work, we focused on the ability of neutrophils—the main cells of the host's immune system to recognize quorum sensing molecules (QSMs) produced by *C. albicans*, especially farnesol (FOH), farnesoic acid (FA), and tyrosol (TR), with emphasis on the neutrophil extracellular traps (NETs) formation in a process called netosis. Our results showed for the first time that only farnesol but not farnesolic acid or tyrosol is capable of activating the NET production. By using selective inhibitors of the NET signaling pathway and analyzing the activity of selected enzymes such as Protein Kinase C (PKC), ERK1/2, and NADPH oxidase, we showed that the Mac−1 and TLR2 receptors are responsible for FOH recognizing and activating the reactive oxygen species (ROS)-dependent netosis pathway.

Keywords: neutrophil extracellular traps; NETs; *Candida albicans*; quorum sensing; farnesol

1. Introduction

Pathogenic microorganisms such as bacteria and fungi are able to successfully attack and colonize the host organism only while living in colonies. Colonies ensure the maintenance of appropriate local environmental conditions, increase local concentrations of many released compounds, such as proteolytic enzymes, and enhance the resistance to the host immune cells [1]. The development of infection is associated with the creation of biofilms - microbial assemblies that cover significant areas of host tissue. A critical factor for the optimal existence of microorganisms within biofilms is proper communication between pathogenic cells. It ensures synchronization of morphological changes, growth, gene expression and secretion of many compounds. The cell-to-cell communication system, called quorum sensing (QS) involves numerous quorum sensing molecules (QSMs), whose presence and concentration in the biofilm regulate biofilm functioning [2]. The first fungal microorganism in which the QSM mechanisms were identified was *Candida albicans*—an opportunistic yeast-like pathogen that resides on the skin and mucous membranes, which, due to a wide range of virulence factors, is responsible for the development of serious and hardly curable infections—candidiases [3–6]. In the properly functioning *C. albicans* QS, the autoregulatory QSMs are involved, including the best known farnesol (FOH) [3], farnesoic acid (FA) [7], and tyrosol (TR) [8,9]. In addition, *C. albicans* secretes phenylethanol and tryptophol, however, whether these two aromatic alcohols can act as QSMs in this fungus still remains to be established [5]. FOH is a sesquiterpene alcohol made up of three isoprene units that is secreted by *C. albicans* into the extracellular space, reaching a concentration of over 50 µM, but the local QSM concentrations may be significantly higher [10,11]. *C. albicans* ATCC 10,231 strain was reported to secrete FA instead of FOH [12]. The presence of QSMs regulates the expression of many genes, including those responsible for the production of yeast virulence factors [13,14]. FOH was shown to work in an autoregulatory fashion, inhibiting the transition of *C. albicans* from the yeast-like to filamentous forms [3], thus blocking the formation of biofilm [15,16]. Its action is contrary to the second QSM-TR, a tyrosine-related alcohol that stimulates hypha production during the early stages of biofilm development [8]. FOH also affects the expression of genes responsible for the protection of *Candida* spp. against oxidative stress [17,18]. Moreover, FOH is used by fungi in the coexistence with *Pseudomonas aeruginosa* where this QSM down-regulates quinolone production by bacteria, thus enabling the coexistence of these two species [19]. Upon contact with the host, FOH presents immunomodulatory properties [20], affecting the efficiency of macrophages by decreasing their phagocytic activity [21], with the stimulation of the inflammatory cytokine expression [22]. FOH is also involved in blocking of monocyte differentiation into immature dendritic cells (DCs) and modulation of the DC's ability to induce T cell proliferation and activation of neutrophils [23].

Neutrophils (PMNs) can identify *C. albicans* and respond very quickly to the appearance of fungal cells by phagocytosis or the release of structures called neutrophil extracellular traps (NETs) [24,25]. However, the mechanism used by neutrophils to select between these two processes is still unknown. NETs are built of DNA backbone decorated with granular proteins like elastase, cathepsin G, proteinase 3 and myeloperoxidase (MPO), responsible for effective killing of pathogens. The process of NET release is also a mechanism of cell death, which results in the rupture of the cell membrane and the release of cellular content into the extracellular space [26]. In contrast, phagocytosis uses membrane tubulovesicular extensions (cytonemes) to capture pathogens without the neutrophil's death [27]. These components of NETs allow to defend against the hyphal form of *C. albicans* cells, which due to their size, cannot be effectively phagocyted [28]. *C. albicans* cells are trapped within the NET structures and then killed by granular enzymes and reactive oxygen species [26,29]. Many studies have indicated that some of *C. albicans'* virulence factors can activate NET release, the process named netosis [28–30]. Among them are glucans and mannans—the components of the fungal cell wall, as well as secreted aspartyl proteases (Saps), all of which can stimulate the netosis. However, the studies showing that the number of NETs significantly increases upon contact with the filamentous form of the pathogen, indicated that the morphology of fungal cells and, consequently, their size can determine the type of neutrophil response [28,30].

Although the influence of FOH on neutrophils has been demonstrated [23] there is no information about the possible netosis activation by QSMs, especially QSMs released by *C. albicans*. Therefore, the aim of this study was to determine the potential of FOH, FA, and TR to trigger NET release and to find the netosis signaling pathway activated by QSMs, as well as to verify their chemotactic properties.

2. Materials and Methods

2.1. Isolation of Neutrophils

Human neutrophils were isolated from EDTA-treated whole blood delivered by the Regional Blood Donation Center, Kraków, Poland, obtained from healthy donors. The neutrophil-containing fraction was isolated by Pancoll gradient separation [30]. The fraction containing neutrophils and erythrocytes was mixed with a solution of polyvinyl alcohol (1%) and incubated for 20 min at room temperature. The upper layer was collected and centrifuged. Erythrocytes were removed by lysis in a hypotonic solution. Cells were washed and resuspended in phosphate buffered saline (PBS). The neutrophil purity was typically >95%, as assessed by forward-scatter and side-scatter flow cytometric analyses.

2.2. Viability Assay

2.2.1. Caspase 3/7 Activity

The cell apoptosis was analyzed by measuring the activity of proapoptotic caspases 3/7. Neutrophils (2×10^5 cells/well), suspended in solutions of FOH (trans,trans–3,7, 11-Trimethyl–2,6,10-dodecatrien–1-ol; Sigma-Aldrich, St. Louis, MO, USA), FA (Echelon Biosciences Inc, Salt Lake City, UT, USA) or TR (Sigma-Aldrich, St. Louis, MO, USA) at variable concentrations, were placed in the wells of a 96-well white microplate and incubated for 1 h at 37 °C, at 5% CO_2. Then, the cells were washed with PBS, and 100 µL of Caspase-Glo® 3/7 Reagent (Caspase-Glo® 3/7 Assay, Promega, Madison, WI, USA) was added to each well, the plate was gently mixed by shaking at 300 rpm for 30 s and the chemiluminescence was measured continuously for 2 h at 37 °C.

2.2.2. Annexin V/Propidium Iodide Analysis (Flow Cytometry)

The disturbance of the cell membrane was monitored using Annexin V (AnV) and propidium iodide (PI). Neutrophils (1×10^6 cells/sample) were placed in an eppendorf tube, washed twice with PBS, and resuspended in solutions of FOH or FA at variable concentrations. Unstimulated cells served as a negative control, and phorbol 12-myristate 13-acetate (PMA)-treated neutrophils represented a positive control. Cells were incubated for 1 h at 37 °C, at 5% CO_2, washed three times with PBS, and stained with propidium iodide and fluorescein isothiocyanate (FITC)-labeled Annexin V for 15 min, according to supplier's instruction (Dead Cell Apoptosis Kit with Annexin V-FITC and PI, Invitrogen, Carlsbad, CA, USA). Then, cells were analyzed with flow cytometry (LSR Fortressa, BD, San Jose, CA, USA).

2.3. Analysis of ROS Production

The production of reactive oxygen species (ROS) by neutrophils was analyzed using chemiluminescence measurements. Neutrophils (2×10^5 cells/well) were suspended in 160 µl of Krebs-Ringer phosphate buffer containing freshly prepared luminol solution (10^{-6} M) and allowed to settle for 15 min at 37 °C, 5% CO_2 in the wells of 96-well white microplate. Then, 10 µl of FOH, FA, or TR were added at variable concentrations. Untreated neutrophils were used as a negative control, and cells stimulated with 25 nM PMA as a positive control. The chemiluminescence of luminol was recorded for one hour with one-second integration time, using a BioTek Synergy H1 microplate reader.

2.4. Analysis of NET Quantity and Image

Neutrophils (2.2×10^5 cells/well) were seeded into the well of 96-wells black microplate in 150 µL of RPMI-1040 and allowed to settle for 15 min at 37 °C, 5% CO_2. Then, neutrophils were stimulated with 150 µL of FOH, FA or TR at variable concentrations in RPMI-1040. Unstimulated cells and cells treated with 25 nM of PMA served as negative and positive controls, respectively. Plates were incubated at 37 °C, 5% CO_2 for 3 h and then analyzed, as follows:

For the visualization of NETs: the samples were fixed with 3.8% paraformaldehyde for 15 min and washed with PBS. Sytox Green (Thermo Fisher, Waltham, MA, USA.) dye was added to each well at the final concentration of 1 µM to visualize extracellular DNA. Imaging was performed using a Nikon Eclipse Ti microscope (Nikon Instruments, Melville, NY, USA).

For extracellular DNA quantification: the cells were washed three times with PBS and then 50 µL micrococcal nuclease (MNase, 1 U/mL) was added to cleave and release small fragments of extracellular DNA, and the microplates were incubated at 37 °C for further 20 min. The enzymatic reaction was stopped by the addition of EDTA solution (100 µg/mL), and after cell centrifugation ($350 \times g$, 5 min) 50 µL of supernatant was transferred into 96-well black microplate containing Sytox Green at a final concentration of 1 µM. Fluorescence was measured using the Biotek Synergy H1 microplate reader at the excitation wavelength of 465 nm and the emission wavelength of 525 nm.

2.5. Identification and Quantification of Myeloperoxidase

Neutrophils (2.2×10^5 cells/well) were seeded into the well of 96-wells black microplate in 150 μL of RPMI-1040 and allowed to settle for 15 min at 37 °C, 5% CO_2. Then, neutrophils were stimulated with 150 μL of FOH at a concentration of 100 μM and 200 μM.

For the visualization of MPO: the samples were fixed with 3.8% paraformaldehyde for 15 min and washed with PBS. 50 μL of 1:100 diluted primary mouse anti-MPO antibodies (Abcam, Cambridge, UK) was added to each well and incubated for a night at 4 °C. Then, cells were washed three times with PBS and incubated with 1:500 diluted secondary Alexa Fluor 555 anti-mouse antibodies (Abcam, Cambridge, UK) for 1 h at 37 °C. Cells were washed two times with PBS, and imaging was performed using a Nikon Eclipse Ti microscope.

For the quantification of MPO: the quantitative determination of MPO was performed using Human MPO ELISA Kit (Wuhan Fine Biotech Co., Ltd., Wuhan, China). The cells were washed three times with PBS and then 50 μL micrococcal nuclease (MNase, 1 U/mL) was added to release DNA-bounded proteins, and the microplates were incubated at 37 °C for further 20 min. After cell centrifugation ($350\times g$, 5 min) 100 μL of supernatant was transferred into anti-MPO pre-coated wells of plate, and the manufacturer's instruction was followed.

2.6. Recognition of Receptors Involved in Netosis

Neutrophils were preincubated with specific antibodies or inhibitors prior to stimulation with *C. albicans* factors. Neutrophils (1×10^6) were preincubated for 30 min at 37 °C in RPMI-1640 medium with 1 μg/mL of blocking antibodies directed against TLR2, TLR4 (Invivogen, Toulouse, France), CD11a, CD11b, CD16, CD18 (BioLegend, San Diego, CA, USA) or isotype control antibody—IgG (Abcam, Cambridge, UK).

2.7. Analysis of Protein Kinase C (PKC)

The activity of PKC was monitored using PepTag® Non-Radioactive Protein Kinase Assays (Promega, Madison, WI, USA). Neutrophils (5×10^6 in 500 μL of PBS per well) were stimulated with 100 μM and 200 μM FOH in 12-well microplate. Negative and positive controls were prepared as described above. After 1 h of incubation at 37 °C, at 5% CO_2, cells were washed with PBS, resuspended in 500 μL of cold PKC extraction buffer, and homogenized in the cold. Lysates were centrifugated for 5 min at 4 °C, $14,000\times g$ and supernatants were purified on diethylaminoethyl (DEAE) cellulose resin. To the reaction solution containing 5 μL of PepTag® PKC Reaction Buffer, 2 μg of PepTag® C1 Peptide, and 5 μL of sonicated PKC Activator, 10 μL of purified samples or 4 μL of Protein Kinase C at concentration of 2.5 μg/mL (as a positive control) were added, followed by incubation at 30 °C for 30 min. Then, the reaction was stopped by placing the tube in a 95 °C heating block for 10 min. 1 μL of 80% glycerol was added to each sample, and then samples were electrophoretically separated on a 0.8% agarose gel at 100 V for 15 min. The phosphorylated peptide migrated to the cathode (+), while the non-phosphorylated peptide migrated to the anode (-). The gel was photographed on a transilluminator.

2.8. Analysis of ERK1/2

The amount of total and phosphorylated ERK1/2 was quantified using SimpleStep ELISA Kit (Abcam, Cambridge, UK). Neutrophils (1×10^6 in 500 μL of PBS per well) were stimulated with 100 μM and 200 μM FOH in 12-well microplate. Negative and positive controls were prepared as described above. After 1 h of incubation at 37 °C in 5% CO_2, cells were lysed using a Cell Extraction Buffer (Abcam, Cambridge, UK). The protein concentration in the lysate was determined using the Bradford assay [31]. Then, 50 μL of lysate was mixed with 50 μL of antibody cocktail (anti-ERK1/2–total or anti-pT202/Y204–phosphorylated ERK1/2 provided by the manufacturer) in wells of SimpleStep pre-coated 96-well microplate, according to manufacturer's instruction. After 1 h of incubation with gentle shaking at room temperature, the wells were washed 3 times with PBS and then TMB (3,3′,5,5′-tetramethylbenzidine) solution was added. After 15 min, the reaction was stopped with a Stop solution, and absorbance at 450 nm was recorded using a BioTek Synergy H1 microplate reader.

2.9. Analysis of Netosis Signaling Pathway

For the analysis of netosis signaling pathway, selected enzyme inhibitors were used. Neutrophils were pre-treated for 30 min prior to stimulation with different inhibitors: 30 µM piceatannol (Syk inhibitor; Sigma-Aldrich, St. Louis, MO, USA), 10 µM PP2 (Src inhibitor; Calbiochem, Darmstadt, Germany), 10 µM UO126 (ERK inhibitor; Cell Signaling Technology, Beverly, MA, USA) or 5 µM DPI (NADPH oxidase inhibitor; Sigma-Aldrich, St. Louis, MO, USA). Then, the cells were stimulated and analyzed as described above.

2.10. Analysis of Neutrophil Chemotaxis

Neutrophil migration was evaluated by the 24-well microchemotaxis chamber technique (Transwell®-Clear inserts, Corning, NY, USA). Neutrophils were labeled for 10 min with 1 µM CellTracker Red solution (Invitrogen, Carlsbad, CA, USA), washed three times with PBS, and placed in the upper compartment of the chamber (1×10^6 cells/well). Samples of FOH (various concentrations of up to 400 µM) or fMLP (1 µM; used as a positive control) were placed in the lower compartment. PBS was used as a negative control. The compartments were separated by a membrane with 3 µm pores. The chambers were incubated at 37 °C in 5% CO_2 atmosphere for 1 h. Neutrophil migration was monitored by fluorescence microscopy (Motic AE31E, MoticEurope, Barcelona, Spain), and the number of cells migrated into the lower compartment of the chamber was quantified.

2.11. Statistical Analysis

Each of the experiments was repeated at least three times, obtaining consistent results. Two replicates were performed in each experiment. The graphs show the results of a single representative experiment.

Statistical analysis was performed with the GraphPad Prism 7 software (GraphPad Software, CA, USA). The statistical significance was assessed by ANOVA and Dunnett's multiple comparisons post-test.

3. Results

3.1. Farnesol but Not Farnesoic Acid or Tyrosol Triggers NET Formation

Neutrophils are the cells with high microbiocidal potential, and their high killing efficiency is due to their ability to recognize many "foreign" molecules released by pathogens. Owing to these properties and because their active cells move under the chemoattractant gradient, neutrophils release their antimicrobial molecules directly at the site of infection. In our current study, we focused on the role of *C. albicans*-released QSMs, in particular FOH.

We verified the neutrophil responses to contact with QSMs released by *C. albicans*, focusing on the PMN ability to release NETs. The stimulation of PMNs with FOH showed the dose-dependent responses with NET release within the whole range of concentrations tested (Figure 1a). The highest level of NETs released by FOH-treated neutrophils was observed for 250 µM FOH, and it reached about 60% of the positive control.

Different results were obtained for FA, a farnesol derivate. PMNs did not release NETs in response to any of the examined concentrations of FA. Although at the concentration of 250 µM the fluorescent signal increased significantly, it was probably a result of cell death induced by this FA concentration. Similar results were observed for TR, the third examined QSM. No released NETs were identified within the entire range of examined TR concentrations.

These quantitative results were confirmed by fluorescence microscopy analysis (Figure 1b), on which Sytox Green-stained neutrophils, stimulated with FOH showed cloud-like structures located around the human cells and composed of green-labeled DNA.

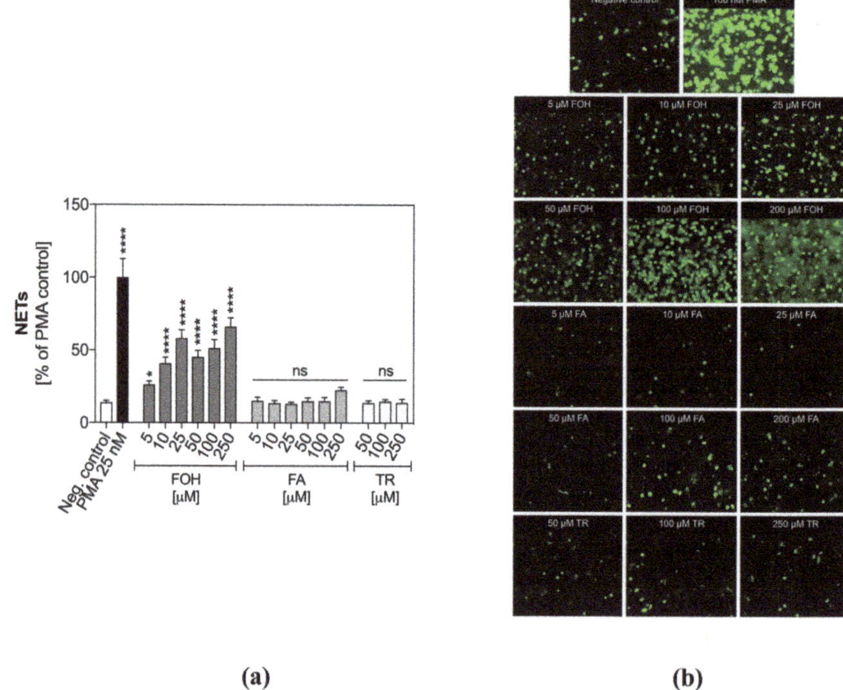

(a) (b)

Figure 1. Release of neutrophil extracellular traps (NETs) by quorum sensing molecule (QSM)-treated neutrophils. Neutrophils were treated with QSMs at variable concentrations for 3 h. Unstimulated cells served as a negative control. (**a**) The released NETs were digested with micrococcal nuclease (MNase) and collected supernatants were stained with Sytox Green and the fluorescence intensity was measured. Data represent the mean fluorescence ± standard error of the mean (S.E.M.). from two replicates. ANOVA and Dunnett's multiple comparisons post-tests were used. Asterisks denote statistical significance ($p > 0.1234$ ns, * $p \leq 0.0332$, **** $p < 0.0001$). (**b**) The extracellular DNA was stained with Sytox Green and visualized with fluorescence microscopy.

To verify the NETs production during FOH treatment, also the extracellular localization of myeloperoxidase was determined, using specific, fluorescent antibodies. During netosis, MPO is moved from granule to the nucleus and then released together with DNA in the form of NETs.

Quantitative analysis of MPO in the samples containing neutrophils treated with FOH, was performed using ELISA. For this purpose, the netting cells were prior washed with PBS, and the extracellular DNA was digested with MNase to liberate bound MPO. In Figure 2a, we showed MPO concentration in the cell supernatants, determined by ELISA. The amount of detected MPO correlated with the DNA quantity, confirming that the observed DNA structures belong to the NETs. Additionally, MPO/DNA complexes were visualized microscopically (Figure 2b). As was shown in the figure, the protein location correlated with DNA clouds released by PMNs, confirming activation of netosis by FOH.

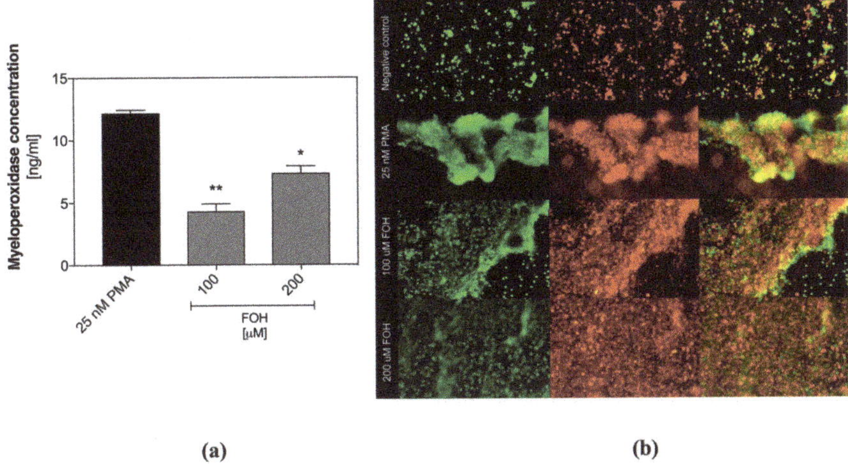

(a)

(b)

Figure 2. Identification of myeloperoxidase in farnesol (FOH)-treated neutrophils. Neutrophils were treated with FOH at a concentration of 100 μM and 200 μM for 3 h. Unstimulated cells served as a negative control. (**a**) The released DNA was digested with MNase, and a concentration of myeloperoxidase (MPO) was analyzed in collected supernatants using ELISA method. Data represent the mean concentration ± S.E.M. from two replicates. ANOVA and Dunnett's multiple comparisons post-tests were used. Asterisks denote statistical significance ($p > 0.1234$ ns, * $p \leq 0.0332$, ** $p \leq 0.0021$). (**b**) The extracellular DNA was stained with Sytox Green, while MPO was identified with primary mouse anti-MPO antibodies and secondary Alexa Fluor 555-labeled anti-mouse antibodies. Samples were visualized with fluorescence microscopy.

3.2. Farnesol Treatment of Neutrophils Does Not Lead to Cell Apoptosis

In order to confirm that the observed effect of the DNA release the cell was associated with the mechanism of netosis, but not cell death like apoptosis, the activation of proapoptotic caspases was analyzed. PMNs were exposed to FOH and FA at the concentration range of 0–1200 μM for one hour, and caspase 3 and 7 activities were measured using the chemiluminometric method (Figure 3).

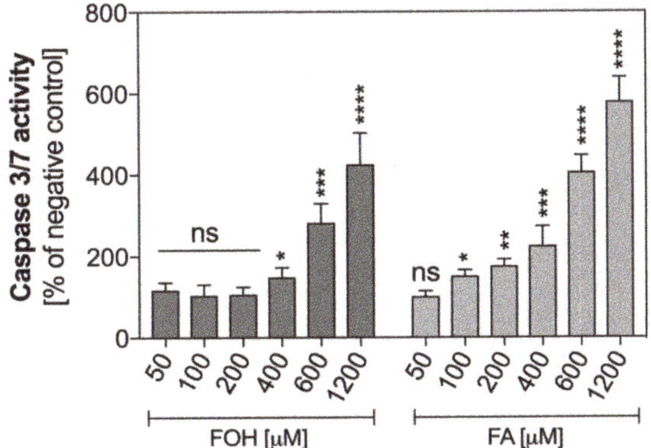

Figure 3. Caspase 3/7 activity in QSM-treated neutrophils. Neutrophils were treated with FOH and farnesoic acid (FA) at variable concentrations, and incubated with Caspase-Glo® 3/7, followed by continuous measurement of chemiluminescence for 2 h. Data represent mean values of luminescence from two replicates ± S.E.M. ANOVA and Dunnett's post-tests were used. Asterisks denote statistical significance ($p > 0.1234$ ns, * $p \leq 0.0332$, ** $p \leq 0.0021$, *** $p \leq 0.0002$, **** $p < 0.0001$).

The results presented in Figure 3 indicated that FOH at the concentration range of 0–200 μM did not activate proapoptotic caspases in neutrophils. However, higher concentrations of FOH led to apoptotic cell death. FA-treated neutrophils showed activation of apoptosis in a dose-dependent manner within the whole tested range of concentrations. This explains the absence of NETs released in the presence of FA, because activation of caspases 3 and 7 inhibits the release of NETs [32].

Besides, the neutrophils were incubated with FOH and FA at concentrations of 100 μM and 200 μM for one hour and then labeled with PI and AnV. The cell viability analysis based on PI and AnV-FITC was performed using flow cytometry. The results (Figure 4a), comparison to the 3/7 caspase analysis, also allow assessing the potential of PMNs for the release of NETs. The changes in the distribution of cell population labeled with PI and AnV (Figure 4b), characteristic to netosis, were previously described and used by Masuda et al. [33].

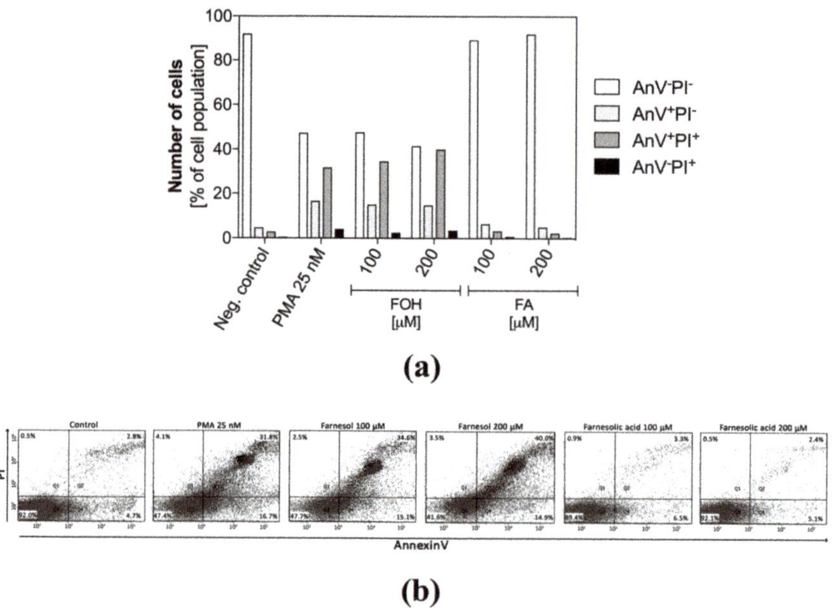

(a)

(b)

Figure 4. Flow cytometric analysis of neutrophil apoptosis. Neutrophils were stimulated with FOH or FA, labeled with annexin V-FITC and propidium iodide, and analyzed by flow cytometry. The results are presented as a percentage ratio of the signal detected for whole cell population and showing no cell death (PI$^-$AnV$^-$), early apoptosis (PI$^-$An$^+$) and late apoptosis (PI$^+$AnV$^+$). Cells stained only with propidium iodide (PI$^+$AnV$^-$) represent the necrotic or NET-forming cells. For each sample, data were collected for 100,000 neutrophils. (**a**) Data are presented as a part of total cell population, (**b**) the diagrams represent AnV and PI cell distribution.

The results showed four groups of cells: AnV$^-$PI$^-$ identified as live; AnV$^+$PI$^-$ identified as early apoptotic; AnV$^+$PI$^+$ identified as apoptotic; AnV$^-$PI$^+$ identified as necrotic. However, the obtained cell distribution patterns, especially for AnV$^+$PI$^+$ cells, were identical for cells in the netosis, represented by PMNs stimulated with PMA. Approximately 35%–40% of FOH-treated neutrophils showed positive labeling for both AnV and PI, similarly to the PMA-treated positive control. This indicated that these cells lost the integrity of the cell membrane, however, the comparison of these results with the activation of caspases led to the conclusion that observed changes did not result from apoptotic cell death. The low percentage of PI-positive neutrophils suggests that DNA released outside the cells was not due to mechanical destruction or necrotic death. The presence of approximately 15% of AnV$^+$PI$^-$ cells suggests that neutrophils were in the ongoing netosis process. In contrast, FA-treated PMNs did not show apoptotic and necrotic cell traits within the tested range of QSM concentrations, within one hour of contact with FA.

3.3. Farnesol Induces Rapid ROS Production

The activation of NADPH oxidase, resulting in the production of ROS is a key step in the ROS-dependent netosis pathway. The chemical stimulation of neutrophils with PMA leads to the release of a high amount of ROS within minutes of activation. We checked the ability of the examined QSMs to activate NADPH oxidase and release ROS. PMNs were treated with selected doses of FOH or FA, and the activity of NADPH oxidase was measured using a chemiluminescence-based assay.

Changes in chemiluminescence intensity over the time showed in Figure 5 were proportional to the amount of ROS produced by PMNs. The stimulation of neutrophils with FOH at the concentration of 100 and 200 µM caused the rapid activation of NADPH oxidase and release of ROS at a time similar to PMA-stimulated cells. The level of ROS released by PMNs treated with 100 µM FOH reached about 25% of the positive control response, while activation with 200 µM FOH resulted in two-fold higher ROS production. Release of ROS by neutrophils correlated with the production of NETs, suggesting that FOH activates the ROS-dependent mechanism of netosis.

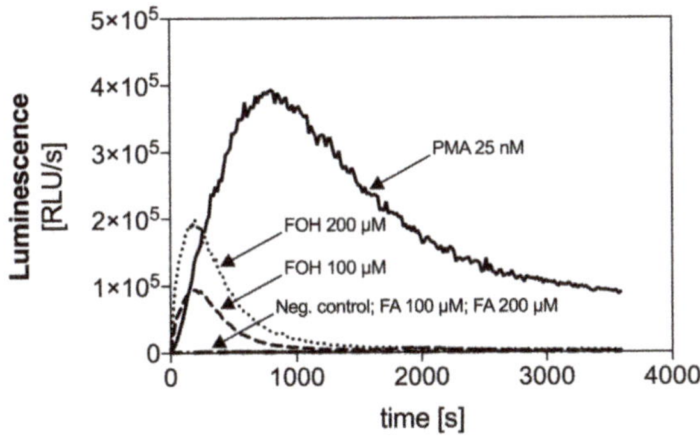

Figure 5. The time course of reactive oxygen species (ROS) generation by neutrophils in response to FOH and FA. ROS production by neutrophils (2×10^5 cells/well) was monitored at 37 °C for 1 h by the luminol chemiluminescence method after suspension of cells in FOH or FA. In the reference samples, the neutrophils were treated with 25 nM phorbol 12-myristate 13-acetate (PMA) or left in Krebs–Ringer phosphate buffer (a negative control).

The response of neutrophils to FA presented relatively low chemiluminescence signal, confirming that this QSM does not participate in NET release.

3.4. Mac-1 and TLR2 Surface Neutrophil Receptors Are Involved in Farnesol-Induced Activation of Netosis

Many of the neutrophil surface receptors are involved in the recognition of molecules derived from pathogenic microorganisms, which leads to activation of the netosis signaling pathway and the NET release. We selected six receptors known to be able to mediate the release of NETs and checked their role in FOH-induced netosis. The receptors were blocked with specific antibodies, and the neutrophils were stimulated with selected concentrations of FOH for three hours. A decrease in the level of fluorescence of Sytox Green-stained DNA suggests the role of this receptor in the activation of netosis. Among selected receptors, we identified that the inhibition of CD11b and CD18 caused a ca. 2.5-fold decrease in the level of released NETs (Figure 6). This result strongly suggests the important role of these receptors in the recognition of FOH and activation of netosis. Moreover, inhibition of the TLR2 receptor caused a reduction of the level of NETs to about 50% of PMA-treated response, also indicating the participation of this receptor in netosis. A small contribution to the activation of

FOH-induced netosis could also be assigned to CD11a receptor whose blockade caused a 20% decrease in the amount of released DNA. Other receptors tested—CD16 and TLR4—did not seem to be essential for FOH-induced netosis.

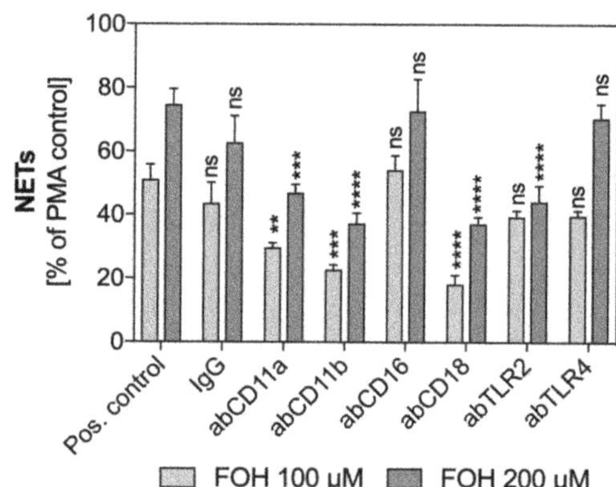

Figure 6. The participation of selected neutrophil receptors in FOH-activated netosis. Neutrophils (2.2×10^5) were preincubated with antibodies (ab, 1 µg/mL) against the selected neutrophil receptors and then netosis was induced for 3 h by 25 nM PMA, 100 µM FOH, and 200 µM FOH. IgG antibody was used as an isotype control. Released NETs were digested with MNase, and collected supernatants were stained with Sytox Green, followed by fluorescence measurements. The results are the means of two replicates ± S.E.M., represented as a percentage relative to the PMA-treated control. ANOVA and Dunnett's post-tests were used. Asterisks denote statistical significance ($p > 0.1234$ ns, ** $p \leq 0.0021$, *** $p \leq 0.0002$, **** $p < 0.0001$).

3.5. Farnesol Leads to the Activation of Protein Kinase C and ERK1/2

PKC plays a crucial role in the netosis signal pathway. We checked the level of PKC activation in lysates of neutrophils previously treated with two concentrations of FOH or FA for one hour. After pre-purification of the lysates on DEAE cellulose, the kinase activity was determined based on the phosphorylation of the synthetic peptide, which was then subjected to electrophoretic separation. Figure 7a presents an electrophoretic separation of a synthetic peptide whose amount in the phosphorylated form determines the level of PKC activation. Figure 7b shows quantitative PKC activity in assayed samples corresponding to the densitometrically analyzed bands of the phosphorylated form of the peptide on an electrophoretic gel.

The results showed that PKC activity in neutrophils treated with FOH increased rapidly, reaching a two-fold higher level than in unstimulated cells, comparable to that obtained for chemically induced (PMA) activation of this enzyme. The PKC activity leads to the activation of subsequent netosis mediators. On the other hand, PMNs treated with FA did not show any changes in PKC activity. The lack of PKC activation by FA confirms that neutrophils do not release NETs in the presence of this QSM.

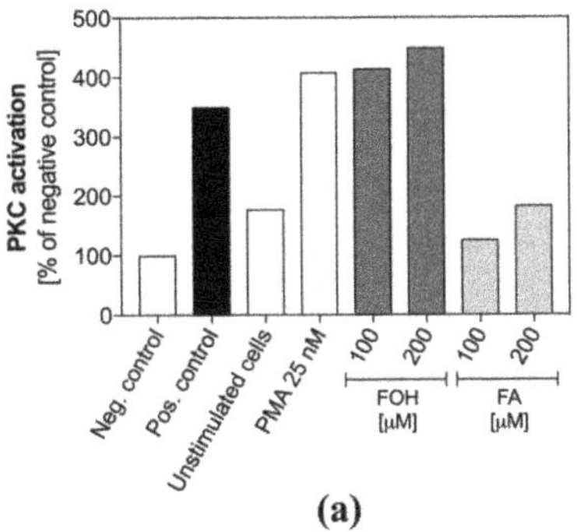

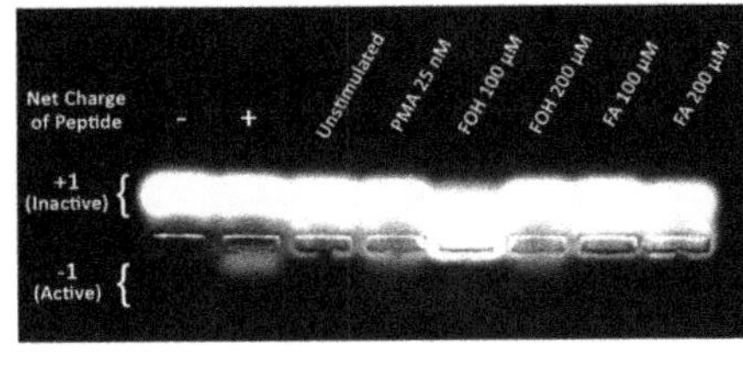

(a) **(b)**

Figure 7. Activation of Protein Kinase C (PKC) in QSM–treated neutrophils. Neutrophils (5×10^5) were stimulated with selected concentrations of FOH, FA, and 25 nM PMA for 1 h. Then, cell lysate was added to the PKC substrate solution-PepTag® C1 Peptide, and after 30 min separated electrophoretically on an agarose gel. Unstimulated cells were negative cellular control, and PMA-treated cells were positive cellular control. Purified PKC enzyme was used for an assay positive control (control of C1 Peptide phosphorylation), negative control was C1 peptide without any PKC enzyme. (**a**) PKC activation as a percentage of phosphorylated C1 peptide, a substrate for PKC. The values represent the densitometrically-analyzed bands on the electrophoretic gel, assigned as "Active" in (**b**).

The results of the analysis of ERK1/2 kinase activation in neutrophils treated with FOH are shown on Figure 8. The activation of ERK1/2 by 100 µM FOH is two-fold higher than in unstimulated cells, but 200 µM FOH caused three-fold greater phosphorylation of this enzyme. These findings suggest that the activation of the signaling pathway by FOH in neutrophils involving ERK1/2 in a dose-dependent manner.

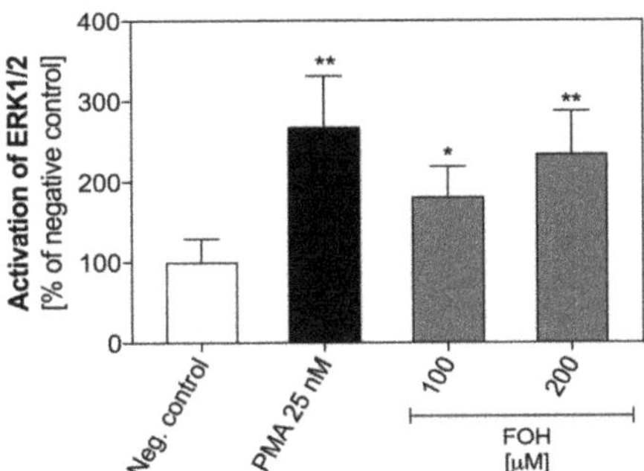

Figure 8. Activation of ERK1/2 in FOH-treated neutrophils. Neutrophil cells (1×10^6 cells/well) were suspended in PBS in 12-well microplate and stimulated with FOH at concentrations of 100 µM and 200 µM. Unstimulated cells served as a negative control, and PMA-treated cells were a positive control. After 1 h, the cells were lysed, and the amount of total and phosphorylated ERK1/2 was quantified using ELISA Kit SimpleStep (Abcam). Data represent the mean values of absorbance ± S.E.M. from two replicates as the percentage ratio of phosphorylated ERK1/2 to total ERK1/2. ANOVA and Tukey post-tests were used. Asterisks denote statistical significance ($p > 0.1234$–ns, * $p \leq 0.0332$, ** $p \leq 0.0021$).

3.6. The ROS-Dependent Netosis Pathway is Activated by Farnesol

Stimulation of surface receptors involved in the induction of netosis leads to the activation of selected mediators of the signaling pathway. We checked the role of the five primary mediators involved in ROS-dependent and ROS-independent netosis pathways. For this purpose, selected mediators were blocked in PMNs using specific inhibitors before neutrophil activation with 200 μM FOH. Fluorescence of Sytox Green-stained extracellular DNA was used to determine NET release.

The results (Figure 9) indicate that each of the tested mediators was involved in FOH-induced netosis, but with a relative variable contribution. Syk and Src kinases co-operated with neutrophil surface receptors, and their involvement in netosis activation appeared to be significant. The inhibition of these proteins caused a 50% decrease in the amount of released NETs. In turn, the role of PI3K in FOH-induced netosis seemed to be less important. PI3K probably played a significant role in the ROS-independent netosis signaling pathway. In our experiments, blockade of this kinase caused a decrease in the amount of extracellular DNA by 20% relative to the control.

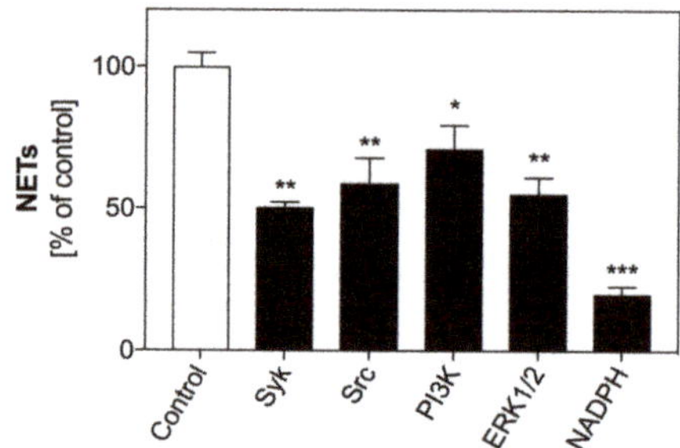

Figure 9. Role of selected signal mediators in activation of netosis by FOH. Neutrophils (2.2×10^5) were preincubated with inhibitors of the indicated signaling mediators: Syk—30 μM piceatannol, Src—10 μM PP2, PI3K—25 μM LY29004, ERK1/2—10 μM U0126, NADPH oxidase—5 μM DPI. Cells were then incubated with FOH at 200 μM concentration for 3 h to induce netosis. Neutrophils not treated with inhibitors but stimulated with FOH served as a control. The data are presented as means ± S.E.M. from two replicates and are expressed as a percentage ratio relative to the control. ANOVA and Tukey post-tests were used. Asterisks denote statistical significance ($p > 0.1234$ ns, * $p \leq 0.0332$, ** $p \leq 0.0021$, *** $p \leq 0.0002$).

ERK1/2 and NADPH oxidase also participate in the activation of the ROS-dependent netosis pathway. The release of NETs depending on ROS production appears to be the primary netosis mechanism involved in neutrophil responses to FOH, as the FOH stimulation of PMNs with blocked ERK1/2 resulted in a 50% reduction of the amount of released NETs. Moreover, NADPH oxidase, which is responsible for the production of ROS in the cells, seems to play the most significant role in the netosis process induced with FOH. Only 20% of DNA was released by neutrophils with the blocked activity of NADPH oxidase compared to the control cells. This result and data showing increased ROS production by neutrophils treated with farnesol confirm that FOH-induced netosis is a ROS-dependent process.

3.7. Farnesol Is a Chemoattractant for Neutrophils

Additionally, we showed that FOH may be a chemoattractant for PMNs. To support this hypothesis, the neutrophils were placed in chambers to measure chemotactic ability, and then the chambers were transferred to the FOH solutions at the concentration within a range of 50 to 400 μM. As the negative control, PBS was used, whereas the positive control was represented by the responses of neutrophils to 1 μM solution of fMLP. The number of cells that passed through the membrane according to the factor gradient was counted after one hour of treatment. The obtained results (Figure 10) showed that FOH is recognized by neutrophils as a chemoattractant, causing the PMN movement toward the concentration gradient. The number of cells that passed through the membrane was proportional to FOH concentration in the range of 50 to 200 μM, that corresponds to the concentration of FOH detected under in vivo conditions [23]. The higher concentrations of FOH did not cause any further increase in neutrophil migration, but anyway the maximal level of neutrophil chemotaxis upon FOH treatment reached 60% of the response to fMLP, the positive control. These results suggest that neutrophils can migrate to the *Candida* infection sites in response to QSMs released by the yeast.

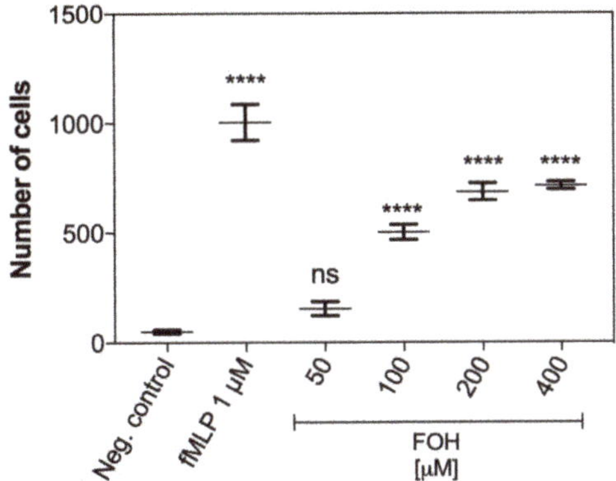

Figure 10. Chemotactic activity of FOH-treated neutrophils. CellTracker Red labeled neutrophil cells (1 × 10⁶ cells/well) were placed into chemotaxis chambers being in contact with different concentration of FOH or 1 µM fML (a positive control). Negative control was PBS. After 1 h of incubation, the chambers were removed, and migrated cells were counted. Data represent the mean number of cells ± S.E.M. from three replicates. ANOVA and Dunnett's multiple comparisons post-tests were used. Asterisks denote statistical significance ($p > 0.1234$ ns, **** $p < 0.0001$).

4. Discussion

Quorum sensing molecules are essential virulence factors of many pathogenic microorganisms-bacteria as well as fungi. The release of QSMs ensures the fast local communication between cells in the infected area, growth synchronization, as well as response to environmental changes of temperature and pH, the presence of biocidal compounds, etc. [34,35].

C. albicans yeast mainly use QSMs to regulate growth, change of morphological form and also create biofilms [36]. However, these molecules have an impact on many host cells, like immune cells, such as macrophages, DCs, and neutrophils [20,23].

Our results presented in this paper indicated an important role of neutrophils in the response to QSMs produced by *C. albicans*, which is based on the release of NETs. We showed that farnesol, one of the three compounds identified as *C. albicans* QSMs (FOH, FA and TR) was responsible for activating the netosis, a finding that had not been presented in the literature previously.

The role of FOH released by *C. albicans* is still not fully understood, but it is known that the presence of this compound inhibits the growth of fungal biofilm, and also blocks the change in the morphological transition of fungal cells from blastospores to filamentous forms. Also, high concentrations of FOH can stimulate the yeast to reverse switch from invasive filamentous hyphae back to blastospore [37]. As we presented in the current work, FOH produced at different local concentrations at the site of infection caused the neutrophil response involving NET release. The finding is important for the host defense against *C. albicans* cells because current knowledge has suggested that the morphological form of the fungus determines the mechanism of neutrophil response [28,30]. Some findings indicated that the size of the fungal cells determines the release of NETs, suggesting that the large, filamentous form of *C. albicans* is responsible for activating the netosis [28]. Other studies indicated that the composition of the cell wall of the filamentous form, as well as the released proteolytic enzymes are crucial for the stimulation of neutrophils to NET production [30,38]. Regardless of the identified NET triggers, all studies pointed that *C. albicans* blastospores generate much smaller amounts of NETs, suggesting that this morphological form of *C. albicans* cells can "hide" from neutrophils and avoid the killing. Perhaps, fungi use FOH to inhibit their cell filamentation and progress of infection, just to survive in milieu infiltrated by neutrophils This situation is dangerous for the host because the 'invisible' to neutrophils intruder cells can survive and under favorable conditions, develop the difficult to treat, secondary infections [39]. Therefore, the ability of neutrophils to recognize FOH, the essential QSM molecule of the fungus, and release NETs in the response to its production at the place of infection, can significantly affect the effectiveness of host defense against *C. albicans* presence. We confirmed the recognition of FOH by neutrophils using chemotaxis analysis, showing that FOH is an efficient chemotactic factor for neutrophils. To date, there is no literature data showing neutrophil migration caused by FOH. However, FOH is known to be a chemoattractant for macrophages [40].

Moreover, given that the microbiocidal activity of NETs covers a certain area of infection, a direct identification of fungal cells by neutrophils is not required, and the presence of FOH may be sufficient.

Studies performed by Leonhardt et al. regarding the effect of FOH on neutrophils did not show any increasing ability of these host cells to phagocyte and kill *C. albicans* cells. However, the viability of *C. albicans* was analyzed after 1 h of contact, while the classic ROS-dependent netosis pathway leads to NET release after about 2–3 h of neutrophil activation [23]. The short time period used in Leonhard's analysis may explain the lack of changes in the fungal cell vitality. The same studies showed an increased FOH concentration-dependent release of elastase, myeloperoxidase, and lactoferrin–granule proteins identified in NETs [23,29]. Thus, our observations of NET release may explain the presence of granule proteins upon neutrophil treatment with FOH in Leonhardt's studies.

Activation of netosis by QSMs has been described in only one case—the *Pseudomonas aeruginosa* bacterium. It was shown that mutations in the quorum-sensing regulatory gene lasR affect the amount and structure of released NETs. In addition, stimulation of neutrophils with purified protein, recombinant endotoxin-free LasA induced NETs in a concentration-dependent manner [41].

The other two analyzed QSMs-FA and TR–did not activate netosis. There are also no literature reports on the impact of these compounds on the functioning of neutrophils. Only TR was identified as a protective agent against phagocytic killing by neutrophils, however, the mechanism of its action is still unknown. One study showed the antioxidant activity of TR [42], which could influence the neutrophil response by blocking ROS production, required for proper functioning of netosis mechanisms. However, other studies showed no antioxidant activity of TR, thus leaving the mechanism of its action on neutrophils unrecognized [18].

The production of extracellular DNA but not apoptosis was demonstrated in this work for neutrophils treated with FOH at the range of concentrations observed locally at the site of *C. albicans* infection. This result is consistent with the observation of Leonhardt et al. [23]. In contrary, we presented that FA is active inducer of neutrophil apoptosis in a dose-dependent manner, the finding that can explain the lack of netosis in neutrophil response to this QSM. These results were confirmed by the cytometric analysis showing the morphological changes of neutrophil cells observed during the FOH-induced netosis process but absent upon treatment with FA.

During the contact of *C. albicans* cells with neutrophils, resulting in NET production, the more common ROS-dependent mechanism of netosis was adopted. The analysis of ROS production by PMNs stimulated with FOH showed that neutrophils release ROS in just a few minutes after activation confirming the ROS-dependent netosis pathway used by neutrophils in response to FOH. In addition, Gilbert et al., identified farnesyl thiotriazole (FTT), a FOH precursor as an activator of NADPH oxidase in neutrophils [43]. However, the production of ROS in response to FA and TR was not observed, confirming a lack of response in the netosis way.

Knowing that FOH is a chemoattractant for neutrophils, and also activates the ROS-dependent netosis pathway, the role of selected surface receptors in activation of netosis by this QSM was analyzed. The results pointed the CD11b/CD18 and TLR2 receptors as being involved in the recognition of FOH and further activation of neutrophils. The CD11b/CD18 receptor engagement in neutrophil chemotaxis and netosis responses to fungal infection was previously demonstrated [30]. Also Leonhardt et al. observed that during stimulation of PMNs by FOH, the level of CD11b receptor on the cell surface increased, while the amount of CD16 receptor decreased [23]. However, Ghosh et al. showed increased

TLR2 and Dectin-1 expression in FOH-treated macrophages [22]. No analogous analysis was performed for neutrophils, however, the effect of FOH on TLR2 may also be significant in PMNs.

Further, the role of known mediators of netosis signaling pathway was verified upon neutrophil treatment with FOH. We showed FOH-induced phosphorylation of PKC, an important signal transducer of netosis. Activation of PKC results in the activation of NADPH oxidase and the production of significant amounts of ROS [44]. This result confirms and explains the role of ROS produced by neutrophils in contact with FOH. There is no literature data on the activation of PKC by FOH in neutrophils; however, in human acute leukemia CEM-C1 cells, the synthesis of diacylglycerol (DAG), a PKC activator, was observed in response to 20 μM FOH [45]. In addition, FTT seems to be also a PKC activator [43].

Inhibition of netosis pathway mediators such as Syk, Src, PI3K, and ERK1/2 caused a decrease in the amount of released NETs. Previously, only the pro-apoptotic activity of FOH was known, leading to reduction of PI3K expression in cells and ERK1/2 in HeLa and DU145 prostate cancer cells [46,47]. In turn, Joo et al. also pointed to the pro-apoptotic effect of FOH on cells, however, by activation of ERK1/2 [48]. However, our results did not show the inhibition of these mediators. In contrary, ERK1/2 kinase activity showed a two-fold increase at the activation of the netosis mechanism during which the apoptosis pathway in the PMNs was blocked.

Our results showed for the first time the role of FOH in the neutrophil recognition of fungal infection at an early stage of microbial invasion. It seems that the regulation of fungal cell morphology by FOH during the progress of fungal infection can also be sensed by the host. Neutrophils, the cells of the first line of host defense can "eavesdrop" the fungal cell communication that uses the quorum sensing molecule and then quickly migrate to the pathogen's habitat and kill or limit its spread by using NETs. The discovery of QSMs that can activate netosis can be of great importance for the developing of effective therapy against early candidiasis.

Author Contributions: Conceptualization, M.R.-K. and M.Z.; methodology, M.R.-K. and M.Z.; conceived and designed the experiments, M.R.-K. and M.Z.; all experiments performed by M.Z., except the data shown in Figure 1b, prepared by K.W.; writing—original draft preparation, M.R.-K. and M.Z.; writing—review and editing, M.R.-K. and M.Z.; funding acquisition M.R.-K.

Funding: This work was funded by a grant from the National Science Centre of Poland (grant number 2015/17/B/NZ6/02078 to MRK).

Acknowledgments: Thanks to Andrzej Kozik for critical discussion during the manuscript preparation.

Conflicts of Interest: The authors declare no conflict of interest.

References

1. Höfs, S.; Mogavero, S.; Hube, B. Interaction of *Candida albicans* with host cells: Virulence factors, host defense, escape strategies, and the microbiota. *J. Microbiol.* **2016**, *54*, 149–169. [CrossRef] [PubMed]

2. Williams, P. Quorum sensing, communication and cross-kingdom signalling in the bacterial world. *Microbiology* **2007**, *153*, 3923–3938. [CrossRef] [PubMed]

3. Hornby, J.M.; Jensen, E.C.; Lisec, A.D.; Tasto, J.J.; Jahnke, B.; Shoemaker, R.; Dussault, P.; Nickerson, K.W. Quorum sensing in the dimorphic fungus *Candida albicans* is mediated by farnesol. *Appl. Environ. Microbiol.* **2001**, *67*, 2982–2992. [CrossRef] [PubMed]

4. Nickerson, K.W.; Atkin, A.L.; Hornby, J.M. Quorum sensing in dimorphic fungi: Farnesol and beyond. *Appl. Environ. Microbiol.* **2006**, *72*, 3805–3813. [CrossRef] [PubMed]

5. Albuquerque, P.; Casadevall, A. Quorum sensing in fungi—A review. *Med. Mycol.* **2012**, *50*, 337–345. [CrossRef] [PubMed]

6. Lim, C.S.-Y.; Rosli, R.; Seow, H.F.; Chong, P.P. *Candida* and invasive candidiasis: Back to basics. *Eur. J. Clin. Microbiol. Infect. Dis.* **2012**, *31*, 21–31. [CrossRef]

7. Oh, K.B.; Miyazawa, H.; Naito, T.; Matsuoka, H. Purification and characterization of an autoregulatory substance capable of regulating the morphological transition in *Candida albicans*. *Proc. Natl. Acad. Sci. USA* **2001**, *98*, 4664–4668. [CrossRef]

8. Alem, M.A.S.; Oteef, M.D.Y.; Flowers, T.H.; Douglas, L.J. Production of tyrosol by *Candida albicans* biofilms and its role in quorum sensing and biofilm development. *Eukaryot. Cell* **2006**, *5*, 1770–1779. [CrossRef]

9. Chen, H.; Fujita, M.; Feng, Q.; Clardy, J.; Fink, G.R. Tyrosol is a quorum-sensing molecule in *Candida albicans*. *Proc. Natl. Acad. Sci.* **2004**, *101*, 5048–5052. [CrossRef]

10. Weber, K.; Schulz, B.; Ruhnke, M. The quorum-sensing molecule E,E-farnesol-its variable secretion and its impact on the growth and metabolism of *Candida* species. *Yeast* **2010**, *27*, 727–739. [CrossRef]

11. Weber, K.; Sohr, R.; Schulz, B.; Fleischhacker, M.; Ruhnke, M. Secretion of E,E-Farnesol and Biofilm Formation in Eight Different *Candida* Species. *Antimicrob. Agents Chemother.* **2008**, *52*, 1859–1861. [CrossRef] [PubMed]

12. Hornby, J.M.; Nickerson, K.W. Enhanced production of farnesol by *Candida albicans* treated with four azoles. *Antimicrob. Agents Chemother.* **2004**, *48*, 2305–2307. [CrossRef] [PubMed]

13. Han, T.L.; Cannon, R.D.; Villas-Bôas, S.G. The metabolic basis of *Candida albicans* morphogenesis and quorum sensing. *Fungal Genet. Biol.* **2011**, *48*, 747–763. [CrossRef] [PubMed]

14. Cho, T.; Aoyama, T.; Toyoda, M.; Nakayama, H.; Chibana, H.; Kaminishi, H. Transcriptional changes in *Candida albicans* Genes by both farnesol and high cell density at an early stage of morphogenesis in N-acetyl-D-glucosamine medium. *Nihon Ishinkin Gakkai Zasshi* **2007**, *48*, 159–167. [CrossRef] [PubMed]

15. Ramage, G.; Saville, S.P.; Wickes, B.L.; López-Ribot, J.L. Inhibition of *Candida albicans* biofilm formation by farnesol, a quorum-sensing molecule. *Appl. Environ. Microbiol.* **2002**, *68*, 5459–5463. [CrossRef] [PubMed]

16. Martins, M.; Henriques, M.; Azeredo, J.; Rocha, S.M.; Coimbra, M.A.; Oliveira, R. Morphogenesis Control in *Candida albicans* and *Candida dubliniensis* through Signaling Molecules Produced by Planktonic and Biofilm Cells. *Eukaryot. Cell* **2007**, *6*, 2429–2436. [CrossRef] [PubMed]

17. Deveau, A.; Piispanen, A.E.; Jackson, A.A.; Hogan, D.A. Farnesol induces hydrogen peroxide resistance in *Candida albicans* yeast by inhibiting the Ras-cyclic AMP signaling pathway. *Eukaryot. Cell* **2010**, *9*, 569–577. [CrossRef]

18. Westwater, C.; Balish, E.; Schofield, D.A. *Candida albicans* -Conditioned Medium Protects Yeast Cells from Oxidative Stress: A Possible Link between Quorum Sensing and Oxidative Stress Resistance. *Eukaryot. Cell* **2005**, *4*, 1654–1661. [CrossRef]

19. Cugini, C.; Calfee, M.W.; Farrow, J.M.; Morales, D.K.; Pesci, E.C.; Hogan, D.A. Farnesol, a common sesquiterpene, inhibits PQS production in *Pseudomonas aeruginosa*. *Mol. Microbiol.* **2007**, *65*, 896–906. [CrossRef]

20. Jung, Y.; Hwang, S.; Sethi, G.; Fan, L.; Arfuso, F.; Ahn, K. Potential Anti-Inflammatory and Anti-Cancer Properties of Farnesol. *Molecules* **2018**, *23*, 2827. [CrossRef]

21. Abe, S.; Tsunashima, R.; Iijima, R.; Yamada, T.; Maruyama, N.; Hisajima, T.; Abe, Y.; Oshima, H.; Yamazaki, M. Suppression of anti-Candida activity of macrophages by a quorum-sensing molecule, farnesol, through induction of oxidative stress. *Microbiol. Immunol.* **2009**, *53*, 323–330. [CrossRef] [PubMed]

22. Ghosh, S.; Howe, N.; Volk, K.; Tati, S.; Nickerson, K.W.; Petro, T.M. *Candida albicans* cell wall components and farnesol stimulate the expression of both inflammatory and regulatory cytokines in the murine RAW264.7 macrophage cell line. *FEMS Immunol. Med. Microbiol.* **2010**, *60*, 63–73. [CrossRef] [PubMed]

23. Leonhardt, I.; Spielberg, S.; Weber, M.; Albrecht-Eckardt, D.; Bläss, M.; Claus, R.; Barz, D.; Scherlach, K.; Hertweck, C.; Löffler, J.; et al. The fungal quorum-sensing molecule farnesol activates innate immune cells but suppresses cellular adaptive immunity. *MBio* **2015**, *6*, e00143. [CrossRef] [PubMed]

24. Netea, M.G.; Joosten, L.A.; van der Meer, J.W.; Kullberg, B.J.; van de Veerdonk, F.L. Immune defence against *Candida* fungal infections. *Nat. Rev. Immunol.* **2015**, *15*, 630–642. [CrossRef]

25. Gazendam, R.P.; Van Hamme, J.L.; Tool, A.T.J.; van Houdt, M.; Verkuijlen, P.J.J.H.; Herbst, M.; Liese, J.G.; Van De Veerdonk, F.L.; Roos, D.; van den Berg, T.K.; et al. Two independent killing mechanisms of *Candida albicans* by human neutrophils: Evidence from innate immunity defects. *Blood* **2014**, *124*, 590–597. [CrossRef]

26. Urban, C.F.; Reichard, U.; Brinkmann, V.; Zychlinsky, A. Neutrophil extracellular traps capture and kill *Candida albicans* yeast and hyphal forms. *Cell. Microbiol.* **2006**, *8*, 668–676. [CrossRef]

27. Galkina, S.I.; Molotkovsky, J.G.; Ullrich, V.; Sud'ina, G.F. Scanning electron microscopy study of neutrophil membrane tubulovesicular extensions (cytonemes) and their role in anchoring, aggregation and phagocytosis. The effect of nitric oxide. *Exp. Cell Res.* **2005**, *304*, 620–629. [CrossRef]

28. Branzk, N.; Lubojemska, A.; Hardison, S.E.; Wang, Q.; Gutierrez, M.G.; Brown, G.D.; Papayannopoulos, V. Neutrophils sense microbe size and selectively release neutrophil extracellular traps in response to large pathogens. *Nat. Immunol.* **2014**, *15*, 1017–1025. [CrossRef]

29. Urban, C.F.; Ermert, D.; Schmid, M.; Abu-Abed, U.; Goosmann, C.; Nacken, W.; Brinkmann, V.; Jungblut, P.R.; Zychlinsky, A. Neutrophil extracellular traps contain calprotectin, a cytosolic protein complex involved in host defense against *Candida albicans*. *PLoS Pathog.* **2009**, *5*, e1000639. [CrossRef]

30. Zawrotniak, M.; Bochenska, O.; Karkowska-Kuleta, J.; Seweryn-Ozog, K.; Aoki, W.; Ueda, M.; Kozik, A.; Rapala-Kozik, M. Aspartic Proteases and Major Cell Wall Components in *Candida albicans* Trigger the Release of Neutrophil Extracellular Traps. *Front. Cell. Infect. Microbiol.* **2017**, *7*, 414. [CrossRef]

31. Bradford, M. A Rapid and Sensitive Method for the Quantitation of Microgram Quantities of Protein Utilizing the Principle of Protein-Dye Binding. *Anal. Biochem.* **1976**, *72*, 248–254. [CrossRef]

32. Kenny, E.F.; Herzig, A.; Krüger, R.; Muth, A.; Mondal, S.; Thompson, P.R.; Brinkmann, V.; von Bernuth, H.; Zychlinsky, A. Diverse stimuli engage different neutrophil extracellular trap pathways. *Elife* **2017**, *6*. [CrossRef] [PubMed]

33. Masuda, S.; Shimizu, S.; Matsuo, J.; Nishibata, Y.; Kusunoki, Y.; Hattanda, F.; Shida, H.; Nakazawa, D.; Tomaru, U.; Atsumi, T.; et al. Measurement of NET formation in vitro and in vivo by flow cytometry. *Cytometry. A* **2017**, *91*, 822–829. [CrossRef] [PubMed]

34. Polke, M.; Leonhardt, I.; Kurzai, O.; Jacobsen, I.D. Farnesol signalling in *Candida albicans*–more than just communication. *Crit. Rev. Microbiol.* **2018**, *44*, 230–243. [CrossRef] [PubMed]

35. Shirtliff, M.E.; Peters, B.M.; Jabra-Rizk, M.A. Cross-kingdom interactions: *Candida albicans* and bacteria. *FEMS Microbiol. Lett.* **2009**, *299*, 1–8. [CrossRef] [PubMed]

36. Madhani, H.D. Quorum Sensing in Fungi: Q&A. *PLoS Pathog.* **2011**, *7*, e1002301.

37. Polke, M.; Jacobsen, I.D. Quorum sensing by farnesol revisited. *Curr. Genet.* **2017**, *63*, 791–797. [CrossRef]

38. Johnson, C.J.; Cabezas-Olcoz, J.; Kernien, J.F.; Wang, S.X.; Beebe, D.J.; Huttenlocher, A.; Ansari, H.; Nett, J.E. The Extracellular Matrix of *Candida albicans* Biofilms Impairs Formation of Neutrophil Extracellular Traps. *PLOS Pathog.* **2016**, *12*, e1005884. [CrossRef]

39. McCarty, T.P.; Pappas, P.G. Invasive Candidiasis. *Infect. Dis. Clin. North Am.* **2016**, *30*, 103–124. [CrossRef]

40. Hargarten, J.C.; Moore, T.C.; Petro, T.M.; Nickerson, K.W.; Atkin, A.L. *Candida albicans* quorum sensing molecules stimulate mouse macrophage migration. *Infect. Immun.* **2015**, *83*, 3857–3864. [CrossRef]

41. Skopelja-Gardner, S.; Theprungsirikul, J.; Lewis, K.A.; Hammond, J.H.; Carlson, K.M.; Hazlett, H.F.; Nymon, A.; Nguyen, D.; Berwin, B.L.; Hogan, D.A.; et al. Regulation of *Pseudomonas aeruginosa*-Mediated Neutrophil Extracellular Traps. *Front. Immunol.* **2019**, *10*, 1–13. [CrossRef] [PubMed]

42. Cremer, J.; Vatou, V.; Braveny, I. 2,4-(hydroxyphenyl)-ethanol, an antioxidative agent produced by *Candida* spp., impairs neutrophilic yeast killing in vitro. *FEMS Microbiol. Lett.* **1999**, *170*, 319–325. [CrossRef] [PubMed]

43. Gilbert, B.A.; Lim, Y.H.; Ding, J.; Badwey, J.A.; Rando, R.R. Farnesyl thiotriazole, a potent neutrophil agonist and structurally novel activator of protein kinase C. *Biochemistry* **1995**, *34*, 3916–3920. [CrossRef] [PubMed]

44. Gray, R.D.; Lucas, C.D.; Mackellar, A.; Li, F.; Hiersemenzel, K.; Haslett, C.; Davidson, D.J.; Rossi, A.G. Activation of conventional protein kinase C (PKC) is critical in the generation of human neutrophil extracellular traps. *J. Inflamm. (Lond).* **2013**, *10*, 12. [CrossRef] [PubMed]

45. Voziyan, P.A.; Haug, J.S.; Melnykovych, G. Mechanism of Farnesol Cytotoxicity: Further Evidence for the Role of PKC-Dependent Signal Transduction in Farnesol-Induced Apoptotic Cell Death. *Biochem. Biophys. Res. Commun.* **1995**, *212*, 479–486. [CrossRef] [PubMed]

46. Park, J.S.; Kwon, J.K.; Kim, H.R.; Kim, H.J.; Kim, B.S.; Jung, J.Y. Farnesol induces apoptosis of DU145 prostate cancer cells through the PI3K/Akt and MAPK pathways. *Int. J. Mol. Med.* **2014**, *33*, 1169–1176. [CrossRef] [PubMed]

47. Wang, Y.-L.; Liu, H.-F.; Shi, X.-J.; Wang, Y. Antiproliferative activity of Farnesol in HeLa cervical cancer cells is mediated via apoptosis induction, loss of mitochondrial membrane potential ($\Lambda\Psi$m) and PI3K/Akt signalling pathway. *J. BUON.* **2018**, *23*, 752–757.

48. Joo, J.H.; Liao, G.; Collins, J.B.; Grissom, S.F.; Jetten, A.M. Farnesol-Induced Apoptosis in Human Lung Carcinoma Cells Is Coupled to the Endoplasmic Reticulum Stress Response. *Cancer Res.* **2007**, *67*, 7929–7936. [CrossRef]

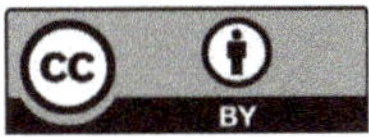

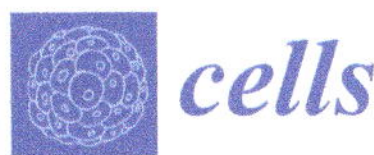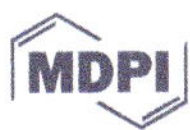

Perspective

Neutrophils and Neutrophil Extracellular Traps Drive Necroinflammation in COVID-19

Bhawna Tomar [1], Hans-Joachim Anders [2], Jyaysi Desai [3] and Shrikant R. Mulay [1,*]

[1]   Division of Pharmacology, CSIR-Central Drug Research Institute, Lucknow 226031, India;
      bhawnatomar415@gmail.com
[2]   Division of Nephrology, Department of Medicine IV University Hospital LMU, 80336 Munich, Germany;
      Hans-Joachim.Anders@med.uni-muenchen.de
[3]   Department of Rheumatology, Leiden University Medical Center, 2333 ZA Leiden, The Netherlands;
      jyaysidesai@gmail.com
*   Correspondence: shrikant.mulay@cdri.res.in

Received: 6 May 2020; Accepted: 30 May 2020; Published: 2 June 2020

Abstract: The COVID-19 pandemic is progressing worldwide with an alarming death toll. There is an urgent need for novel therapeutic strategies to combat potentially fatal complications. Distinctive clinical features of severe COVID-19 include acute respiratory distress syndrome, neutrophilia, and cytokine storm, along with severe inflammatory response syndrome or sepsis. Here, we propose the putative role of enhanced neutrophil infiltration and the release of neutrophil extracellular traps, complement activation and vascular thrombosis during necroinflammation in COVID-19. Furthermore, we discuss how neutrophilic inflammation contributes to the higher mortality of COVID-19 in patients with underlying co-morbidities such as diabetes and cardiovascular diseases. This perspective highlights neutrophils as a putative target for the immunopathologic complications of severely ill COVID-19 patients. Development of the novel therapeutic strategies targeting neutrophils may help reduce the overall disease fatality rate of COVID-19.

Keywords: SARS-CoV-2; coronavirus; neutrophils; NETs; complement; thrombosis; MERS-CoV; necroinflammation

---

1. Introduction

The novel severe acute respiratory syndrome coronavirus (SARS-CoV)-2 was first discovered in Wuhan, China, and believed to have transmitted from bats to humans [1]. The SARS-CoV-2 has higher human-to-human transmission capabilities compared to the SARS-CoV and Middle East respiratory syndrome coronavirus (MERS-CoV) and has resulted in a pandemic. The World Health Organization has named the disease COVID-19: coronavirus disease-2019; since it was first reported in December 2019. Although SARS-CoV-2 affects lungs at first, it can extend to many organs, including the heart, kidneys, gut, blood vessels, and the brain [2].

The SARS-CoV-2 is closely related to the SARS-CoV since they have 80% similarity in genome sequence and seven conserved non-structural domains identified by protein sequence analysis [3,4]. Moreover, they both have a similar receptor-binding domain, and therefore both use the same cell entry receptor, i.e. angiotensin-converting enzyme II (ACE2) [5]. Subsequently, viral replication in combination with the subsequent antiviral immune response both contribute to the severity of COVID-19, which in some patients involves cytokine storm followed by severe inflammatory response syndrome (SIRS), sepsis, multi-organ failure, and death [6]. However, little is known about the immune pathomechanisms that trigger the cytokine storm during COVID-19. We propose that as part of the first line of the innate immune defense, neutrophils are critical for the exacerbation of the immune response, and that neutrophil extracellular traps (NETs)-related necroinflammation plays a central role in the development of the cytokine storm, sepsis and multi-organ failure during COVID-19.

2. ACE2 and Neutrophils

ACE2, a homolog of ACE and central negative regulator of the renin-angiotensin system is a type 1 integral membrane glycoprotein monocarboxypeptidase that converts angiotensin-II (AngII) to Ang-(1–7) and is constitutively expressed by the epithelial cells of the lungs, kidney, heart, and intestines on the outer surface [5,7]. Ang-(1–7) is a vasodilator that mediates anti-inflammatory, anti-proliferative, and anti-fibrotic effects through the Mas receptor [8]. Using ACE2-mutant mice, Imai, et al. demonstrated protective functions of ACE2 in acute respiratory distress syndrome (ARDS) [7]. They observed that ACE2 negatively regulates AngII, and thus, increases vascular permeability, lung edema, and the infiltration of neutrophils, partially mediated by the angiotensin 1 receptor (AT1R) [7]. Interestingly, SARS-CoV-infected mice or mice receiving injections of SARS-CoV spike protein showed an aggravated phenotype compared to ACE2-mutant mice, suggesting the contribution of ACE2 beyond being a mere receptor for SARS-CoV [9]. Similar to SARS-CoV, upon binding to ACE2, SARS-CoV-2 enters cells along with ACE2 leading to reduced ACE2 expression on the cell surface [5]. Therefore, the loss of ACE2 might contribute to the severity of ARDS during COVID-19 by increasing AngII- and AT1R-mediated vascular permeability, lung edema, and neutrophils infiltration [10].

How does ACE2 regulate the infiltration of neutrophils mechanistically? Sodhi et al. demonstrated that attenuation of pulmonary ACE2 activity leads to activation of des-Arg9 bradykinin (DABK)/ bradykinin receptor B1 (BKB1R) axis, the release of pro-inflammatory chemokines e.g., C-X-C motif chemokine ligand 5 (CXCL5), macrophage inflammatory protein-2 (MIP2), CXCL1, and tumor necrosis factor (TNF)-α from airway epithelia, increased neutrophil infiltration, and exaggerated endotoxin-induced lung inflammation and injury [11]. The dynamic variation of pulmonary ACE2 was found essential to control neutrophilic inflammation, i.e., a balanced reduction of ACE2 while encountering a bacterial lung infection to recruit inflammatory neutrophils to combat the infection and later its recovery to restrict neutrophil accumulation to alleviate the inflammation by limiting interleukin (IL)-17 signaling by reducing STAT3 pathway activity [12]. Thus, ACE2 prevents the infiltration of neutrophils at the injury or infection site.

3. SARS-CoV-2, Neutrophils, and Necroinflammation in COVID-19

An increased neutrophil-to-lymphocyte ratio predicts severe illness in the early stage of SARS-CoV-2 infection, whereas neutrophilia frequently develops in COVID-19 patients in intensive care units [6,13–16]. Being part of the first line of innate immune defense, neutrophils have been thought to have protective roles during bacterial or fungal infections, where they kill bacteria or fungi by phagocytosis as well as NET formation [16]. However, their role in viral infections remains unclear. In murine SARS-CoV infection, neutrophils were dispensable for antibody-mediated clearance of SARS-CoV from pulmonary cells as well as the survival of SARS-CoV-infected mice [17,18]. On the other hand, continuous infiltration of neutrophils at the site of infection and their degranulation and release of NETs in response to microbial stimuli to raise an immune response produces exaggerated cytokines and chemokine that might result in the "cytokine storm" and contribute to the ARDS, SIRS and sepsis development during COVID-19 [6,14,19]. Higher levels of interleukin (IL)-1β, interferon-γ, CXCL10, monocyte chemoattractant protein-1, granulocyte colony-stimulating factor, monocyte inhibitory protein-1, and TNF-α were observed in COVID-19 patients requiring ICU admission [6,14]. A lung autopsy from a patient who succumbed to COVID-19 revealed an extensive neutrophil infiltration in pulmonary capillaries with extravasation into the alveolar space displaying acute capillaritis, as well as neutrophilic mucositis of the trachea indicating inflammation to the entire airway [20]. Moreover, SARS-CoV-2 infection of endothelial cells and the accumulation of inflammatory cells induced endothelitis in multiple organs, which may contribute to the systemic impaired microcirculatory function during COVID-19 [21] and to the phenomenon of the "happy hypoxia" [22].

The SARS-CoV accessory protein open reading frames SARS3a induced multimodal necrotic cell death in epithelial cells [23]. Interestingly, SARS3a is conserved in SARS-CoV-2 [4], suggesting the engagement of similar pathomechanisms during COVID-19. Cellular necrosis as well as NET formation results in the release of several intracellular danger-associated molecular patterns that activate the pattern recognition receptors on the surrounding immune and non-immune cells resulting in more production of inflammatory cytokines and chemokines [24]. The release of NETs disperses histones, DNA, and granule proteins, such as myeloperoxidase, neutrophil elastase, cathepsin G, and proteinase 3, which results in severe tissue destruction, setting up the auto-amplification loop of necroinflammation [24,25] (Figure 1).

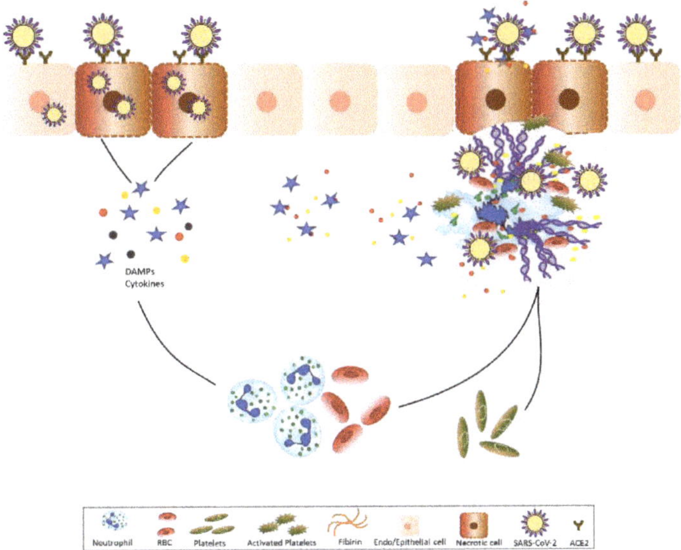

Figure 1. Neutrophils and neutrophil extracellular traps drive necroinflammation in COVID-19. The severe acute respiratory syndrome coronavirus-2 (SARS-CoV-2) binds to ACE2 and enter epithelial as well as endothelial cells along with it leading to reduced ACE2 expression that stimulates neutrophil recruitment. Subsequently, neutrophils undergo degranulation and NET formation releasing intracellular danger-associated molecular patterns, e.g., DNA, histones, neutrophil elastase that activate the pattern recognition receptors on surrounding immune and non-immune cells to induce cytokine secretion. The extracellular DNA released by NETs activates platelets and aggregated NETs provide a scaffold for binding of erythrocytes and activated platelets that promote thrombus formation. The extracellular histones present on NETs induce necrosis in epithelial or endothelial cells leading to the release of associated molecular patterns. This sets up an auto-amplification loop of necroinflammation that aggravate the disease severity during COVID-19. SARS-CoV-2 = severe acute respiratory syndrome coronavirus 2, ACE2 = angiotensin-converting enzyme 2, NET = neutrophil extracellular traps, DAMPs = danger-associated molecular patterns.

NETing neutrophils tend to form larger aggregates called "AggNETs" that drive the formation of thrombi in blood vessels [26]. Interestingly, high incidences of venous thrombosis are reported in COVID-19 [27]. The extracellular DNA released by NETs activates the platelets, and the AggNETs provide a scaffold for binding of the erythrocytes and activated platelets, which further promote the NET formation and set up a vicious cycle propagating thrombus formation [26]. NETs also activate the complement system. Myeloperoxidase, cathepsin G, and proteinase 3 activate properdin, factor B, and C3, three components of the alternative pathway required to induce the complement cascade [28]. Activated neutrophils also express properdin, factor B, and C3, suggesting an important role of neutrophils in complement activation. Of note, activation of the complement system has been reported in the severe COVID-19 patients [27]. Together, neutrophils infiltration and NETs formation drive necroinflammation during coronavirus infections (Table 1).

Table 1. Evidence for neutrophil-mediated necroinflammation in coronavirus infections.

Virus	Evidence for Involvement of Neutrophils	Reference
SARS-CoV-2	High levels of markers of NETs, e.g., cell free-DNA, myeloperoxidase-DNA, and citrullinated histone 3 in sera from severely ill patients	[19]
	High neutrophil-to-lymphocyte ratio cause ARDS in patients	[13,15,29]
	Neutrophil infiltration in pulmonary capillaries with extravasation into the alveolar space	[20]
	High neutrophil-to-lymphocyte ratio and D-dimer levels in patients	[30]
SARS-CoV	C3 mediated neutrophil recruitment during disease progression in mice	[31]
	Neutrophils infiltration in lungs during the late phase of infection in mice	[32]
	Neutrophils count correlate with the cytokine storm in patients	[33]
	Higher levels of neutrophil chemokine IL-8 found in patients	[34]
	Neutrophilia is associated with the severity of disease in patients	[35]
MERS-CoV	Neutrophil-mediated innate inflammatory response in human DPP4 knock-in mice	[36]
	Increased neutrophils contribute to leukocytosis, an indicator of disease severity and fatality in patients	[37]
	Increased release of ROS caused extensive pulmonary lesions and increased the disease severity in marmosets	[38]

SARS-CoV = severe acute respiratory syndrome coronavirus, MERS-CoV = Middle East respiratory syndrome coronavirus, NET = neutrophil extracellular trap, ARDS = acute respiratory distress syndrome, C3 = complement factor 3, ROS = reactive oxygen species.

4. Diabetes, SARS-CoV-2, and Neutrophils

Many prevalent co-morbidities increase the severity and mortality of COVID-19 [14,27,39–41]. One of the most distinctive co-morbidities is diabetes mellitus [6]. Out of 1099 cases reported by Guan et al., 16.2% of patients with severe disease had a higher prevalence of diabetes compared to 5.7% of patients with the non-severe disease [14]. Case fatality was higher in COVID patients with diabetes [42]. This may be attributed to the dysfunctional innate immunity, as well as the exaggerated pro-inflammatory cytokine response in patients with diabetes [43]. Furthermore, higher glucose levels glycosylate and shed ACE2 [44] may contribute to the severity of ARDS during COVID-19 by increasing vascular permeability, edema, and neutrophils infiltration in DM patients. On the other hand, it was believed that patients with diabetes treated with ACE inhibitors and angiotensin-receptor blockers may develop increased ACE2 expression, which could further facilitate the cell entry of SARS-CoV-2 and aggravate the infection [40]. However, a recent study reported no association with the likelihood of COVID-19 positive test or severity of COVID-19 with renin-angiotensin system inhibitors [45]. Hyperglycemia in diabetes primes neutrophils to release NETs that might further contribute to the cytokine storm, SIRS, and sepsis in COVID-19 [43]. Besides, sugar-activated neutrophils produce S100 Calcium-binding proteins A8/A9 (S100A8/A9) that increased the production of thrombopoietin in the liver and subsequent thrombocytosis [46], which might contribute to thrombus formation in COVID-19. Th17-associated cytokine production promoted disease-predictive inflammation in DM [47]. Interestingly, a higher number of CCR6+ TH17 cells were found in the peripheral blood of COVID-19 patients, suggesting critical involvement of TH17 response [48]. Together, neutrophil-mediated cytokine storm leads to sepsis and subsequent multi-organ failure to aggravate the severity of COVID-19 disease.

5. Cardiovascular Diseases, SARS-CoV-2, and Neutrophils

Cardiovascular diseases, including coronary heart disease, cardiomyopathy, arrhythmias, myocardial injury, and hypertension are other distinctive co-morbidities of COVID-19 that have higher overall mortality rates [14,42,49]. Especially, the extent of myocardial injury correlated with cardiac dysfunction, arrhythmias, and fatal outcome of COVID-19 [49]. ACE2 exerts vasodilatory effects through Ang-(1–7) and the Mas receptor [8]. Therefore downregulation of ACE2 upon SARS-CoV-2 cell entry induces vasoconstriction and subsequent hypertension. Subsequent ACE2-mediated neutrophil infiltration, as well as NET formation, might be responsible for the exaggerated inflammatory response, which in turn contributes to the development of cardiovascular diseases, e.g., thrombosis, atherosclerosis, and endothelial injury, etc. One in five hospitalized COVID-19 patients showed increased troponin, brain natriuretic peptide, lymphopenia, and inflammation markers, such as c-reactive protein, IL-1β, and IL-6 in the early course of the disease suggesting cardiac injury [49,50]. Recently, NET-related endothelial cell injury was reported to contribute to vascular pathology in pulmonary hypertension [39]. Moreover, IL-1β promoted the thrombus formation via NET-associated tissue factor during atheroembolic events during cardiovascular diseases [51,52]. Furthermore, increased neutrophil elastase activity was reported to contribute to obesity, insulin resistance, and related inflammation [53]. Interestingly, the presence of obesity in metabolic associated fatty liver disease increased the severity of COVID-19 six-fold [41]. All these reports indicate the involvement of neutrophils and related necroinflammation in the pathology and severity of COVID-19.

6. Summary and Perspectives

To summarize, neutrophils play a central role in the immunopathology of COVID-19. SARS-CoV-2 infection, as well as downregulation of ACE2 upon the cell entry of SARS-CoV-2 triggers neutrophil infiltration in the lungs. Necrotic cell death of alveolar epithelial cells, as well as NET formation, releases damage-associated molecular patterns and alarmins in the surrounding extracellular space, which induce production of pro-inflammatory cytokines and vice versa, setting up a loop of necroinflammation that is responsible for the cytokine storm and sepsis. NETting neutrophils cause endothelial injury and necroinflammation via complement activation, as well as promote the venous thrombus formation during COVID-19. Underlying co-morbidities in COVID-19 patients, e.g., diabetes and cardiovascular diseases enhance the neutrophilic inflammation and thereby severity of COVID-19. Therefore, the development of novel therapeutic strategies targeted at neutrophils, e.g., inhibitors of neutrophil recruitment or NET formation may help reduce the overall disease mortality rate of COVID-19.

Author Contributions: S.R.M. conceived the idea. B.T., H.-J.A., J.D., S.R.M. wrote the manuscript. All authors have read and agreed to the published version of the manuscript.

Funding: This research was funded by grants from the Department of Biotechnology, Government of India (BT/RLF/Re-entry/01/2017) and Council of Scientific and Industrial Research (CSIR), India to S.R.M. and the Deutsche Forschungsgemeinschaft (AN372/14-3, 23-1, and 24-1) to H.-J.A.

Acknowledgments: This manuscript has CDRI communication number 10074.

Conflicts of Interest: The authors declare no conflict of interest.

References

1. Zhou, P.; Yang, X.L.; Wang, X.G.; Hu, B.; Zhang, L.; Zhang, W.; Si, H.R.; Zhu, Y.; Li, B.; Huang, C.L.; et al. A pneumonia outbreak associated with a new coronavirus of probable bat origin. *Nature* **2020**, *579*, 270–273. [CrossRef] [PubMed]
2. Wadman, M.; Couzin-Frankel, J.; Kaiser, J.; Matacic, C. A rampage through the body. *Science* **2020**, *368*, 356–360. [PubMed]

3. Lu, R.; Zhao, X.; Li, J.; Niu, P.; Yang, B.; Wu, H.; Wang, W.; Song, H.; Huang, B.; Zhu, N.; et al. Genomic characterisation and epidemiology of 2019 novel coronavirus: Implications for virus origins and receptor binding. *Lancet* **2020**, *395*, 565–574. [CrossRef]

4. Wrapp, D.; Wang, N.; Corbett, K.S.; Goldsmith, J.A.; Hsieh, C.L.; Abiona, O.; Graham, B.S.; McLellan, J.S. Cryo-EM structure of the 2019-nCoV spike in the prefusion conformation. *Science* **2020**, *367*, 1260–1263. [CrossRef] [PubMed]

5. Hoffmann, M.; Kleine-Weber, H.; Schroeder, S.; Kruger, N.; Herrler, T.; Erichsen, S.; Schiergens, T.S.; Herrler, G.; Wu, N.H.; Nitsche, A.; et al. SARS-CoV-2 Cell Entry Depends on ACE2 and TMPRSS2 and Is Blocked by a Clinically Proven Protease Inhibitor. *Cell* **2020**, *181*, 271–280.e278. [CrossRef] [PubMed]

6. Huang, C.; Wang, Y.; Li, X.; Ren, L.; Zhao, J.; Hu, Y.; Zhang, L.; Fan, G.; Xu, J.; Gu, X.; et al. Clinical features of patients infected with 2019 novel coronavirus in Wuhan, China. *Lancet* **2020**, *395*, 497–506. [CrossRef]

7. Imai, Y.; Kuba, K.; Rao, S.; Huan, Y.; Guo, F.; Guan, B.; Yang, P.; Sarao, R.; Wada, T.; Leong-Poi, H.; et al. Angiotensin-converting enzyme 2 protects from severe acute lung failure. *Nature* **2005**, *436*, 112–116. [CrossRef]

8. Xu, J.; Fan, J.; Wu, F.; Huang, Q.; Guo, M.; Lv, Z.; Han, J.; Duan, L.; Hu, G.; Chen, L.; et al. The ACE2/Angiotensin-(1-7)/Mas Receptor Axis: Pleiotropic Roles in Cancer. *Front. Physiol.* **2017**, *8*, 276. [CrossRef]

9. Kuba, K.; Imai, Y.; Rao, S.; Gao, H.; Guo, F.; Guan, B.; Huan, Y.; Yang, P.; Zhang, Y.; Deng, W.; et al. A crucial role of angiotensin converting enzyme 2 (ACE2) in SARS coronavirus-induced lung injury. *Nat. Med.* **2005**, *11*, 875–879. [CrossRef]

10. Eguchi, S.; Kawai, T.; Scalia, R.; Rizzo, V. Understanding Angiotensin II Type 1 Receptor Signaling in Vascular Pathophysiology. *Hypertension* **2018**, *71*, 804–810. [CrossRef]

11. Sodhi, C.P.; Wohlford-Lenane, C.; Yamaguchi, Y.; Prindle, T.; Fulton, W.B.; Wang, S.; McCray, P.B., Jr.; Chappell, M.; Hackam, D.J.; Jia, H. Attenuation of pulmonary ACE2 activity impairs inactivation of des-Arg(9) bradykinin/BKB1R axis and facilitates LPS-induced neutrophil infiltration. *Am. J. Physiol. Lung Cell. Mol. Physiol.* **2018**, *314*, L17–L31. [CrossRef] [PubMed]

12. Sodhi, C.P.; Nguyen, J.; Yamaguchi, Y.; Werts, A.D.; Lu, P.; Ladd, M.R.; Fulton, W.B.; Kovler, M.L.; Wang, S.; Prindle, T., Jr.; et al. A Dynamic Variation of Pulmonary ACE2 Is Required to Modulate Neutrophilic Inflammation in Response to Pseudomonas aeruginosa Lung Infection in Mice. *J. Immunol.* **2019**, *203*, 3000–3012. [CrossRef] [PubMed]

13. Liu, Y.; Du, X.; Chen, J.; Jin, Y.; Peng, L.; Wang, H.H.X.; Luo, M.; Chen, L.; Zhao, Y. Neutrophil-to-lymphocyte ratio as an independent risk factor for mortality in hospitalized patients with COVID-19. *J. Infect.* **2020**. [CrossRef] [PubMed]

14. Guan, W.J.; Ni, Z.Y.; Hu, Y.; Liang, W.H.; Ou, C.Q.; He, J.X.; Liu, L.; Shan, H.; Lei, C.L.; Hui, D.S.C.; et al. Clinical Characteristics of Coronavirus Disease 2019 in China. *N. Engl. J. Med.* **2020**, *382*, 1708–1720. [CrossRef]

15. Lagunas-Rangel, F.A. Neutrophil-to-lymphocyte ratio and lymphocyte-to-C-reactive protein ratio in patients with severe coronavirus disease 2019 (COVID-19): A meta-analysis. *J. Med. Virol.* **2020**. [CrossRef]

16. Németh, T.; Sperandio, M.; Mócsai, A. Neutrophils as emerging therapeutic targets. *Nat. Rev. Drug Discov.* **2020**, *19*, 253–275. [CrossRef]

17. Yasui, F.; Kohara, M.; Kitabatake, M.; Nishiwaki, T.; Fujii, H.; Tateno, C.; Yoneda, M.; Morita, K.; Matsushima, K.; Koyasu, S.; et al. Phagocytic cells contribute to the antibody-mediated elimination of pulmonary-infected SARS coronavirus. *Virology* **2014**, *454–455*, 157–168. [CrossRef]

18. Channappanavar, R.; Fehr, A.R.; Vijay, R.; Mack, M.; Zhao, J.; Meyerholz, D.K.; Perlman, S. Dysregulated Type I Interferon and Inflammatory Monocyte-Macrophage Responses Cause Lethal Pneumonia in SARS-CoV-Infected Mice. *Cell Host Microbe* **2016**, *19*, 181–193. [CrossRef]

19. Zuo, Y.; Yalavarthi, S.; Shi, H.; Gockman, K.; Zuo, M.; Madison, J.A.; Blair, C.N.; Weber, A.; Barnes, B.J.; Egeblad, M.; et al. Neutrophil extracellular traps in COVID-19. *JCI Insight* **2020**. [CrossRef]

20. Barnes, B.J.; Adrover, J.M.; Baxter-Stoltzfus, A.; Borczuk, A.; Cools-Lartigue, J.; Crawford, J.M.; Daßler-Plenker, J.; Guerci, P.; Huynh, C.; Knight, J.S.; et al. Targeting potential drivers of COVID-19: Neutrophil extracellular traps. *J. Exp. Med.* **2020**, *217*, e20200652. [CrossRef]

21. Varga, Z.; Flammer, A.J.; Steiger, P.; Haberecker, M.; Andermatt, R.; Zinkernagel, A.S.; Mehra, M.R.; Schuepbach, R.A.; Ruschitzka, F.; Moch, H. Endothelial cell infection and endotheliitis in COVID-19. *Lancet* **2020**, *395*, 1417–1418. [CrossRef]

22. Couzin-Frankel, J. The mystery of the pandemic's 'happy hypoxia'. *Science* **2020**, *368*, 455–456. [CrossRef]

23. Yue, Y.; Nabar, N.R.; Shi, C.S.; Kamenyeva, O.; Xiao, X.; Hwang, I.Y.; Wang, M.; Kehrl, J.H. SARS-Coronavirus Open Reading Frame-3a drives multimodal necrotic cell death. *Cell Death Dis.* **2018**, *9*, 904. [CrossRef]

24. Linkermann, A.; Stockwell, B.R.; Krautwald, S.; Anders, H.J. Regulated cell death and inflammation: An auto-amplification loop causes organ failure. *Nat. Rev. Immunol.* **2014**, *14*, 759–767. [CrossRef]

25. Mulay, S.R.; Linkermann, A.; Anders, H.J. Necroinflammation in Kidney Disease. *J. Am. Soc. Nephrol.* **2016**, *27*, 27–39. [CrossRef]

26. Nakazawa, D.; Desai, J.; Steiger, S.; Müller, S.; Devarapu, S.K.; Mulay, S.R.; Iwakura, T.; Anders, H.J. Activated platelets induce MLKL-driven neutrophil necroptosis and release of neutrophil extracellular traps in venous thrombosis. *Cell Death Discov.* **2018**, *4*, 6. [CrossRef]

27. Llitjos, J.F.; Leclerc, M.; Chochois, C.; Monsallier, J.M.; Ramakers, M.; Auvray, M.; Merouani, K. High incidence of venous thromboembolic events in anticoagulated severe COVID-19 patients. *J. Thromb. Haemost.* **2020**. [CrossRef]

28. de Bont, C.M.; Boelens, W.C.; Pruijn, G.J.M. NETosis, complement, and coagulation: A triangular relationship. *Cell. Mol. Immunol.* **2019**, *16*, 19–27. [CrossRef]

29. Liu, J.; Liu, Y.; Xiang, P.; Pu, L.; Xiong, H.; Li, C.; Zhang, M.; Tan, J.; Xu, Y.; Song, R.; et al. Neutrophil-to-lymphocyte ratio predicts critical illness patients with 2019 coronavirus disease in the early stage. *J. Transl. Med.* **2020**, *18*, 206. [CrossRef]

30. Fu, J.; Kong, J.; Wang, W.; Wu, M.; Yao, L.; Wang, Z.; Jin, J.; Wu, D.; Yu, X. The clinical implication of dynamic neutrophil to lymphocyte ratio and D-dimer in COVID-19: A retrospective study in Suzhou China. *Thromb. Res.* **2020**, *192*, 3–8. [CrossRef]

31. Gralinski, L.E.; Sheahan, T.P.; Morrison, T.E.; Menachery, V.D.; Jensen, K.; Leist, S.R.; Whitmore, A.; Heise, M.T.; Baric, R.S. Complement Activation Contributes to Severe Acute Respiratory Syndrome Coronavirus Pathogenesis. *mBio* **2018**, *9*, e01753-18. [CrossRef] [PubMed]

32. Chen, J.; Lau, Y.F.; Lamirande, E.W.; Paddock, C.D.; Bartlett, J.H.; Zaki, S.R.; Subbarao, K. Cellular immune responses to severe acute respiratory syndrome coronavirus (SARS-CoV) infection in senescent BALB/c mice: CD4+ T cells are important in control of SARS-CoV infection. *J. Virol.* **2010**, *84*, 1289–1301. [CrossRef] [PubMed]

33. Huang, K.J.; Su, I.J.; Theron, M.; Wu, Y.C.; Lai, S.K.; Liu, C.C.; Lei, H.Y. An interferon-gamma-related cytokine storm in SARS patients. *J. Med. Virol.* **2005**, *75*, 185–194. [CrossRef] [PubMed]

34. Wong, C.K.; Lam, C.W.; Wu, A.K.; Ip, W.K.; Lee, N.L.; Chan, I.H.; Lit, L.C.; Hui, D.S.; Chan, M.H.; Chung, S.S.; et al. Plasma inflammatory cytokines and chemokines in severe acute respiratory syndrome. *Clin. Exp. Immunol.* **2004**, *136*, 95–103. [CrossRef]

35. Wong, R.S.; Wu, A.; To, K.F.; Lee, N.; Lam, C.W.; Wong, C.K.; Chan, P.K.; Ng, M.H.; Yu, L.M.; Hui, D.S.; et al. Haematological manifestations in patients with severe acute respiratory syndrome: Retrospective analysis. *BMJ* **2003**, *326*, 1358–1362. [CrossRef]

36. Li, K.; Wohlford-Lenane, C.L.; Channappanavar, R.; Park, J.E.; Earnest, J.T.; Bair, T.B.; Bates, A.M.; Brogden, K.A.; Flaherty, H.A.; Gallagher, T.; et al. Mouse-adapted MERS coronavirus causes lethal lung disease in human DPP4 knockin mice. *Proc. Natl. Acad. Sci. USA* **2017**, *114*, 3119–3128. [CrossRef]

37. Min, C.K.; Cheon, S.; Ha, N.Y.; Sohn, K.M.; Kim, Y.; Aigerim, A.; Shin, H.M.; Choi, J.Y.; Inn, K.S.; Kim, J.H.; et al. Comparative and kinetic analysis of viral shedding and immunological responses in MERS patients representing a broad spectrum of disease severity. *Sci. Rep.* **2016**, *6*, 25359. [CrossRef]

38. Baseler, L.J.; Falzarano, D.; Scott, D.P.; Rosenke, R.; Thomas, T.; Munster, V.J.; Feldmann, H.; de Wit, E. An Acute Immune Response to Middle East Respiratory Syndrome Coronavirus Replication Contributes to Viral Pathogenicity. *Am. J. Pathol.* **2016**, *186*, 630–638. [CrossRef]

39. Aldabbous, L.; Abdul-Salam, V.; McKinnon, T.; Duluc, L.; Pepke-Zaba, J.; Southwood, M.; Ainscough, A.J.; Hadinnapola, C.; Wilkins, M.R.; Toshner, M.; et al. Neutrophil Extracellular Traps Promote Angiogenesis: Evidence From Vascular Pathology in Pulmonary Hypertension. *Arterioscler. Thromb. Vasc. Biol.* **2016**, *36*, 2078–2087. [CrossRef]

40. Fang, L.; Karakiulakis, G.; Roth, M. Are patients with hypertension and diabetes mellitus at increased risk for COVID-19 infection? *Lancet. Respir. Med.* **2020**, *8*, e21. [CrossRef]

41. Zheng, K.I.; Gao, F.; Wang, X.B.; Sun, Q.F.; Pan, K.H.; Wang, T.Y.; Ma, H.L.; Liu, W.Y.; George, J.; Zheng, M.H. Obesity as a risk factor for greater severity of COVID-19 in patients with metabolic associated fatty liver disease. *Metabolism* **2020**, 154244. [CrossRef] [PubMed]

42. Wu, Z.; McGoogan, J.M. Characteristics of and Important Lessons From the Coronavirus Disease 2019 (COVID-19) Outbreak in China: Summary of a Report of 72 314 Cases From the Chinese Center for Disease Control and Prevention. *Jama* **2020**. [CrossRef] [PubMed]

43. Wong, S.L.; Demers, M.; Martinod, K.; Gallant, M.; Wang, Y.; Goldfine, A.B.; Kahn, C.R.; Wagner, D.D. Diabetes primes neutrophils to undergo NETosis, which impairs wound healing. *Nat. Med.* **2015**, *21*, 815–819. [CrossRef]

44. Salem, E.S.; Grobe, N.; Elased, K.M. Insulin treatment attenuates renal ADAM17 and ACE2 shedding in diabetic Akita mice. *Am. J. Physiol. Renal. Physiol.* **2014**, *306*, F629–F639. [CrossRef]

45. Reynolds, H.R.; Adhikari, S.; Pulgarin, C.; Troxel, A.B.; Iturrate, E.; Johnson, S.B.; Hausvater, A.; Newman, J.D.; Berger, J.S.; Bangalore, S.; et al. Renin-Angiotensin-Aldosterone System Inhibitors and Risk of Covid-19. *N. Engl. J. Med.* **2020**. [CrossRef]

46. Kraakman, M.J.; Lee, M.K.; Al-Sharea, A.; Dragoljevic, D.; Barrett, T.J.; Montenont, E.; Basu, D.; Heywood, S.; Kammoun, H.L.; Flynn, M.; et al. Neutrophil-derived S100 calcium-binding proteins A8/A9 promote reticulated thrombocytosis and atherogenesis in diabetes. *J. Clin. Investig.* **2017**, *127*, 2133–2147. [CrossRef]

47. Nicholas, D.A.; Proctor, E.A.; Agrawal, M.; Belkina, A.C.; Van Nostrand, S.C.; Panneerseelan-Bharath, L.; Jones, A.R.t.; Raval, F.; Ip, B.C.; Zhu, M.; et al. Fatty Acid Metabolites Combine with Reduced β Oxidation to Activate Th17 Inflammation in Human Type 2 Diabetes. *Cell Metab.* **2019**, *30*, 447–461. [CrossRef]

48. Wu, D.; Yang, X.O. TH17 responses in cytokine storm of COVID-19: An emerging target of JAK2 inhibitor Fedratinib. *J. Microbiol. Immunol. Infect.* **2020**. [CrossRef]

49. Guo, T.; Fan, Y.; Chen, M.; Wu, X.; Zhang, L.; He, T.; Wang, H.; Wan, J.; Wang, X.; Lu, Z. Cardiovascular Implications of Fatal Outcomes of Patients With Coronavirus Disease 2019 (COVID-19). *JAMA Cardiol.* **2020**. [CrossRef]

50. Chapman, A.R.; Bularga, A.; Mills, N.L. High-Sensitivity Cardiac Troponin Can Be an Ally in the Fight Against COVID-19. *Circulation* **2020**, *141*, 1733–1735. [CrossRef]

51. Yadav, V.; Chi, L.; Zhao, R.; Tourdot, B.E.; Yalavarthi, S.; Jacobs, B.N.; Banka, A.; Liao, H.; Koonse, S.; Anyanwu, A.C.; et al. Ectonucleotidase tri(di)phosphohydrolase-1 (ENTPD-1) disrupts inflammasome/ interleukin 1beta-driven venous thrombosis. *J. Clin. Investig.* **2019**, *129*, 2872–2877. [CrossRef]

52. Liberale, L.; Holy, E.W.; Akhmedov, A.; Bonetti, N.R.; Nietlispach, F.; Matter, C.M.; Mach, F.; Montecucco, F.; Beer, J.H.; Paneni, F.; et al. Interleukin-1beta Mediates Arterial Thrombus Formation via NET-Associated Tissue Factor. *J. Clin. Med.* **2019**, *8*, 2072. [CrossRef]

53. Mansuy-Aubert, V.; Zhou, Q.L.; Xie, X.; Gong, Z.; Huang, J.Y.; Khan, A.R.; Aubert, G.; Candelaria, K.; Thomas, S.; Shin, D.J.; et al. Imbalance between neutrophil elastase and its inhibitor α1-antitrypsin in obesity alters insulin sensitivity, inflammation, and energy expenditure. *Cell Metab.* **2013**, *17*, 534–548. [CrossRef]

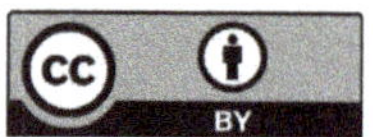

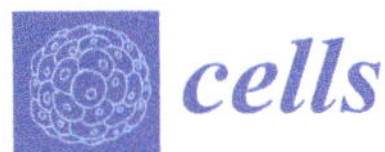 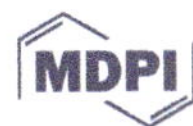

Article

Neutrophil Extracellular Traps in the Pathogenesis of Equine Recurrent Uveitis (ERU)

Leonie Fingerhut [1,2,3], Bernhard Ohnesorge [3], Myriam von Borstel [4], Ariane Schumski [1], Katrin Strutzberg-Minder [5], Matthias Mörgelin [6], Cornelia A. Deeg [7], Henk P. Haagsman [8], Andreas Beineke [9], Maren von Köckritz-Blickwede [1,2,*] and Nicole de Buhr [1,2,*]

[1] Department of Physiological Chemistry, University of Veterinary Medicine Hannover, Bünteweg 17, D-30559 Hannover, Germany; leonie.fingerhut@tiho-hannover.de (L.F.); Ariane.Schumski@med.uni-muenchen.de (A.S.)
[2] Research Center for Emerging Infections and Zoonoses (RIZ), University of Veterinary Medicine Hannover, Bünteweg 17, D-30559 Hannover, Germany
[3] Clinic for Horses, University of Veterinary Medicine Hannover, Bünteweg 9, D-30559 Hannover, Germany; bernhard.ohnesorge@tiho-hannover.de
[4] Tierärztliche Gemeinschaftspraxis für Pferde Wedemark, Lange Loh 15, D-30900 Wedemark, Germany; info@pferdepraxis-wedemark.de
[5] IVD Gesellschaft für Innovative Veterinärdiagnostik mbH (IVD GmbH), Albert-Einstein-Str. 5, D-30926 Seelze, Germany; strutzberg@ivd-gmbh.de
[6] Colzyx AB, Medicon Village, SE-223 81 Lund, Sweden; matthias@colzyx.com
[7] Chair of Animal Physiology, Department of Veterinary Sciences, LMU Munich, Lena Christ Str. 48, D-82152 Martinsried, Germany; Cornelia.Deeg@lmu.de
[8] Department of Infectious Diseases & Immunology, Faculty of Veterinary Medicine, Utrecht University, Yalelaan 1, 3584 CL Utrecht, The Netherlands; H.P.Haagsman@uu.nl
[9] Department of Pathology, University of Veterinary Medicine Hannover, Bünteweg 17, D-30559 Hannover, Germany; andreas.beineke@tiho-hannover.de
* Correspondence: maren.von.koeckritz-blickwede@tiho-hannover.de (M.v.K.-B.); nicole.de.buhr@tiho-hannover.de (N.d.B.); Tel.: +49-511-953-6119 (N.d.B.)

Received: 27 October 2019; Accepted: 22 November 2019; Published: 27 November 2019

Abstract: Equine recurrent uveitis (ERU) is considered one of the most important eye diseases in horses and typically appears with relapsing inflammatory episodes without systemic effects. Various disorders have been described as an initial trigger, including infections. Independent of the initiating cause, there are numerous indications that ERU is an immune-mediated disease. We investigated whether neutrophil extracellular traps (NETs) are part of the ERU pathogenesis. Therefore, vitreous body fluids (VBF), sera, and histological sections of the eye from ERU-diseased horses were analyzed for the presence of NET markers and compared with horses with healthy eyes. In addition, NET formation by blood derived neutrophils was investigated in the presence of VBF derived from horses with healthy eyes versus ERU-diseased horses using immunofluorescence microscopy. Interestingly, NET markers like free DNA, histone-complexes, and myeloperoxidase were detected in higher amounts in samples from ERU-diseased horses. Furthermore, in vitro NET formation was higher in neutrophils incubated with VBF from diseased horses compared with those animals with healthy eyes. Finally, we characterized the ability of equine cathelicidins to induce NETs, as potential NET inducing factors in ERU-diseased horses. In summary, our findings lead to the hypothesis that ERU-diseased horses develop more NETs and that these may contribute to the pathogenesis of ERU.

Keywords: NETs; equine recurrent uveitis; horse; cathelicidin

1. Introduction

Equine recurrent uveitis (ERU) is considered one of the most important eye diseases in horses, affecting between 2 and 25 percent of animals [1–4]. Common clinical findings include corneal haze, aqueous flare, pupil miosis, and opacified vitreous body fluid (VBF) with deposits. This serofibrinous and lymphoplasmacellular inflammation often results in chronic alterations such as synechiae, cataracts, lens luxation, retinal detachment, and phthisis bulbi [5–7]. Eventually, the cumulative degeneration of ocular structures can lead to blindness. Thus, a diagnosis can be made when a horse is presented with relapsing uveitic findings without systemic effects. This disease can be divided into three different types, the most typical in Europe being the posterior form affecting predominantly vitreous body, retina, and choroid [7]. The initial cause of the uveitis remains obscure, but genetic and autoimmune components were found [8–10]. In a genome-wide association study, a single nucleotide polymorphism on chromosome 20 was discovered to be associated with ERU [11]. Additionally, *Leptospira* spp. can be detected in about 60 percent of the patients [12–15]. Whether those pathogens cause the destruction of the blood-retina barrier or the barrier is destroyed first, thus enabling pathogens to enter the immune-privileged organ, is under discussion [16]. The treatment options range from immunosuppressive medication to different surgical procedures, for instance, vitrectomy. Hereby, vitreous body fluid is exchanged in a minimally invasive way by buffered salt solution with or without antibiotics.

As autoimmune processes are discussed as being part of ERU, it is of interest that a defense mechanism of neutrophils, neutrophil extracellular traps (NETs) formation, is described as being involved in autoimmune diseases [17–19]. Besides phagocytosis and degranulation, NET formation is another strategy of neutrophils against invading pathogens, also referred to as NETosis [20]. NET formation was explained mainly by two different mechanisms [21–24]. The 'suicidal' NETosis is a synonym for the lytic NET release, leading to dead neutrophils after several hours. The 'vital' NETosis is characterized by the rapid release of NETs, and neutrophils undergoing this mechanism are still able to phagocyte or degranulate [25]. NET release by viable cells is mediated by a vesicular mechanism and reactive oxygen independent [23]. Furthermore, NET release by viable cells in the form of mitochondrial DNA has been described. NETs, independent of the mechanism, consist of decondensed chromatin, histones, antimicrobial peptides (AMPs), and granule proteins [21,22]. The contained AMPs play an important role in the formation and antimicrobial function of NETs. These components build web-like structures to entrap and kill microbes [21]. Host nucleases are crucial for maintaining the balance between NET formation and elimination, and hence for preventing accumulation of NETs [26]. On the other hand, a detrimental role of NETs has been detected in non-infectious conditions, such as autoimmune or chronic diseases, thrombosis, and cancer. For instance, NETs contribute to the pathogenesis of systemic lupus erythematosus, psoriasis, or rheumatoid arthritis by autoantigen exposition [18,27,28]. Moreover, the involvement of NETs and associated proteins in bacterial keratitis owing to *Pseudomonas aeruginosa* ocular biofilms and in the ocular graft-versus-host disease dry eye in humans, with both diseases affecting the ocular surface, has been proven [29,30]. Barliya et al. [31] demonstrated intraocular NET induction through cytokines, namely interleukin-8 (IL-8) and tumor necrosis factor α (TNF-α), in a murine model. Furthermore, they showed the occurrence of NETs in human vitreous body fluid and other ocular components in proliferative diabetic retinopathy, to a higher extent in more severe cases [31]. The existence of NETs in VBF of such patients, as well as in diabetic rats, has recently been confirmed by Wang et al. [32]. Whether NETs contribute to the pathogenesis of ERU has not yet been investigated.

Thus, it seems obvious to assume a potential role of NETs or the associated AMPs in the pathogenesis of ERU. Interestingly, the closest genes to the single nucleotide polymorphism found to be linked with ERU are IL-17A and IL-17F [11]. This proinflammatory family of cytokines was recently reported to modulate NET formation and AMP production [27,33]. Furthermore, IL-17 occurs with an elevated tissue expression in human autoimmune uveitis [34]. Chen et al. [35] suggest an inductive effect of IL-17 on the expression of the human cathelicidin LL-37. Cathelicidins are a subtype of AMPs and three different sequences can be found in equine bone marrow RNA, referred to as eCATH 1-3. However, only two pro-peptides are cleaved inside neutrophils into the mature peptides eCATH 2 and 3 [36].

The aim of this study was to first clarify the appearance of NETs during ERU, as well as the involvement of associated AMPs in the pathogenesis of this commonly occurring disease. The focus within the AMPs was on the equine cathelicidins owing to their possible connection to IL-17 and the genetic components of ERU.

2. Materials and Methods

2.1. Samples

In the conducted experiments, samples from two different clinics were analyzed. In study part I, serum samples obtained in Munich, Germany, were investigated in quantitative measurements of free DNA and nuclease activity, comparing healthy eyes of horses with those of ERU-diseased horses (Figure 1). Furthermore, these serum samples were used in an ELISA for equine cathelicidins (Figure A2a). All other experiments (study part II) were performed using vitreous body fluid (VBF) and blood samples for neutrophil isolation from Hannover, Germany.

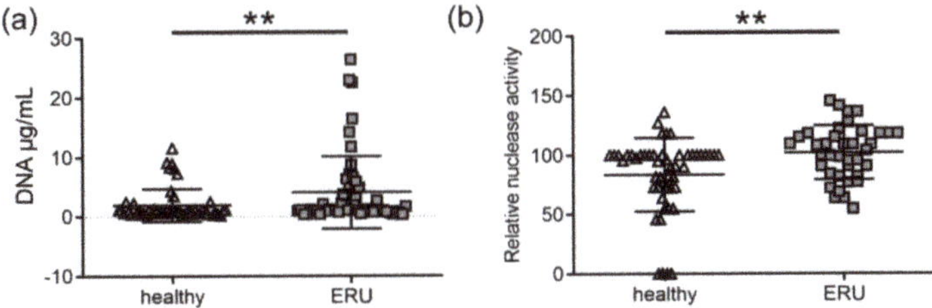

Figure 1. Free extracellular DNA and relative nuclease activity in serum. The amounts of free extracellular DNA (**a**) and relative nuclease activity (**b**) were analyzed in serum from 52 equine recurrent uveitis (ERU) patients and 51 eye-healthy control animals (study part I, Munich). In (**a**), a Pico Green assay was used. Significantly more free DNA was detected in the ERU serum compared with the control serum. In (**b**), the relative nuclease activity was calculated to a control digestion with DNase I. The individual values and the mean value of the respective groups are given. In the ERU serum, a significantly higher nuclease activity was observed compared with the control serum. In (**a,b**) the individual values and the mean value ± SD of the respective groups are shown (** $p < 0.01$, two-tailed Mann–Whitney test).

2.1.1. Study Part I (Munich)

The serum samples included in the analysis of free DNA and nuclease activity were obtained from horses vitrectomized owing to diagnosis of ERU at the Equine Hospital of the Faculty of Veterinary Medicine, LMU Munich in Munich, Germany, until 2012. The control samples were taken from those animals with healthy eyes. The study protocol for obtaining blood samples from ERU cases in the quiescent stage of the disease and controls (both obtained from the Equine Clinic, LMU Munich) was permitted by the Ethical Committee of Upper Bavaria's Regional Government (Regierung von Oberbayern; permit number: ROB-55.2Vet-2532.Vet_03-17-88). All experiments were performed in accordance with the relevant guidelines and regulations. The samples were stored at −20 °C until further analysis.

2.1.2. Study Part II (Hannover)

Blood Samples for Neutrophil Isolation

Blood collection from healthy horses was approved by Lower Saxony State Office for Consumer Protection and Food Safety (LAVES) (Niedersächsisches Landesamt für Verbraucherschutz und Lebensmittelsicherheit) under nos. 12A243 and 18A302 for study part II. Fresh equine neutrophils were isolated from these lithium-heparinized blood samples.

VBF Samples Obtained from Vitrectomy Patients and Healthy Horses

The VBF samples of ERU-diseased horses included in the NET induction assay, ELISA to detect equine cathelicidins, and electron microscopy evaluation were obtained from horses vitrectomized between 2016 and 2018 at the Clinic for Horses of the University of Veterinary Medicine Hannover, Germany. The pre-examinations, treatment, and surgical procedure were performed as previously published by von Borstel et al. and Baake et al. [6,37]. Remnant VBF samples from diagnostic procedures were used in this study. The control samples were derived post mortem from horses without ophthalmologic findings indicating ERU, which had been euthanized because of other reasons between 2016 and 2017. The euthanasia of these horses had been approved and registered by the local Animal Welfare Officer in accordance with the German Animal Welfare Law under number TiHo-T-2016-4. The eyes from these horses were enucleated and freed from the surrounding tissues, and VBF was extracted with a 5 mL syringe through a cross-opening cut into the eye. These patients are described in more detail in Table A1. Signalment and clinical data were obtained from the medical records.

The samples of ERU-diseased horses were chosen randomly from a collection of samples taken between 2016 and 2019. Inclusion criteria were a positive microscopic agglutination test (MAT) for intraocular leptospiral antibodies and a positive result of a polymerase chain reaction (PCR) detecting leptospiral DNA. This analysis is routinely conducted in VBF that is completely exchanged and collected in all ERU-diseased horses during vitrectomy. The VBF of included control horses was analyzed in a similar manner and VBF was included if negative MAT and PCR results were found. The samples were stored at −80 °C until further analysis. MAT and PCR were conducted at IVD GmbH, Seelze, Germany.

Samples Obtained from Enucleations

The paraffin sections and vitreous body fluid for NET detection ex vivo and in situ were received from eyes that had been enucleated at the Clinic for Horses of the University of Veterinary Medicine Hannover, Germany, in 2019 as part of curative surgery. A description of signalment, pathological findings, and the results of the screening for *Leptospira* by MAT and PCR are displayed in Table A2. Signalment and clinical data were obtained from the medical records. The eyes were freed from the surrounding tissues and 1-5 mL VBF was extracted with a 5 mL syringe through a cross-opening cut into the eye. VBF was immediately put on slides (8 mm, Thermo Fisher, Waltham, MA, USA CB00080RA120) coated beforehand with 0.01% poly-L-lysine (Sigma-Aldrich, St. Louis, MO, USA P4707) for 20 min. They were then centrifuged for five minutes at 370 g at room temperature and afterwards fixated with paraformaldehyde (Science Services E15710-250) to a final concentration of 4%. To fixate the eye, it was flushed first with phosphate-buffered formalin (10%, 3×5 mL) by injection through a needle (21G, WDT 07391) at the opposite side of the first insertion and then put in formalin and fixed for two to four days. Samples were dehydrated in a graded series of ethanol and embedded via xylene in paraffin wax and cut into 4 μm sections with a microtome. Slides were deparaffinised and hydrated through descending concentrations of ethanol. Afterwards, sections were stained with hematoxylin-eosin (HE, hemalaun according to Delafield) following a routine protocol. Histology slices were examined with a standard light microscope.

2.2. Pico Green Assay

The amount of free DNA in serum of horses with healthy eyes and ERU-diseased horses was evaluated by a Pico Green assay using a plate reader (FLUOStar, Optima) in study part I. Therefore, 1:200 in Tris-EDTA buffer solution (TE) diluted PicoGreen (Quant-iT PicoGreen Invitrogen, Carlsbad, CA, USA P11496) was mixed 1:2 with serum in a 96 black flat bottom well plate (BRANDplates® 781608). A dilution series of calf thymus DNA (Sigma-Aldrich D3664, 1 mg/mL) was used for a standard curve. The plate was measured after a five minute incubation period at room temperature in the dark.

2.3. Nuclease Activity Assay

2.3.1. Quantitative Measurement

The nuclease activity in serum was examined in study part I by mixing 7.5 µg of calf thymus DNA (Sigma-Aldrich D3664, 1 mg/mL) with 10 µL serum and 40 µL Tris. Respective controls were included in each run. As negative control of 7.5 µg of calf thymus DNA was mixed with 50 µL Tris, as positive control of 7.5 µg of calf thymus DNA was mixed with 40 µL Tris and 10 µL DNaseI (2 U/mL). Samples were incubated for six hours at 37 °C. Afterwards, intact DNA was precipitated with phenol-chloroform. The DNA was visualized on 1% agarose gel containing Roti®-GelStain (Carl Roth 3865.1) by gel electrophoresis. The relative nuclease activity was determined by comparison with a standard row of nuclease activity (DNaseI 0, 0.015, 0.03, 0.06, 0.125, 0.25, 0.5, and 1 U/mL, respectively).

2.3.2. Qualitative Measurement

The nuclease activity in serum and VBF of healthy controls and ERU patients were examined in study part II by mixing 0.5 µg of calf thymus DNA (Sigma-Aldrich D3664, 1 mg/mL) with 50 µL of the sample (serum or VBF). This was then incubated at 37 °C for 20 h. Afterwards, 1% agarose gel electrophoresis was conducted with DNA staining with Roti®-GelStain (Carl Roth 3865.1). A 1 kb marker (Invitrogen 1 kb Plus DNA Ladder 10787-018, 1 µg/µL), as well as a negative and positive control with Hank's Balanced Salt Solution (GIBCO®HBSS 14025050) and 0.5 µg calf thymus DNA, with or without 0.5 µL micrococcal nuclease (Sigma-Aldrich N5386, 1 Units/µL), were added.

2.4. PMN Isolation

In study part II, fresh equine neutrophils were isolated from lithium-heparinized blood using Biocoll density gradient and lysis of erythrocytes. All steps were performed in duplicate. Thereby, the blood was diluted 2.5:1 in phosphate-buffered saline (Sigma-Aldrich P5493-1L, 10× PBS diluted in endotoxin-free water to 1× concentrated), layered onto the Biocoll (Biochrom AG L6115, 1.077 g/mL), and then centrifuged for 20 min at 400 *g* at room temperature without using a centrifuge brake. Afterwards, the supernatant was removed and cold endotoxin-free 0.2% NaCl-solution was added to the sediment for 30 s and carefully inverted. The lysis of the erythrocytes was then stopped by adding cold endotoxin-free 1.6% NaCl-solution. This was then centrifuged at 250 *g* for six minutes at 4 °C. The lysis step was repeated once or twice depending on the clarity of the obtained pellet. The two pellets were finally pooled and resuspended in cold Roswell Park Memorial Institute medium (RPMI, gibco 11835063).

2.5. NET Induction

Within study part II, fresh isolated blood-derived equine neutrophils were seeded in a concentration of 2×10^6 cells mL^{-1} (2×10^5 cells per well) on slides (8 mm, Thermo Fisher CB00080RA120), which had previously been coated for 20 min with 0.01% poly-L-lysine (Sigma-Aldrich P4707). Then, 100 µL stimulus was added to each well and incubated for 240 min at 37 °C with 5% CO_2. The well plate was then centrifuged for five minutes with 370 g at room temperature and, afterwards, the samples were fixated with paraformaldehyde (Science Services E15710-250, final concentration of 3.2%) and stored at 4 °C. The examined stimuli included the equine cathelicidins (eCATH 1, eCATH 2, eCATH 3 [38]), each in a 5 µM and 10 µM concentration, in different environments. The first set-up analyzed the equine cathelicidins in the presence of RPMI (gibco 11835063), using RPMI alone as a negative control and methyl-β-cyclodextrin (Sigma-Aldrich C4555-1G, final 10 mM) diluted in RPMI as a positive control. The next five independent experiments were conducted in the presence of VBF from the control horses with healthy eyes, with an additional control of VBF alone. The methyl-β-cyclodextrin was hereby diluted in VBF. A set-up of seven independent experiments using VBF obtained from ERU patients was also performed.

2.6. Immunofluorescence Staining of NETs

The samples in study part II were permeabilized for five minutes with Triton X-100 (Sigma-Aldrich T8787-50ML) for the co-staining of DNA/histone-1 and myeloperoxidase as NET markers. Then, they were blocked for 20 min with 3% normal donkey serum (Sigma-Aldrich D9663-10ML), 3% cold water fish gelatine (Sigma-Aldrich G7041-100G), 1% bovine serum albumin (Albumin fraction V, Roth 2923225), and 0.05% Tween20 (Roth 9127.2) in 1× phosphate-buffered saline (PBS, Sigma-Aldrich P5493-1l, 10× PBS diluted to 1× PBS in distilled water). Afterwards, the samples were incubated for one hour with a monoclonal mouse anti-DNA/histone-1 antibody (Millipore, Burlington, MA, USA MAB3864, 0.55 mg/mL) diluted 1:1000 in blocking buffer and a rabbit anti-human myeloperoxidase antibody (Dako A0398, 3.2 mg/mL) diluted 1:300 in blocking buffer. Isotype controls were incubated with an IgG2α antibody from murine myeloma (Sigma-Aldrich M5409-.1MG, 0.2 mg/mL) diluted 1:364 in blocking buffer and IgG from rabbit serum (Sigma-Aldrich I5006, 10.4 mg/mL) diluted 1:975 in blocking buffer. After washing, a goat anti-mouse DyLight 488 antibody (Thermo Scientific 35503, 1 mg/mL) diluted 1:1000 and a goat anti-rabbit Alexa 633 antibody (Thermo Scientific A 21070, 2 mg/mL) diluted 1:500, both in blocking buffer, were used to perform the secondary staining for one hour in the dark. After washing, staining with aqueous Hoechst 33342 (Thermo Fisher 62249, 1:1000 in aqua dist.) was carried out for ten minutes. The slides were washed and embedded in ProLong®Gold antifade reagent (Invitrogen P36930).

2.7. Immunofluorescence Staining of Paraffin Sections

The paraffin sections of study part II were handled as described by de Buhr et al. [39]. Briefly, after dewaxing, rehydration, permeabilization, and blocking, the staining was performed for one hour with a monoclonal mouse anti-DNA/histone-1 antibody (Millipore MAB3864, 0.55 mg/mL) diluted 1:100 and rabbit anti-human myeloperoxidase antibody (Dako A0398, 3.2 mg/mL) diluted 1:300 or rabbit anti-elastase antibody (Abcam, Cambridge, UK Ab1876, 10 mg/mL) diluted 1:50, with all dilutions in blocking buffer. An isotype control staining was achieved by using IgG2α from murine myeloma (Sigma-Aldrich M5409-.1MG, 0.2 mg/mL) and IgG from rabbit serum (Sigma-Aldrich I5006, 10.4 mg/mL) in adjusted concentrations. Goat anti-mouse DyLight 488 (Thermo Scientific 35503, 1 mg/mL, 1:1000) and goat anti-rabbit Alexa 633 (Thermo Scientific A 21070, 2 mg/mL, 1:500) antibodies, both diluted in blocking buffer, were utilized for the secondary staining for one hour in the dark. The samples were then washed, embedded in ProLong®Gold with 4′,6-diamidino-2-phenylindole (DAPI) (Thermo Fisher P36931), and covered with a cover slip (Roth H878).

2.8. Immunofluorescence Microscopy and Analysis of NETs

A Leica TCS SP5 AOBS confocal inverted-base fluorescence microscope with an HCX PL APO 40× 0.75–1.25 oil immersion objective and an HCX PL APO lambda blue × 63 1.40 oil immersion UV objective was used to record the samples in study part II. The settings were adjusted with respective isotype controls. For the NET induction assays, in each sample, a minimum of six randomly selected images per independent experiment were taken and used for quantifying the activated NET-positive cells. On the basis of the inhomogeneous structure and size of nuclei in horse neutrophils, the size of nuclei was not used as a parameter for the NET-positive cells. Instead, a cell was defined as positive when the nucleus of the cell showed a positive signal for DNA/histone-1 staining as NET marker. For each individual experiment and horse, a respective negative control was analyzed in parallel.

2.9. ELISA for eCATH

Serum from study part I and VBF samples of horses with healthy eyes and ERU-diseased horses from study part II were examined with a Horse Cathelicidin Antimicrobial Peptide ELISA Kit (Biozol, Eching, Germany ASB-OKEH03902) in accordance with the manufacturer's recommendations for evaluating the amount of equine cathelicidins in those samples.

2.10. Electron Microscopy

Fresh isolated blood-derived equine neutrophils were put in Eppendorf tubes at a concentration of 1×10^6 cells per tube and centrifuged for five minutes at 400 g at room temperature. After the supernatant was pipetted off, 100 µL VBF of one animal with healthy eyes (study part II) or 100 µL RPMI (gibco 11835063) was added to the pellet. Then, 10 µM of equine cathelicidins (eCATH 1 or 2, see above), diluted in VBF or RPMI, was added in a 2:1 ratio. This was incubated for 240 min at 37 °C with 5% CO_2. The subsequent steps were additionally performed with 2 mL VBF of one ERU-diseased horse from study part II. The samples were centrifuged for five minutes at 400 g at room temperature, after which the supernatant was discarded and 250 µL 2.5% (vol/vol) glutaraldehyde in 0.1 M sodium cacodylate (pH 7.2) was added to the pellet. They were then post fixed with 1% osmium tetroxide (wt/vol) and 0.15 M sodium cacodylate (pH 7.2) for 1 h at 4 °C, washed, and further processed for electron microscopy.

For transmission electron microscopy, the fixed and washed samples were subsequently dehydrated in ethanol and further processed for standard Epon embedding. Sections were cut with an LKB ultratome and mounted on Formvar-coated copper grids. The sections were post fixed with uranyl acetate and lead citrate and examined in a Philips/FEI CM100 BioTwin transmission electron microscope operated at a 60-kV accelerating voltage. Images were recorded with a Gatan Multiscan 791 charge-coupled device camera.

The ultrathin sections were stained with uranyl acetate (Laurylab, Saint Fons, France) and lead citrate (Laurylab). Immunolabeling of thin sections after antigen unmasking with sodium metaperiodate (Merck) [40] with gold-labeled anti-TNFα (BBInternational, Cardiff, UK) was performed as described previously [41], with the modification that Aurion-BSA (Aurion, Wageningen, The Netherlands) was used as a blocking agent.

2.11. Statistical Analysis

Data were analyzed using Excel 2010 and 2016 (Microsoft) and GraphPad Prism version 8.0.1. (GraphPad Software). Normal distribution of data was verified using the Kolmogorov-Smirnov normality test (GraphPad software, San Diego, CA, USA) prior to statistical analysis. Differences between groups were analyzed as described in the figure legends (* $p < 0.05$, ** $p < 0.01$, *** $p < 0.001$, **** $p < 0.0001$).

3. Results

3.1. More NET Markers in Serum of ERU-Diseased Horses

To test whether NETs could contribute to the pathogenesis of ERU, an initial screening for NET markers using serum from ERU-diseased horses and animals with healthy eyes was performed. As NETs consist of DNA, the amount of free DNA was evaluated by a Pico Green assay in the serum. Hereby, it needs to be taken into account that free DNA in serum might originate from sources other than neutrophils [42,43]. Thus, the results only represent first indications of the possible presence of NETs in ERU-diseased horses. The average amount of free DNA was significantly different with

4.0 ± 6.1 µg/mL in the ERU serum and 1.9 ± 2.7 µg/mL in the serum of horses with healthy eyes (Figure 1a). As mentioned in the introduction, NET formation is often associated with an increased release of nucleases by the host in order to maintain a balance between NET formation and NET elimination [26]. An analysis of nuclease activity in the same serum also revealed a significant difference between samples from horses with healthy eyes and ERU-diseased horses. In the ERU serum, a significantly higher relative nuclease activity of 102 ± 22.6 was observed, compared with 83.5 ± 31.2 in the control serum (Figure 1b). However, this finding harbored a first suspicion that NETs contribute to the pathogenesis of ERU-diseased horses.

3.2. NET Detection Ex Vivo

In order to confirm the presence of NETs in the eyes of ERU-diseased horses, we performed a series of immunofluorescence stainings for NET markers in VBF. The NETs were identified through a positive signal for DNA/histone-1-complexes and a colocalization of the signal with myeloperoxidase. NET structures were present ex vivo in the VBF of two of three ERU patients (Figure 2), but not in those animals with healthy eyes. All eyes were additionally examined histologically to confirm or exclude ERU (Table A2). As shown in Figure 3, several of the activated cells formed vesicles rather than NET fibers containing DNA/histone-1-complexes. This vesicular release is a special form of extracellular trap formation shown in vitro in cases of response to *Staphylococcus aureus* in human neutrophils [23], and is induced by *Listeria* in murine microglia [44].

We additionally examined VBF of one ERU-diseased horse (horse H) via transmission electron microscopy for a more detailed analysis of NET-releasing cells ex vivo. Hereby, H3-cit and elastase were labeled by immunogold staining. As shown in Figure 4, neutrophils were detected with clear signs of NETosis, for example, disruption of the nuclear membrane and release of extracellular traps. Besides cells undergoing NETosis, the formation of nuclear vesicles positive for H3-cit and elastase in neutrophils that were found inside the VBF of ERU-diseased horses was also confirmed. The magnified pictures in Figure 4e show the vesicular NET formation in several neutrophils.

The presence of NET markers and neutrophils during NETosis in VBF from ERU-diseased horses confirmed our hypothesis that NETs play a role in ERU pathogenesis.

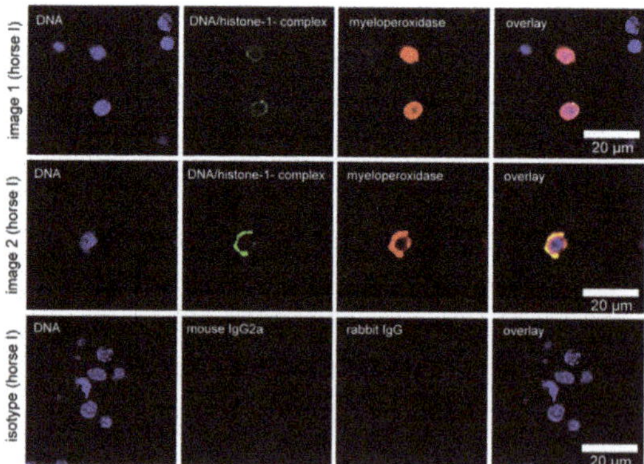

Figure 2. Ex vivo neutrophil extracellular trap (NET) detection in vitreous body fluid (VBF) of ERU-diseased horses (study part II, Hannover). The VBF of enucleated eyes from ERU-diseased horses was analyzed after cytospin and immunofluorescence staining with a confocal microscope. NET staining for immunofluorescence microscopy of the cells contained in the VBF was conducted (blue = DNA (Hoechst), green = DNA/histone-1-complexes, and red = myeloperoxidase). Representative images of cells from one animal (horse I) are shown in rows 1 and 2. Cells in image one are stained in the center of the cells, whereas in image 2, the staining of DNA/histone-1-complexes and myeloperoxidase surrounds the cell. The respective isotype control is presented in row 3.

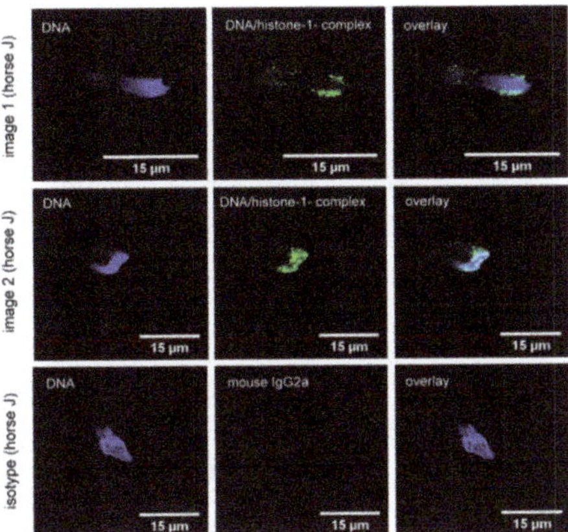

Figure 3. Ex vivo NET detection in VBF of ERU-diseased horses (study part II, Hannover). The VBF of enucleated eyes from ERU-diseased horses was analyzed for cells and NET markers after cytospin and immunofluorescence staining with a confocal microscope (blue = DNA, green = DNA/histone-1-complexes). Images of different cells from one animal (horse J) are shown in images 1 and 2, where the activated cells formed vesicles rather than NET fibers. The respective isotype is presented in row 3.

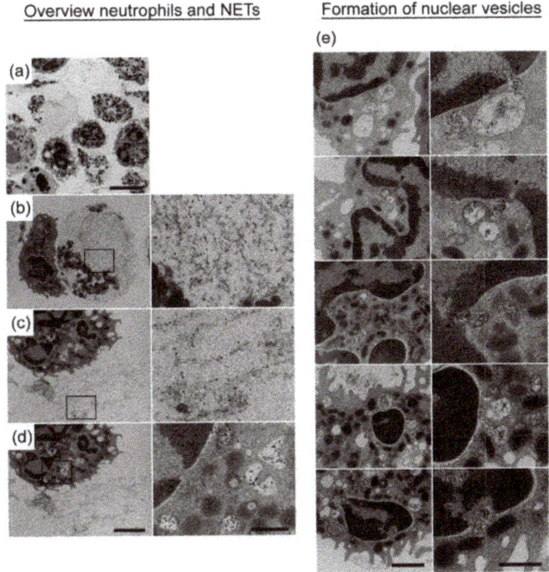

Figure 4. Ex vivo NET detection via transmission electron microscopy in VBF of an ERU-diseased horse (study part II, Hannover). The VBF of an enucleated eye from an ERU-diseased horse (horse H) was analyzed with a transmission electron microscope. (**a**) overview, (**b**) neutrophil during NETosis (**c**) neutrophil with an extracellular trap, and (**d**) neutrophil with nuclear vesicles. In (**a–d**), the right column displays respective magnifications with immunogold labeling (5 nm gold/H3-cit, 10 nm gold/elastase). (**e**) All images show the formation of H3-cit and elastase positive nuclear vesicles (5 nm gold/H3-cit, 10 nm gold/elastase). Arrows mark the formation of nuclear vesicles. On the right-hand side, the right column displays respective magnifications. Scale bar size: (**a**) = 5 μm, (**b–d**) left-hand side = 2 μm, (**b,d**) right-hand side = 200 nm, (**e**) left-hand side = 1 μm, and (**e**) right-hand side = 500 nm.

3.3. More Activated Neutrophils in ERU-Diseased Horses Despite Nuclease Activity

To obtain a deeper insight into the influence of VBF on NET formation, we exposed fresh neutrophils isolated from healthy horses to VBF from animals with healthy eyes compared with ERU-diseased horses. A significant increase in the percentage of activated cells could be identified in VBF of the ERU-diseased horses compared with those with healthy eyes (Figure 5a,b). The incubation of neutrophils with methyl-β-cyclodextrin diluted in VBF, serving as positive control, also led to a significantly higher NET formation in ERU-diseased horses compared with those with healthy eyes.

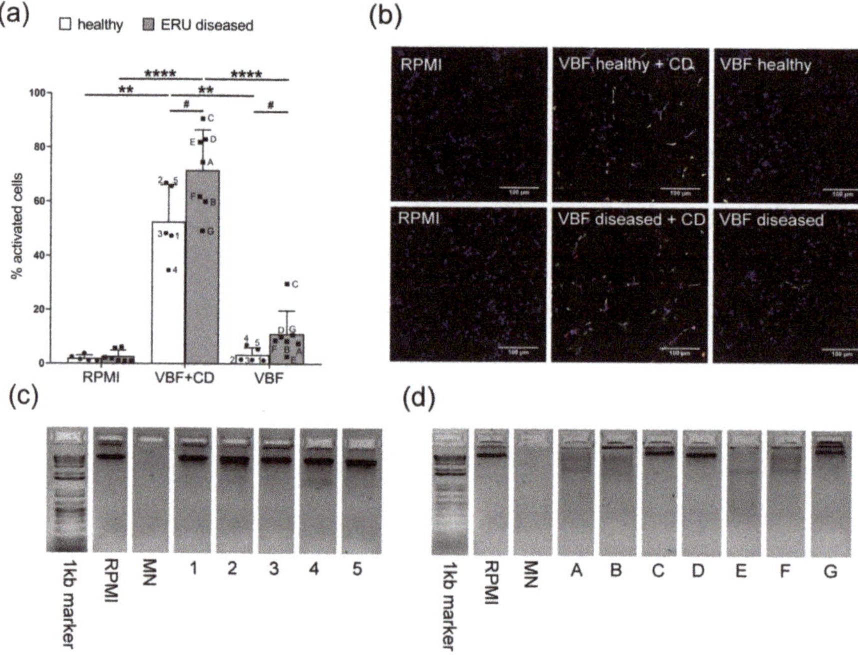

Figure 5. Activation of neutrophils by VBF of horses with healthy eyes and ERU-diseased horses (VBF diseased) and respective nuclease activities (study part II, Hannover). (**a**) After a 240 min incubation period of fresh isolated blood derived neutrophils with VBF, significantly more activated neutrophils were detected in samples from ERU-diseased horses. Roswell Park Memorial Institute medium (RPMI) was used as negative control, with methyl-β-cyclodextrin (CD) diluted in VBF as positive control. The bars represent mean ± SD of five (healthy eyes) or seven (ERU-diseased) independent experiments. Statistical analysis: # represents results of a one-tailed unpaired student's *t*-test; * represents results of one-way analysis of variance (ANOVA), followed by Tukey's multiple comparison test. *p*-values of # $p < 0.05$, ** $p < 0.005$, and **** $p < 0.0001$ were considered significant. (**b**) Representative images (horses 3 and E) of immunofluorescence analysis are presented (blue = Hoechst, green = DNA/histone-1-complexes, red = myeloperoxidase). The respective isotype control stainings and single channel pictures are shown in Figure A1. (**c**,**d**) The corresponding nuclease activities in the VBF samples were analyzed by a qualitative DNase activity test. The results of horses with healthy eyes are shown in (**c**) and of ERU-diseased horses in (**d**). RPMI was used as a negative control and micrococcal nuclease (MN) as a positive control.

As host nucleases are important for NET elimination and might also be present in the VBF, we evaluated their corresponding activities in the VBF samples by means of a DNase activity test. The numbers and letters below the gels and in the graph indicate the corresponding samples tested at the same time for NET formation. While the VBF of horses with healthy eyes were all negative, most of the VBF of ERU-diseased horses showed distinct nuclease activity (Figure 5c,d). These data are in good accordance with the detected increased nuclease values in sera from ERU-diseased horses shown in Figure 1. Although this difference between the amount of activated cells in VBF compared with VBF without nuclease activity was not significant, a tendency for higher nuclease activity in VBF of ERU-diseased horses was detectable ($p = 0.068$). However, it is important to highlight that a high amount of NET formation was found in neutrophils treated with VBF of ERU-diseased horses, despite the presence of the shown higher nuclease activity. These data again confirmed that NETs might play a role during ERU pathogenesis.

3.4. Influence of Equine Cathelicidins

3.4.1. NET Induction with Equine Cathelicidins

After having demonstrated the presence of NETs in ERU-diseased horses, we aimed to analyze possible NET-inducing factors during ERU pathogenesis. Because cathelicidins are described as an NET-inducing factor in humans [45], and because the cathelicidin-modulating factor IL-17 is linked to ERU [11], it may be assumed that cathelicidins might be involved in NET formation in ERU-diseased horses. Therefore, we focused on further characterizing the impact of equine cathelicidins on NET release in horses (Figure 6). Fresh isolated blood derived neutrophils from donors with healthy eyes were incubated with three different eCATH at amounts of 5 µM and 10 µM. These concentrations were chosen because human cathelicidin has been shown to induce NETs in human neutrophils in such concentrations [45]. After a 240 min incubation period with RPMI and eCATH, the cathelicidins eCATH 1 and 2 induced significantly more NETs compared with a negative control with RPMI alone (Figure 6a). Moreover, a concentration of 10 µM activated more cells than 5 µM. However, eCATH 3 did not make any difference, independent of the concentration used. Similarly, as shown ex vivo in VBF (Figure 3), several of the activated cells formed vesicles rather than NET fibers (Figure 6c). The results of an analysis of equine neutrophils incubated over 120 min with eCATH 1, 10 µM diluted in RPMI via transmission electron microscopy, and neutrophils incubated only in RPMI are depicted in Figure 6d. Again, neutrophils during NETosis and with extracellular traps were detected. Furthermore, nuclear vesicles positive for H3-cit and elastase were found. With these results, a potential influence of eCATH 1 and 2 on NET formation in horses was suggested.

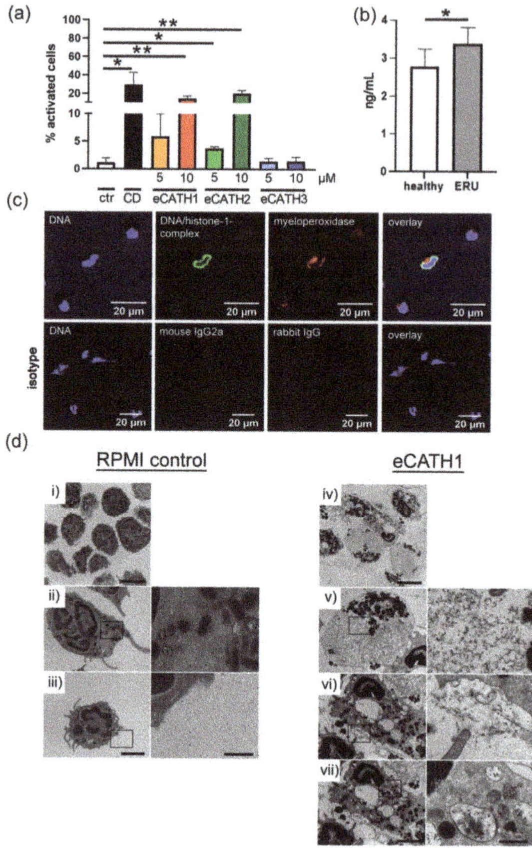

Figure 6. Influence of equine cathelicidins (eCATH) 1-3. (**a**) After a 240 min incubation period, eCATH 1 and 2 activated neutrophils in RPMI depending on the quantity used, whereas eCATH 3 did not lead to activation. The bars represent mean ± SD of three independent experiments. A one-tailed paired *t*-test was conducted. *p* values of * *p* < 0.05 and ** *p* < 0.01 compared with control were considered significant. (**b**) Equine cathelicidins in VBF. The amounts of equine cathelicidins in VBF of ERU-diseased (*n* = 7) and controls with healthy eyes (*n* = 5) were analyzed using a commercial ELISA. A significant increase in equine cathelicidins in VBF of ERU-diseased horses was observed. The bars represent mean ± SD. A one-tailed unpaired *t*-test was performed. *p* values of * *p* < 0.05 compared with control were considered significant. In (**c**), representative immunofluorescence images of equine neutrophils stimulated with eCATH are presented, in this case with eCATH 2 and 10 μM in RPMI (blue = Hoechst, green = DNA/histone-1-complexes, red = myeloperoxidase). The respective isotype control stainings are included. In (**d**), transmission electron microscopy images of equine neutrophils are shown. Control images from neutrophils incubated for 120 min in RPMI are presented on the left-hand side. Neutrophils stimulated with eCATH 1 (10 μM in RPMI) for 120 min are presented on the right-hand side. An overview is given in (i) and (iv). The right column in each group displays respective magnifications with immunogold labeling (5 nm gold/H3-cit, 10 nm gold/elastase). (ii) shows an intact neutrophil with elastase positive granular. (iii) shows the intact outer membrane of an unstimulated neutrophil. (v) presents a neutrophil with a high amount of H3-cit and elastase positive content in the cytosol. (vi) shows the release of an extracellular trap that is H3-cit and elastase positive. (vii) depicts a neutrophil with H3-cit and elastase positive nuclear vesicles. Scale bar size: (i) and (iv) = 5 μm, (all others) left-hand side = 2 μm, (all others) right-hand side = 200 nm.

3.4.2. More Cathelicidins in VBF of ERU-Diseased Horses

After showing the impact of eCATH 1 and 2 on horse neutrophils in vitro, we subsequently investigated their concentrations in VBF of horses with healthy eyes and ERU patients. For this purpose, we performed a horse cathelicidin antimicrobial peptide ELISA with VBF samples from animals with healthy eyes and ERU patients (Figure 6b). The values of ERU-diseased animals showed a significantly higher amount of cathelicidins. The mean values hereby were 2.8 ng/mL for the horses with healthy eyes and 3.3 ng/mL for the diseased horses. However, these concentrations were distinctly lower than that used in NET induction assays. No difference was seen for serum levels of cathelicidins (Figure A2a).

4. Discussion

Numerous indications of an immune-mediated pathogenesis were reported in ERU. As neutrophil infiltration was characterized during the course of this disease [46–48], we investigated their contribution in terms of NET production in ERU patients. Our results demonstrate that significantly more NET markers are present in serum of ERU-diseased horses compared with horses with healthy eyes (Figure 1). However, these markers are not specific for NETs and could also originate, for example, from necrotic or apoptotic cells, or be present owing to diverse pathological states [42,43]. Other serum NET markers, such as myeloperoxidase, neutrophil elastase, myeloid-related protein, or nucleosome levels, exist, but free DNA was shown to be the most promising among these serum NET markers [49]. Another possibility would be to perform a serum analysis for H3-cit, which is considered as the most specific marker [50,51]. Nevertheless, we subsequently focused on more specific NET markers together with the visualization of the cells inside the affected eye. Such NET markers as H3-cit, DNA/histone complexes, and myeloperoxidase or elastase are present in activated neutrophils or nuclear vesicles of VBF from most ERU-diseased horses (Figures 2–4) and their VBF activates more neutrophils than VBF of horses with healthy eyes (Figure 5a). We did not find NET markers in VBF of every diseased horse, which might be because of the sample size or the fact that neutrophils are rather involved in the onset of the disease than in the later phases [46]. Our samples for the ex vivo NET detection were all derived from horses with several reported acute phases in their history, leading to a recurrent condition with eye damage, so the eye had to be removed for therapeutical reasons at a later stage of the disease. This chronic state of ERU, when the eye was removed, is described as being characterized by lymphoplasmatic cells [46], which was confirmed in our histopathological examinations (Table A2). Owing to this stage of the disease, we might not have found NET fibers in the three ERU-diseased horses included in the in situ analysis. However, in the Appendix A (Figure A3), we show an in situ analysis derived from a horse with acute uveitis (no ERU). This horse shows clear NET fibers inside the ciliary body, demonstrating the possibility of NET release inside this tissue during acute phases of inflammation.

In summary, our findings lead to the hypothesis that ERU-diseased horses develop more NET markers and that NETs may contribute to the pathogenesis thereof. This is in accordance with studies in which a pathological component of NETs was already found in other diseases. For instance, autoimmune antibodies against intracellular antigens bind NETs as they are exposing intracellular components to the extracellular space [52]. Such antibodies were, for example, detected in rheumatoid arthritis, in this particular case against citrullinated histone [27]. Furthermore, autoantibodies themselves can in turn induce NETs, leading to a vicious circle of NETosis and autoantibody production, maintaining the inflammation [27]. Among others, protein excess through release of neutrophil elastase and an activation of the complement system by non-degraded NET particles are described mechanisms [53]. Nevertheless, NETosis also appears as a mixed blessing with both beneficial and detrimental effects at once. This was described by Thanabalasuriar et al. [29] in a *Pseudomonas aeruginosa* ocular surface infection. By building up a dead zone underneath the biofilm, NETs limit the bacterial dissemination into the brain, but coincidently cause a more severe ocular clinic. Hence, a detrimental effect of NETs also arising in ERU is plausible.

Besides clear signs of NETosis, hints of vesicular release of NETs were also detectable in ERU-diseased horses. The vesicular NET formation was described as a vital NET formation [23].

This mechanism was identified as a response of neutrophils to the presence of *Staphylococcus aureus*. With the present study, we identified a similar picture ex vivo as well as in vitro in the VBF of an ERU-diseased horse and after eCATH stimulation in vitro (Figures 3–5). Interestingly, by means of electron microscopy (EM) analysis, the different forms of NET formation were identified in the same sample. Alongside the vesicular NET formation, neutrophils with a clear NET release and a membrane disruption were identified. Therefore, this leads to the hypothesis that neutrophils are primed or programmed in different ways, eventually by different stimuli during ERU pathogenesis.

As potential NET inducing factors, we investigated the amount and effects of the equine cathelicidins 1-3 (Figure 6), because of the described genetic link of the cathelicidin-modulating factor IL-17 to ERU [11]. Antimicrobial peptides in general and cathelicidins specifically have been reported to induce NETosis and stabilize NETs [54]. A detrimental effect thereof can be seen in mice, where cathelicidin in NETs promotes atherosclerosis through activation of plasmacytoid dendritic cells [55]. Additionally, defects in processing, expression, or function were found in several human inflammatory skin diseases. Hereby, an overexpression can be just as detrimental as a deficient antimicrobial barrier function caused by downregulation [56].

In horses, three different cathelicidin sequences have been identified at the RNA level, but only two mature peptides [36]. However, we performed the assays with all three equine cathelicidins, as the likelihood of an eCATH 1 expression under specific conditions or in other cell types than myeloid cells was suggested by Bruhn et al. [57]. Our results show that eCATH 1 and 2, but not eCATH 3, have the ability to activate neutrophils to form NETs in RPMI (Figure 6a), as already shown for the human cathelicidin LL-37 in human neutrophils [45]. The varying results between the cathelicidins could be owing to their molecular structure. The coding regions of the eCATH peptides have different lengths and no significant sequence homology [58]. In particular, eCATH 3 has a low hydrophobic part, thus explaining its poor effects [36]. The equine cathelicidins have also been reported to be different regarding their antimicrobial properties. A synthetic eCATH 1 was hereby most bactericidal, followed by eCATH 2. The reaction of eCATH 3 is highly dependent on its environment, as it effectively combats pathogens in low salt concentrations, but shows an inhibited activity in physiologic salt medium [36]. Interestingly, the used low-ionic media contained a salt concentration of 100 mM NaCl, similar to the RPMI used in our experiments (103 mM). Nonetheless, we still have not discovered a NET inducing activity for eCATH 3 in RPMI. This is in line with the finding that bactericidal activity of cationic antimicrobial peptides does not always correlate with the NET-inducing or NET-stabilizing activity, as shown by Neumann et al. [45,54]. An influence of sodium chloride has likewise been reported for the interaction between DNA and LL-37 in humans. Salt promotes the dissociation of LL-37 from extracellular DNA through interference of the ionic interactions between DNA phosphate groups and amino acids of the AMP [59]. The amount of sodium chloride in equine VBF is 17.7% higher [60] than in RPMI, but still only about a third of the lowest amount tested by Lande et al. [59]. Moreover, the pH is an influencing factor on the activity of several human AMPs, including the human cathelicidin LL-37, where an acidic surrounding reduces the function [54,61]. In line with this discussion is the finding that the NET-inducing effect of eCATH 1 and 2 is lost in the presence of VBF of healthy or diseased horses (Figure A2b,c). Thus, it still remains questionable if the eCATH does in fact contribute to NET induction in ERU-diseased horses. To investigate this in detail, the effects of an inhibitor of eCATH on NET formation could be examined, but no effective antibodies are currently available.

Additionally, the NET-inducing capacity of eCATH 1 and 2 was evident at higher concentrations (5 µM and 10 µM) compared with the measured lower amounts of eCATH in the VBF. However, it has to be mentioned that these measured samples were derived from eyes in sub-clinical stages. The actual amounts inside an acutely inflamed eye are likely to be much higher, as the expression of LL-37 is induced during inflammation [62], leading, for example, to median levels up to 300 µM in psoriatic skin lesions [63]. On the basis of these results, we assume that besides cathelicidins, other factors, such as pathogens, might also contribute to NET formation during ERU.

One possible major contributor to the pathogenesis of ERU is *Leptospira*, which can be found in about 60% [12–14] of ERU-diseased horses and, importantly, not in VBF of horses with healthy eyes. Nothing is known about their influence in the context of NETs in ERU so far. However, as *Leptospira* have been proven to induce NETs, for example, in humans, mice, and cattle [64,65], their impact on equine neutrophils remains to be determined. According to our data, there is neither a link between the *Leptospira* titer (Table A1) and the percentage of activated cells in the NET induction assay (Figure A2b,c), nor to the nuclease activity. The horse with the lowest titer even induced the highest percentage of NETs. This corresponds with the finding that both *Leptospira* positive and negative horses develop all degrees of severity of this disease [14]. All samples were positive for the serovar Grippotyphosa, which is in accordance with data describing it as being the most widely distributed serovar in Europe [13,14,66]. Nevertheless, there could be a connection between the amount of NETs in acutely inflamed eyes and living *Leptospira* inside the inflamed VBF, as our samples were derived during clinically quiescent periods. In humans, a concentration-dependent induction of NETs was found [64].

Regardless of their initiating trigger, the involvement of NETs leads to treatment options not yet included in the current therapy approaches of ERU. In other diseases regarding NETosis, the application of DNase, heparin, or anti-VEGF was successful. DNase degrades extracellular DNA and is thus able to clear NETs [67]. An impairment of this enzyme has been shown to contribute to disease progression, such as lupus nephritis [18]. For instance, DNase treatment is established in cystic fibrosis therapy in humans [53]. Additionally, DNase eye drops had beneficial effects in dry eye disease, like significantly reduced corneal defects and mucoid debris [67,68]. Barliya et al. [31] have proven a decreasing effect of DNase ex vivo, treating NETs in cryosections of murine eyes inflamed owing to injection of IL-8 or TNF-α. Consequently, they discuss a potential therapeutic use of DNase in intraocular inflammatory processes. Another approach to degrade NETs in an ocular disease has been performed in ocular graft-versus-host disease using heparin [30]. This drug removes histones from NETs owing to its high negative charge, resulting in destabilization [30]. In a sub-anticoagulant dose, it not only reduced the clinical symptoms and led to fewer amounts of inflammatory cytokines, but also increased cell proliferation. Furthermore, a decrease in NET formation in proliferative diabetic retinopathy has been demonstrated after intraocular anti-VEGF injection [32].

Administering these drugs could consequently help to show the extent to which NETs contribute to the development of ERU and whether a DNase or heparin treatment could be used as a new therapy. Nevertheless, beforehand, further studies using in vivo experiments or complex 3D culture system, which closely mimic the cellular interactions in the host, are needed. For this purpose, a 3D cell culture system should be used to separate the blood from the VBF compartment of the eye. Thereby, the blood-retina barrier, over which the neutrophils need to migrate, would be mimicked. In humans, the retinal pigment epithelium cell line ARPE-19 has already been used on filters to simulate this barrier [69]. Nevertheless, as the presented study focused on ERU in horses, an equine system is needed to investigate this aspect in the future. Additionally, a cell culture system could prospectively enable specific knock-outs of antimicrobial peptide production via CRISPR/Cas. Furthermore, in this line, a conceivable detrimental effect of NETs on the retinal barrier could be investigated with this system. NETs could probably act detrimentally towards this epithelial barrier, as they also display a destructive impact on other epithelial tissue. For instance, NETs cause cell death in lung epithelial cells in a concentration-dependent manner [70]. As this effect was independent of DNase treatment, but dependent to varying degrees on anti-histone antibodies, polysialic acid, and MPO inhibitor, Saffarzadeh et al. [70] suggest a mediation of cytotoxicity mainly by histones and MPO instead of the DNA components of NETs. This corresponds to the finding that NETs lead to corneal and conjunctival epitheliopathy, which was treatable with heparin [30].

In conclusion, our data suggest an involvement of NETs within the pathogenesis of ERU. Meanwhile, the equine cathelicidins seem to not be the determining factor, but only a contributing one. The association of NETs with eye diseases remains an important field that has yet to be investigated. Thereby, attention should be given to molecular processes in regards to the development of future therapeutic approaches, as recommended by Estúa-Acosta et al. [71]. Possible molecular processes to focus on would be the signaling pathways and clearance of NETs during these ocular pathologies [71]. Furthermore, the discussed open questions should be answered in the future using complex 3D cell culture system that mimic cellular interactions in the host.

Author Contributions: Conceptualization, N.d.B., M.v.K.-B., and B.O.; methodology, N.d.B., M.v.K.-B., and B.O.; validation, N.d.B., L.F., and B.O.; formal analysis, N.d.B., M.v.K.-B., and L.F.; investigation, N.d.B., L.F., K.S.-M., A.B., M.M., and A.S.; resources, B.O., H.P.H., M.v.B., and C.A.D.; data curation, N.d.B., L.F., and B.O.; writing—original draft preparation, L.F. and N.d.B.; writing—review and editing, all authors; visualization, L.F., N.d.B., M.M., and M.v.K.-B.; supervision, N.d.B., M.v.K.-B., and B.O.; project administration, N.d.B., M.v.K.-B., and B.O.; funding acquisition, N.d.B., M.v.K.-B., and B.O.

Funding: This research was funded by the German Research Foundation (DFG), grant numbers BU 3523/1-1, OH 166/2-1, and KO 3552/8-1. This publication was supported by the DFG and the University of Veterinary Medicine Hannover, Foundation and LMU Munich within the funding program Open Access Publishing.

Acknowledgments: We are grateful to the staff at the BioEM Lab, Biozentrum, University of Basel, the Core Facility for Integrated Microscopy (CFIM), Panum Institute, University of Copenhagen, and the Microscopy Facility at the Department of Biology, Lund University, for providing highly innovative environments for electron microscopy. We wish to thank Cinzia Tiberi (BioEM lab) and Ola Gustafsson (Microscopy Facility) for their skilful work, and Carola Alampi (BioEM lab), Mohamed Chami (BioEM lab), and Klaus Qvortrup (FCIM) for their practical help with electron microscopy.

Conflicts of Interest: The authors declare no conflict of interest. The funders had no role in the design of the study; in the collection, analyses, or interpretation of data; in the writing of the manuscript; or in the decision to publish the results.

Appendix A

Table A1. Horses included in the neutrophil extracellular trap (NET) induction assay. ERU, equine recurrent uveitis.

Number	Diagnosis	Age	Breed	Gender	*Leptospira* Titer
1	healthy eye	16	Westphalian	mare	MAT −, PCR −
2	healthy eye	9	Trakehner	gelding	MAT −, PCR −
3	healthy eye	3	Hanoverian	gelding	MAT −, PCR −
4	healthy eye	15–20	Dutch warmblood	mare	MAT −, PCR −
5	healthy eye	23	Icelandic horse	mare	MAT −, PCR −
A	ERU	9	Hanoverian	mare	MAT +, PCR + (400 *Australis*, 100 *Bratislava*, 3200 *Atumnalis*, 1600 *Grippotyphosa*, >3200 *Pomona*, 3200 *Altodouro*, 400 *Hardjo*)
B	ERU	16	Icelandic horse	mare	MAT +, PCR + (>3200 *Grippotyphosa*, 800 *Icterohaemorrhagiae*)
C	ERU	6	Icelandic horse	mare	MAT +, PCR + (400 *Grippotyphosa*)
D	ERU	8	Alt-Oldenburger and Ostfriesen	gelding	MAT +, PCR + (1600 *Grippotyphosa*)
E	ERU	11	Icelandic horse	mare	MAT +, PCR + (3200 *Grippotyphosa*)
F	ERU	4	Hanoverian	mare	MAT +, PCR + (>3200 *Grippotyphosa*)
G	ERU	10	Trotter	gelding	MAT +, PCR + (3200 *Grippotyphosa*)

MAT = microscopic agglutination test, PCR = polymerase chain reaction.

Table A2. Horses included in the ex vivo, histological, or electron microscopy examination.

Number	Diagnosis	Age	Breed	Gender	*Leptospira* titer	Pathological Findings
6	ERU-free, retrobulbar mass	25	Partbred Arabian	mare	MAT −, PCR −	healthy eye
7	ERU-free, chronic keratitis	20	Hanoverian	gelding	PCR −, MAT −	retinal detachment with atrophy
8	ERU-free, glaucoma	26	Westphalian	gelding	PCR −, MAT −	retinal folds with focal atrophy, focal erosion of corneal epithel, hyalinisation of ligamentum pectinatum
H	ERU	11	Hanoverian	gelding	MAT −, PCR +	lymphoplasmacellular panophthalmia
I	ERU	20	Pinto	gelding	MAT +, PCR − (1600 *Grippotyphosa*)	lymphoplasmacellular panophthalmia
J	ERU	13	Oldenburger	gelding	MAT +, PCR − (800 *Grippotyphosa*)	phthisis bulbi, chronic-degenerative and reactive changes
U1	acute uveitis	13	Paint Horse	gelding	MAT −, no PCR	hypopyon and retinal detachment

MAT = microscopic agglutination test, PCR = polymerase chain reaction.

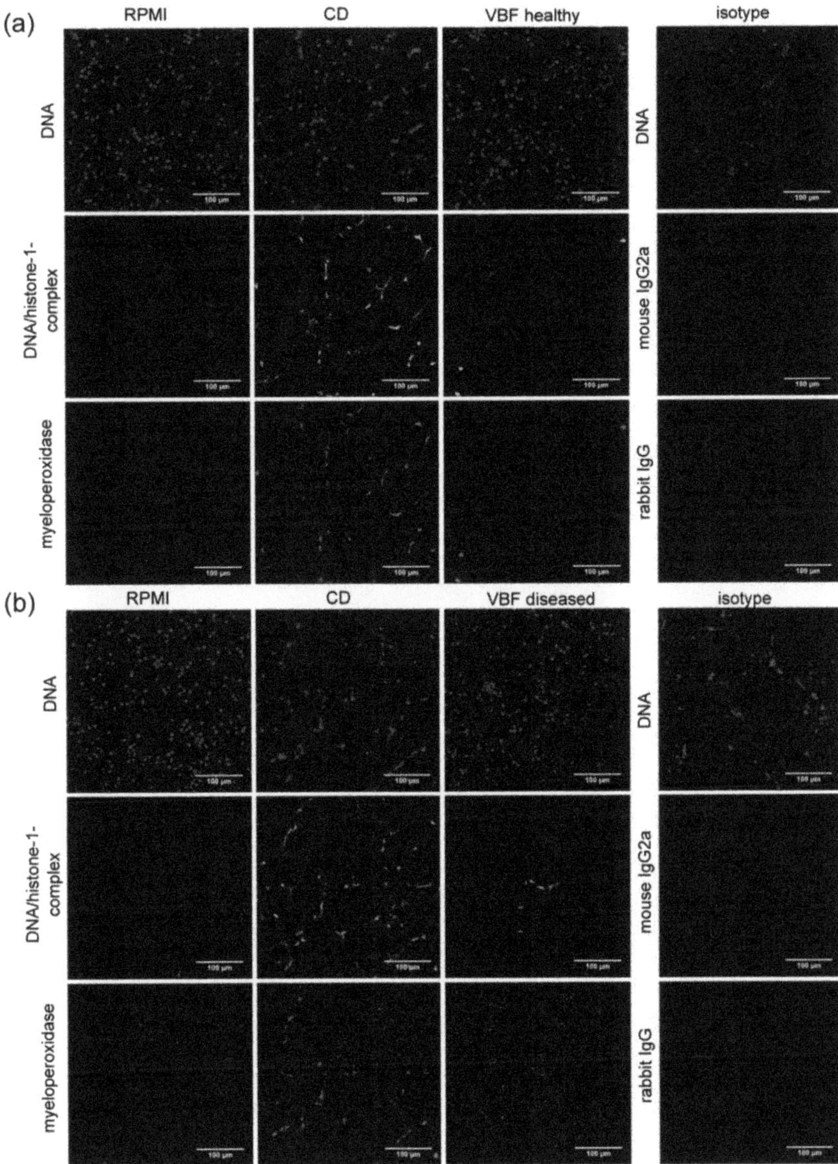

Figure A1. Activation of neutrophils by VBF of horses with healthy eyes and ERU-diseased horses. Fresh isolated blood-derived neutrophils were incubated for 240 min with VBF. RPMI was used as negative control, with methyl-β- cyclodextrin (CD) diluted in VBF as positive control. (**a**) shows the single channel pictures and isotype control of representative immunofluorescence pictures of a horse with healthy eyes (horse 3). In (**b**), the corresponding images of an ERU-diseased horse (horse E) are included. Blue staining represents DNA (Hoechst), green indicates DNA/histone-1-complexes, and red indicates myeloperoxidase.

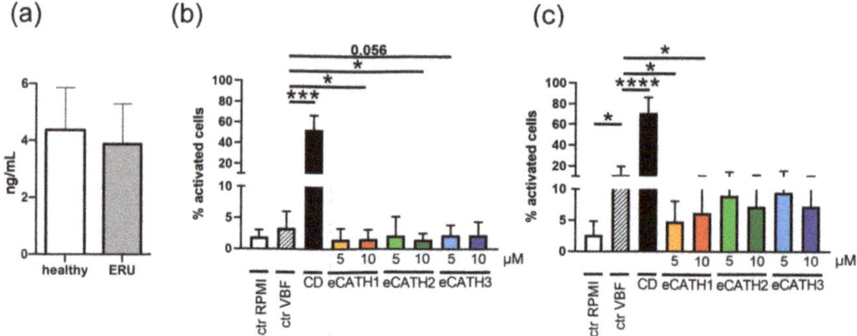

Figure A2. Equine cathelicidins (eCATH) as a potential NET inducing factor. (**a**) shows the amount of eCATH in serum from ERU patients (n = 50) and control horses with healthy eyes (*n* = 20), analyzed using a commercial ELISA. No significant decrease in eCATH in serum of ERU-diseased horses was observed. The bars represent mean ± SD. A one-tailed unpaired *t*-test was conducted. In (**b**,**c**), the activation of neutrophils by eCATH 1–3 in VBF is depicted. After 240 min incubation, none of the cathelicidins induced NETs in vitreous body fluid from horses with healthy eyes (**b**) or ERU-diseased horses (**c**). They rather reduced the amount of NETs compared with VBF alone. A significantly higher percentage of activated cells in VBF of ERU patients compared with samples with healthy eyes was detected. The bars represent mean ± SD of five (healthy eyes) and seven (ERU-diseased) independent experiments. A one-tailed paired *t*-test was conducted. *p*-values of * $p < 0.05$ and ** $p < 0.01$ compared with the control were considered significant.

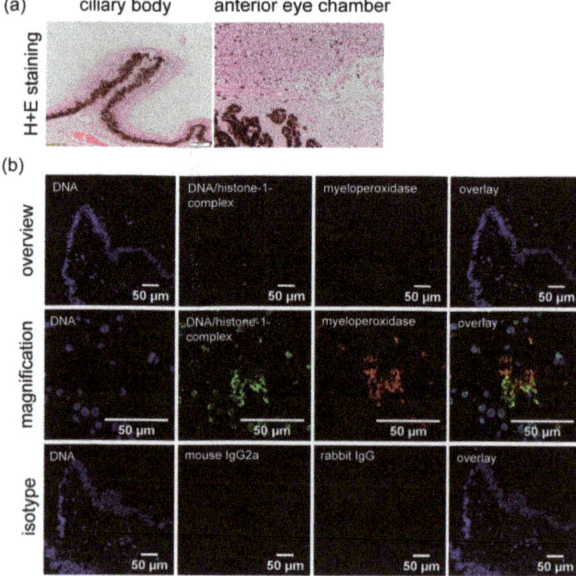

Figure A3. In situ NET detection in a histological eye section of a horse with acute uveitis. NET structures are present in the ciliary body of a uveitis patient (horse U1). (**a**) The corresponding hematoxylin-eosin (H+E) section of the ciliary body to the pictures in (**b**) is presented. The H+E section of the anterior eye chamber of this horse confirms the uveitis by showing a neutrophil, in part lymphohistiocytic infiltration in the area of the chamber angle. (**b**) NETs are hereby identified through colocalization of DNA (blue, Dapi), DNA/histone-1-complexes (green), and myeloperoxidase (red). The respective isotype control staining is included.

References

1. Schwink, K.L. Equine Uveitis. *Vet. Clin. North Am. Equine Pract.* **1992**, *8*, 557–574. [CrossRef]
2. Lowe, R.C. Equine uveitis: A UK perspective. *Equine Vet. J.* **2010**, *42*, 46–49. [CrossRef]
3. Gilger, B.C.; Deeg, C. *Equine Ophthalmology*, 2nd ed.; Gilger, B.C., Ed.; Elsevier: Saint Louis, MO, USA, 2011; ISBN 9781437708462.
4. Szemes, P.; Gerhards, H. Untersuchungen zur Prävalenz der equinen rezidivierenden Uveitis im Großraum Köln-Bonn. *Prakt Tierarzt* **2000**, *81*, 408–420.
5. Gerhards, H.; Wollanke, B. Diagnosis and therapy of uveitis in horses. *Pferdeheilkd. Equine Med.* **2001**, *17*, 319–329. [CrossRef]
6. Von Borstel, M.; Oppen, V.; Frühauf, G.; Boevé, D.; Ohnesorge, B. Langzeitergebnisse der Pars-plana-Vitrektomie bei equiner rezidivierender Uveitis. *Pferdeheilkunde* **2005**, *21*, 13–18. [CrossRef]
7. Gilger, B.C. Equine recurrent uveitis: The viewpoint from the USA. *Equine Vet. J. Suppl.* **2010**, *37*, 57–61. [CrossRef]
8. Deeg, C.a.; Kaspers, B.; Gerhards, H.; Thurau, S.R.; Wollanke, B.; Wildner, G. Immune responses to retinal autoantigens and peptides in equine recurrent uveitis. *Investig. Ophthalmol. Vis. Sci.* **2001**, *42*, 393–398.
9. Zipplies, J.K.; Hauck, S.M.; Eberhardt, C.; Hirmer, S.; Amann, B.; Stangassinger, M.; Ueffing, M.; Deeg, C.A. Miscellaneous vitreous-derived IgM antibodies target numerous retinal proteins in equine recurrent uveitis. *Vet. Ophthalmol.* **2012**, *15*, 57–64. [CrossRef]
10. Regan, D.P.; Aarnio, M.C.; Davis, W.S.; Carmichael, K.P.; Vandenplas, M.L.; Lauderdale, J.D.; Moore, P.a. Characterization of cytokines associated with Th17 cells in the eyes of horses with recurrent uveitis. *Vet. Ophthalmol.* **2012**, *15*, 145–152. [CrossRef]
11. Kulbrock, M.; Lehner, S.; Metzger, J.; Ohnesorge, B.; Distl, O. A Genome-Wide Association Study Identifies Risk Loci to Equine Recurrent Uveitis in German Warmblood Horses. *PLoS ONE* **2013**, *8*, e71619. [CrossRef]
12. Kulbrock, M.; von Borstel, M.; Rohn, K.; Distl, O.; Ohnesorge, B. Occurrence and severity of equine recurrent uveitis in warmblood horses - A comparative study. *Pferdeheilkd. Equine Med.* **2016**, *29*, 27–36. [CrossRef]
13. Dorrego-Keiter, E.; Tóth, J.; Dikker, L.; Sielhorst, J.; Schusser, G.F. Ritz Kultureller Nachweis von Leptospiren in Glaskörperflüssigkeit und Antikörpernachweis gegen Leptospiren in Glaskörperflüssigkeit und Serum von 225 Pferden mit equiner rezidivierender Uveitis (ERU). *Berl. Munch. Tierarztl. Wochenschr.* **2016**, *129*, 209–215.
14. Von Borstel, M.; Oey, L.; Strutzberg-Minder, K.; Boeve, M.H.; Ohnesorge, B. Direct and indirect detection of leptospires in vitreal samples of horses with ERU. *Pferdeheilkd. Equine Med.* **2010**, *26*, 219–225. [CrossRef]
15. Vincent, A.T.; Schiettekatte, O.; Goarant, C.; Neela, V.K.; Bernet, E.; Thibeaux, R.; Ismail, N.; Mohd Khalid, M.K.N.; Amran, F.; Masuzawa, T.; et al. Revisiting the taxonomy and evolution of pathogenicity of the genus Leptospira through the prism of genomics. *PLoS Negl. Trop. Dis.* **2019**, *13*, e0007270. [CrossRef] [PubMed]
16. Kulbrock, M.; Distl, O.; Ohnesorge, B. A Review of Candidate Genes for Development of Equine Recurrent Uveitis. *J. Equine Vet. Sci.* **2013**, *33*, 885–892. [CrossRef]
17. Pieterse, E.; van der Vlag, J. Breaking Immunological Tolerance in Systemic Lupus Erythematosus. *Front. Immunol.* **2014**, *5*, 1–8. [CrossRef]
18. Hakkim, A.; Furnrohr, B.G.; Amann, K.; Laube, B.; Abed, U.A.; Brinkmann, V.; Herrmann, M.; Voll, R.E.; Zychlinsky, A. Impairment of neutrophil extracellular trap degradation is associated with lupus nephritis. *Proc. Natl. Acad. Sci. USA* **2010**, *107*, 9813–9818. [CrossRef]
19. De Buhr, N.; von Köckritz-Blickwede, M. How Neutrophil Extracellular Traps Become Visible. *J. Immunol. Res.* **2016**, *2016*, 4604713. [CrossRef]
20. Steinberg, B.E.; Grinstein, S. Unconventional Roles of the NADPH Oxidase: Signaling, Ion Homeostasis, and Cell Death. *Sci. STKE* **2007**, *2007*, pe11. [CrossRef]
21. Brinkmann, V.; Reichard, U.; Goosmann, C.; Fauler, B.; Uhlemann, Y.; Weiss, D.S.; Weinrauch, Y.; Zychlinsky, A. Neutrophil extracellular traps kill bacteria. *Science* **2004**, *303*, 1532–1535. [CrossRef]
22. Fuchs, T.A.; Abed, U.; Goosmann, C.; Hurwitz, R.; Schulze, I.; Wahn, V.; Weinrauch, Y.; Brinkmann, V.; Zychlinsky, A. Novel cell death program leads to neutrophil extracellular traps. *J. Cell Biol.* **2007**, *176*, 231–241. [CrossRef] [PubMed]

23. Pilsczek, F.H.; Salina, D.; Poon, K.K.H.; Fahey, C.; Yipp, B.G.; Sibley, C.D.; Robbins, S.M.; Green, F.H.Y.; Surette, M.G.; Sugai, M.; et al. A Novel Mechanism of Rapid Nuclear Neutrophil Extracellular Trap Formation in Response to Staphylococcus aureus. *J. Immunol.* **2010**, *185*, 7413–7425. [CrossRef]

24. Yousefi, S.; Mihalache, C.; Kozlowski, E.; Schmid, I.; Simon, H.U. Viable neutrophils release mitochondrial DNA to form neutrophil extracellular traps. *Cell Death Differ.* **2009**, *16*, 1438–1444. [CrossRef]

25. Yipp, B.G.; Petri, B.; Salina, D.; Jenne, C.N.; Scott, B.N.V.; Zbytnuik, L.D.; Pittman, K.; Asaduzzaman, M.; Wu, K.; Meijndert, H.C.; et al. Infection-induced NETosis is a dynamic process involving neutrophil multitasking in vivo. *Nat. Med.* **2012**, *18*, 1386–1393. [CrossRef]

26. Sonawane, S.; Khanolkar, V.; Namavari, A.; Chaudhary, S.; Gandhi, S.; Tibrewal, S.; Jassim, S.H.; Shaheen, B.; Hallak, J.; Horner, J.H.; et al. Ocular surface extracellular DNA and nuclease activity imbalance: A new paradigm for inflammation in dry eye disease. *Investig. Ophthalmol. Vis. Sci.* **2012**, *53*, 8253–8263. [CrossRef] [PubMed]

27. Khandpur, R.; Carmona-Rivera, C.; Vivekanandan-Giri, A.; Gizinski, A.; Yalavarthi, S.; Knight, J.S.; Friday, S.; Li, S.; Patel, R.M.; Subramanian, V.; et al. NETs are a source of citrullinated autoantigens and stimulate inflammatory responses in rheumatoid arthritis. *Sci. Transl. Med.* **2013**, *5*, 1–24. [CrossRef]

28. Giaglis, S.; Hahn, S.; Hasler, P. "The NET Outcome": Are Neutrophil Extracellular Traps of Any Relevance to the Pathophysiology of Autoimmune Disorders in Childhood? *Front. Pediatr.* **2016**, *4*, 1–8. [CrossRef]

29. Thanabalasuriar, A.; Scott, B.N.V.; Peiseler, M.; Willson, M.E.; Zeng, Z.; Warrener, P.; Keller, A.E.; Surewaard, B.G.J.; Dozier, E.A.; Korhonen, J.T.; et al. Neutrophil Extracellular Traps Confine Pseudomonas aeruginosa Ocular Biofilms and Restrict Brain Invasion. *Cell Host Microbe* **2019**, *25*, 526–536. [CrossRef]

30. An, S.; Raju, I.; Surenkhuu, B.; Kwon, J.E.; Gulati, S.; Karaman, M.; Pradeep, A.; Sinha, S.; Mun, C.; Jain, S. Neutrophil extracellular traps (NETs) contribute to pathological changes of ocular graft-vs.-host disease (oGVHD) dry eye: Implications for novel biomarkers and therapeutic strategies. *Ocul. Surf.* **2019**, *17*, 589–614. [CrossRef]

31. Barliya, T.; Dardik, R.; Nisgav, Y.; Dachbash, M.; Gaton, D.; Kenet, G.; Ehrlich, R.; Weinberger, D.; Livnat, T. Possible involvement of NETosis in inflammatory processes in the eye: Evidence from a small cohort of patients. *Mol. Vis.* **2017**, *23*, 922–932.

32. Wang, L.; Zhou, X.; Yin, Y.; Mai, Y.; Wang, D.; Zhang, X. Hyperglycemia Induces Neutrophil Extracellular Traps Formation Through an NADPH Oxidase-Dependent Pathway in Diabetic Retinopathy. *Front. Immunol.* **2019**, *9*, 1–14. [CrossRef] [PubMed]

33. Kolls, J.K.; McCray, P.B.; Chan, Y.R. Cytokine-mediated regulation of antimicrobial proteins. *Nat. Rev. Immunol.* **2008**, *8*, 829–835. [CrossRef] [PubMed]

34. Chi, W.; Yang, P.; Li, B.; Wu, C.; Jin, H.; Zhu, X.; Chen, L.; Zhou, H.; Huang, X.; Kijlstra, A. IL-23 promotes CD4+ T cells to produce IL-17 in Vogt-Koyanagi-Harada disease. *J. Allergy Clin. Immunol.* **2007**, *119*, 1218–1224. [CrossRef] [PubMed]

35. Chen, X.; Takai, T.; Xie, Y.; Niyonsaba, F.; Okumura, K.; Ogawa, H. Human antimicrobial peptide LL-37 modulates proinflammatory responses induced by cytokine milieus and double-stranded RNA in human keratinocytes. *Biochem. Biophys. Res. Commun.* **2013**, *433*, 532–537. [CrossRef]

36. Skerlavaj, B.; Scocchi, M.; Gennaro, R.; Risso, A.; Zanetti, M. Structural and Functional Analysis of Horse Cathelicidin Peptides. *Antimicrob. Agents Chemother.* **2001**, *45*, 715–722. [CrossRef]

37. Baake, E.I.A.; von Borstel, M.; Rohn, K.; Boevé, M.O.B. Long-term ophthalmologic examinations of eyes with equine recurrent uveitis after pars plana vitrectomy. *Pferdeheilkd. Equine Med.* **2019**, *35*, 220–233. [CrossRef]

38. Coorens, M.; Scheenstra, M.R.; Veldhuizen, E.J.A.; Haagsman, H.P. Interspecies cathelicidin comparison reveals divergence in antimicrobial activity, TLR modulation, chemokine induction and regulation of phagocytosis. *Sci. Rep.* **2017**, *7*, 40874. [CrossRef]

39. De Buhr, N.; Bonilla, M.C.; Pfeiffer, J.; Akhdar, S.; Schwennen, C.; Kahl, B.C.; Waldmann, K.; Valentin-Weigand, P.; Hennig-Pauka, I.; von Köckritz-Blickwede, M. Degraded neutrophil extracellular traps promote the growth of Actinobacillus pleuropneumoniae. *Cell Death Dis.* **2019**, *10*, 657. [CrossRef]

40. Stirling, J.W.; Graff, P.S. Antigen unmasking for immunoelectron microscopy: Labeling is improved by treating with sodium ethoxide or sodium metaperiodate, then heating on retrieval medium. *J. Histochem. Cytochem.* **1995**, *43*, 115–123. [CrossRef]

41. Roth, J. Post-embedding cytochemistry with gold-labelled reagents: A review. *J. Microsc.* **1986**, *143*, 125–137. [CrossRef]

42. Aucamp, J.; Bronkhorst, A.J.; Badenhorst, C.P.S.; Pretorius, P.J. The diverse origins of circulating cell-free DNA in the human body: A critical re-evaluation of the literature. *Biol. Rev.* **2018**, *93*, 1649–1683. [CrossRef] [PubMed]

43. Butt, A.N.; Swaminathan, R. Overview of Circulating Nucleic Acids in Plasma/Serum. *Ann. N. Y. Acad. Sci.* **2008**, *1137*, 236–242. [CrossRef] [PubMed]

44. Wang, C.; Wang, Y.; Shi, X.; Tang, X.; Cheng, W.; Wang, X.; An, Y.; Li, S.; Xu, H.; Li, Y.; et al. The TRAPs From Microglial Vesicles Protect Against Listeria Infection in the CNS. *Front. Cell. Neurosci.* **2019**, *13*, 1–17. [CrossRef] [PubMed]

45. Neumann, A.; Berends, E.T.M.; Nerlich, A.; Molhoek, E.M.; Gallo, R.L.; Meerloo, T.; Nizet, V.; Naim, H.Y.; von Köckritz-Blickwede, M. The antimicrobial peptide LL-37 facilitates the formation of neutrophil extracellular traps. *Biochem. J.* **2014**, *464*, 3–11. [CrossRef]

46. Labelle, P. The Eye. In *Pathologic Basis of Veterinary Disease*; Zachary, J.F., Ed.; Elsevier: Saint Louis, MO, USA, 2017; pp. 1265–1318. ISBN 978-0323357753.

47. Gilger, B.C.; Malok, E.; Cutter, K.V.; Stewart, T.; Horohov, D.W.; Allen, J.B. Characterization of T-lymphocytes in the anterior uvea of eyes with chronic equine recurrent uveitis. *Vet. Immunol. Immunopathol.* **1999**, *71*, 17–28. [CrossRef]

48. Brandes, K.; Wollanke, B.; Niedermaier, G.; Brem, S.; Gerhards, H. ERU vitreal examination with ultrastructural detection of leptospira. *J. Vet. Med.* **2007**, *275*, 270–275. [CrossRef]

49. Lee, K.H.; Cavanaugh, L.; Leung, H.; Yan, F.; Ahmadi, Z.; Chong, B.H.; Passam, F. Quantification of NETs-associated markers by flow cytometry and serum assays in patients with thrombosis and sepsis. *Int. J. Lab. Hematol.* **2018**, *40*, 392–399. [CrossRef]

50. Grilz, E.; Mauracher, L.M.; Posch, F.; Königsbrügge, O.; Zöchbauer-Müller, S.; Marosi, C.; Lang, I.; Pabinger, I.; Ay, C. Citrullinated histone H3, a biomarker for neutrophil extracellular trap formation, predicts the risk of mortality in patients with cancer. *Br. J. Haematol.* **2019**, *186*, 311–320.

51. Vallés, J.; Lago, A.; Santos, M.T.; Latorre, A.M.; Tembl, J.I.; Salom, J.B.; Nieves, C.; Moscardó, A. Neutrophil extracellular traps are increased in patients with acute ischemic stroke: Prognostic significance. *Thromb. Haemost.* **2017**, *117*, 1919–1929. [CrossRef]

52. Sørensen, O.E.; Borregaard, N. Neutrophil extracellular traps—The dark side of neutrophils. *J. Clin. Investig.* **2016**, *126*, 1612–1620. [CrossRef]

53. Gray, R.; McCullagh, B.; McCray, P. NETs and CF Lung Disease: Current Status and Future Prospects. *Antibiotics* **2015**, *4*, 62–75. [CrossRef] [PubMed]

54. Neumann, A.; Völlger, L.; Berends, E.T.M.; Molhoek, E.M.; Stapels, D.A.C.; Midon, M.; Friães, A.; Pingoud, A.; Rooijakkers, S.H.M.; Gallo, R.L.; et al. Novel Role of the Antimicrobial Peptide LL-37 in the Protection of Neutrophil Extracellular Traps against Degradation by Bacterial Nucleases. *J. Innate Immun.* **2014**, *6*, 860–868. [CrossRef] [PubMed]

55. Doring, Y.; Manthey, H.D.; Drechsler, M.; Lievens, D.; Megens, R.T.; Soehnlein, O.; Busch, M.; Manca, M.; Koenen, R.R.; Pelisek, J.; et al. Auto-Antigenic Protein-DNA Complexes Stimulate Plasmacytoid Dendritic Cells to Promote Atherosclerosis. *Circulation* **2012**, *125*, 1673–1683. [CrossRef] [PubMed]

56. Reinholz, M.; Ruzicka, T.; Schauber, J. Cathelicidin LL-37: An Antimicrobial Peptide with a Role in Inflammatory Skin Disease. *Ann. Dermatol.* **2012**, *24*, 126–135. [CrossRef] [PubMed]

57. Bruhn, O.; Grötzinger, J.; Cascorbi, I.; Jung, S. Antimicrobial peptides and proteins of the horse—Insights into a well-armed organism. *Vet. Res.* **2011**, *42*, 1–22. [CrossRef] [PubMed]

58. Scocchi, M.; Bontempo, D.; Boscolo, S.; Tomasinsig, L.; Giulotto, E.; Zanetti, M. Novel cathelicidins in horse leukocytes. *FEBS Lett.* **1999**, *457*, 459–464. [CrossRef]

59. Lande, R.; Gregorio, J.; Facchinetti, V.; Chatterjee, B.; Wang, Y.H.; Homey, B.; Cao, W.; Wang, Y.H.; Su, B.; Nestle, F.O.; et al. Plasmacytoid dendritic cells sense self-DNA coupled with antimicrobial peptide. *Nature* **2007**, *449*, 564–569. [CrossRef]

60. McLaughlin, B.G.; McLaughlin, P.S. Equine vitreous humor chemical concentrations: Correlation with serum concentrations, and postmortem changes with time and temperature. *Can. J. Vet. Res.* **1988**, *52*, 476–480.

61. Johansson, J.; Gudmonsson, G.H.; Rottenberg, M.E.; Berndt, K.; Agerberth, B. Conformation-dependent Antibacterial Activity of the Naturally Occurring Human Peptide LL-37. *J. Biol. Chem.* **1998**, *273*, 3718–3724. [CrossRef]

62. Kościuczuk, E.M.; Lisowski, P.; Jarczak, J.; Strzałkowska, N.; Jóźwik, A.; Horbańczuk, J.; Krzyzewski, J.; Zwierzchowski, L.; Bagnicka, E. Cathelicidins: Family of antimicrobial peptides. A review. *Mol. Biol. Rep.* **2012**, *39*, 10957–10970. [CrossRef]

63. Ong, P.Y.; Ohtake, T.; Brandt, C.; Strickland, I.; Boguniewicz, M.; Ganz, T.; Gallo, R.L.; Leung, D.Y.M. Endogenous Antimicrobial Peptides and Skin Infections in Atopic Dermatitis. *N. Engl. J. Med.* **2002**, *347*, 1151–1160. [CrossRef]

64. Scharrig, E.; Carestia, A.; Ferrer, M.F.; Cédola, M.; Pretre, G.; Drut, R.; Picardeau, M.; Schattner, M.; Gómez, R.M. Neutrophil Extracellular Traps are Involved in the Innate Immune Response to Infection with Leptospira. *PLoS Negl. Trop. Dis.* **2015**, *9*, e0003927. [CrossRef] [PubMed]

65. Wilson-Welder, J.H.; Frank, A.T.; Hornsby, R.L.; Olsen, S.C.; Alt, D.P. Interaction of bovine peripheral blood polymorphonuclear cells and Leptospira species; innate responses in the natural bovine reservoir host. *Front. Microbiol.* **2016**, *7*, 1–14. [CrossRef] [PubMed]

66. Tömördy, E.; Hässig, M.; Spiess, B.M. The outcome of pars plana vitrectomy in horses with equine recurrent uveitis with regard to the presence or absence of intravitreal antibodies against various serovars of Leptospira interrogans. *Pferdeheilkunde* **2010**, *26*, 251–254. [CrossRef]

67. Mun, C.; Gulati, S.; Tibrewal, S.; Chen, Y.-F.; An, S.; Surenkhuu, B.; Raju, I.; Buwick, M.; Ahn, A.; Kwon, J.-E.; et al. A Phase I/II Placebo-Controlled Randomized Pilot Clinical Trial of Recombinant Deoxyribonuclease (DNase) Eye Drops Use in Patients with Dry Eye Disease. *Transl. Vis. Sci. Technol.* **2019**, *8*, 10. [CrossRef]

68. Tibrewal, S.; Sarkar, J.; Jassim, S.H.; Gandhi, S.; Sonawane, S.; Chaudhary, S.; Byun, Y.S.; Ivanir, Y.; Hallak, J.; Horner, J.H.; et al. Tear fluid extracellular dna: Diagnostic and therapeutic implications in dry eye disease. *Investig. Ophthalmol. Vis. Sci.* **2013**, *54*, 8051–8061. [CrossRef]

69. Mannermaa, E.; Reinisalo, M.; Ranta, V.-P.; Vellonen, K.-S.; Kokki, H.; Saarikko, A.; Kaarniranta, K.; Urtti, A. Filter-cultured ARPE-19 cells as outer blood–retinal barrier model. *Eur. J. Pharm. Sci.* **2010**, *40*, 289–296. [CrossRef]

70. Saffarzadeh, M.; Juenemann, C.; Queisser, M.A.; Lochnit, G.; Barreto, G.; Galuska, S.P.; Lohmeyer, J.; Preissner, K.T. Neutrophil Extracellular Traps Directly Induce Epithelial and Endothelial Cell Death: A Predominant Role of Histones. *PLoS ONE* **2012**, *7*, e32366. [CrossRef]

71. Estúa-Acosta, G.A.; Zamora-Ortiz, R.; Buentello-Volante, B.; García-Mejía, M.; Garfias, Y. Neutrophil Extracellular Traps: Current Perspectives in the Eye. *Cells* **2019**, *8*, 979. [CrossRef]

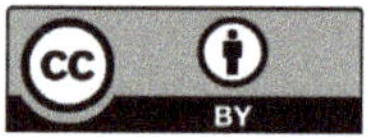

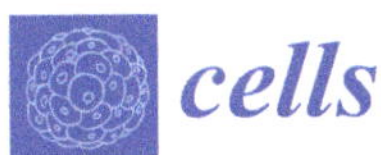 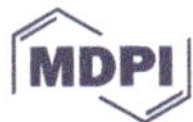

Review

Neutrophil Extracellular Traps and Cardiovascular Diseases: An Update

Aldo Bonaventura [1,2,*], Alessandra Vecchié [1,2], Antonio Abbate [1] and Fabrizio Montecucco [3,4]

[1] Pauley Heart Center, Division of Cardiology, Department of Internal Medicine, Virginia Commonwealth University, 1200 E Marshall St, Richmond, VA 23298, USA; alessandra.vecchie@vcuhealth.org (A.V.); antonio.abbate@vcuhealth.org (A.A.)

[2] First Clinic of Internal Medicine, Department of Internal Medicine, University of Genoa, viale Benedetto XV 6, 16132 Genoa, Italy

[3] First Clinic of Internal Medicine, Department of Internal Medicine and Centre of Excellence for Biomedical Research (CEBR), University of Genoa, viale Benedetto XV 6, 16132 Genoa, Italy; fabrizio.montecucco@unige.it

[4] IRCCS Ospedale Policlinico San Martino Genova—Italian Cardiovascular Network, Largo R. Benzi 10, 16132 Genoa, Italy

* Correspondence: aldo.bonaventura@vcuhealth.org or aldo.bonaventura@edu.unige.it

Received: 24 December 2019; Accepted: 15 January 2020; Published: 17 January 2020

Abstract: Neutrophil extracellular traps (NETs) are formed by decondensed chromatin, histones, and neutrophil granular proteins and have a role in entrapping microbial pathogens. NETs, however, have pro-thrombotic properties by stimulating fibrin deposition, and increased NET levels correlate with larger infarct size and predict major adverse cardiovascular (CV) events. NETs have been involved also in the pathogenesis of diabetes, as high glucose levels were found to induce NETosis. Accordingly, NETs have been described as drivers of diabetic complications, such as diabetic wound and diabetic retinopathy. Inflammasomes are macromolecular structures involved in the release of pro-inflammatory mediators, such as interleukin-1, which is a key mediator in CV diseases. A crosstalk between the inflammasome and NETs is known for some rheumatologic diseases, while this link is still under investigation and not completely understood in CV diseases. In this review, we summarized the most recent updates about the role of NETs in acute myocardial infarction and metabolic diseases and provided an overview on the relationship between NET and inflammasome activities in rheumatologic diseases, speculating a possible link between these two entities also in CV diseases.

Keywords: NETs; neutrophils; NLRP3 inflammasome; IL-1β; cardiovascular disease; inflammation; diabetes; obesity

---

1. Introduction

Neutrophils are the most abundant effector cells of the innate immune system [1]. Apart from their defensive role against infections, neutrophils have acquired a distinct role in the pathophysiology of many cardiovascular (CV) diseases [2]. The most important mechanism for their phagocytic and antimicrobial activity is the release of granular products (i.e., metalloproteinase [MMP]-8 and -9, myeloperoxidase [MPO], neutrophil gelatinase-associated lipocalin [NGAL], and neutrophil elastase [NE]) [2,3]. More recently, neutrophil extracellular traps (NETs) have been recognized as an additional mechanism of defense through a process called NETosis [4,5]. NETs are made up of chromatin decorated with histones, proteases, and granular proteins through which neutrophils can block and catch up invading microorganisms [6,7] (Figure 1). The presence of granular proteins is an essential requirement for NET formation since both NE knockout mice and MPO-deficient patients were found to produce a lesser amount of NETs [8,9]. Indeed, in experimental studies, mice unable to activate NETosis showed a higher susceptibility to infectious diseases [10]. NETs, however, have been recognized as important drivers also in the pathophysiology of CV diseases [2,11,12].

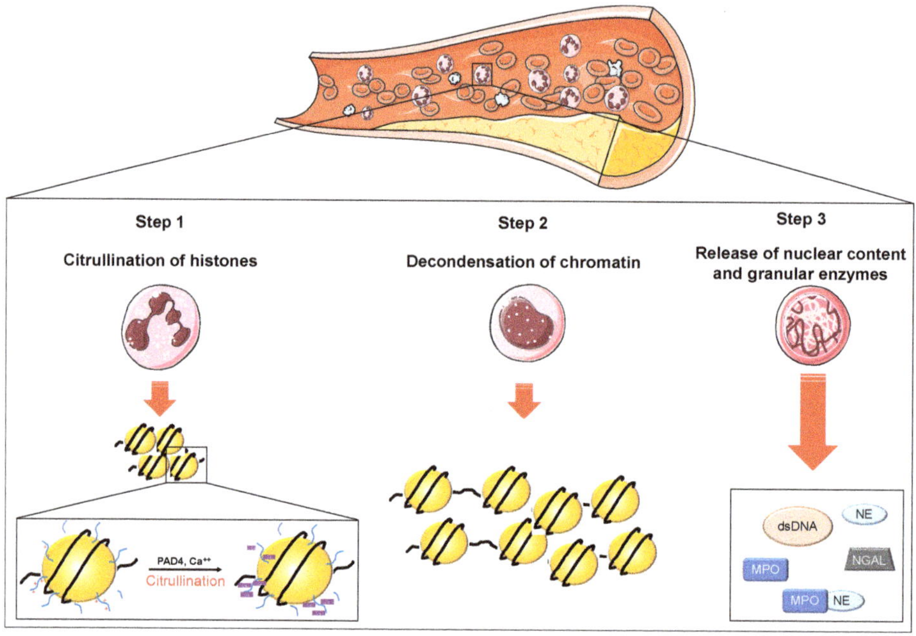

Figure 1. Overview of NETosis. NETosis occurs through the release of neutrophil extracellular traps (NETs) and represents an additional mechanism of defense. The cascade of events leading to NETosis include the histone tail citrullination of positively charged arginine residues mediated by the calcium-dependent PAD4 (Step 1), that leads to chromatin decondensation (Step 2). After this, the nuclear envelope destroys, the granule content enters the nucleus followed by the release of the nuclear material along with granular enzymes (Step 3). Legend. Ca++: calcium. Cit: citrullinated histone tail. dsDNA: double-stranded deoxyribonucleic acid. PAD4: peptidylarginine deiminase type 4. MPO: myeloperoxidase. NE: neutrophil elastase. NGAL: neutrophil gelatinase-associated lipocalin.

Inflammasomes are intracellular, macromolecular complexes that sense dangers and trigger a local or systemic inflammatory response through the release of cytokines belonging to the interleukin (IL)-1 family [13]. In particular, the NACHT, LRR, and PYD domain-containing protein 3 (NLRP3) inflammasome is thought to act as a central player in the setting of acute myocardial infarction (AMI) and heart failure [13]. A crosstalk between the inflammasome and NETs was described in different settings, with NETs able to prime macrophages to produce IL-1 through the NLRP3 inflammasome, thus amplifying the inflammatory response [14], although this interplay is less understood in CV diseases.

In this review, we aim to summarize the most recent findings concerning the role of NETs in AMI and metabolic diseases (particularly diabetes and obesity). In addition, we provide some information on the relationship between NET and inflammasome activities in rheumatologic diseases, speculating a possible link between these two entities in CV diseases.

2. Review Criteria

This narrative review is based on original articles and reviews published over the last years and retrieved through PubMed using the following search terms (or combination of terms): NETs, neutrophils, NE, MPO, inflammation, NLRP3 inflammasome, acute myocardial infarction, ST elevation myocardial infarction, obesity, type 1 diabetes, type 2 diabetes, and outcomes. Only English-language papers were included. Additional papers identified from the reference list of the retrieved articles were also considered.

3. NETs in Acute Myocardial Infarction

Acute myocardial infarction (AMI) is triggered in most cases by the erosion/rupture of a coronary atherosclerotic plaque, followed by the formation of a thrombus occluding the artery [15]. Although monocytes and macrophages are known to play an essential role, in recent years neutrophils have also been described to be involved in atherothrombosis [16,17], as demonstrated by their accumulation in coronary thrombi [18] and their predictive role in acute coronary events [19,20]. As well, neutrophils and NETs were described in animal models of ischemia/reperfusion injury (IRI) along with the beneficial effect of DNase in mitigating the IRI and the no-reflow phenomenon [21].

NETs play a central role in thrombosis by promoting fibrin deposition and formation of fibrin networks [22]. Following the interaction between platelets and neutrophils at the site of plaque rupture during STEMI, NETs were recognized to express functional tissue factor and to induce platelet activation and further thrombin generation, thus increasing the thrombogenic potential of NETs [23] (Figure 2). Importantly, the integrity of the deoxyribonucleic acid (DNA) scaffold was proved as a necessary condition for the tissue factor to be expressed on NETs from infarct-related coronary arteries [23]. Despite the presence of NETs in developing thrombi, human intact NETs did not show any pro-coagulant property in vitro in contrast to single histones able to induce thrombin generation in a platelet-dependent way [24]. This probably depends on the neutralization of the negative charge of DNA on the NET surface. Additionally, it is now clear that activated platelets can present high-mobility group box 1 (HMGB1) to neutrophils and stimulate these cells to form NETs [25] (Figure 2). More recently, a concept emerged following the discovery that toll-like receptor (TLR)-2 stimulation along with NETs trapped within the fibrin strands might have a role in plaque erosion through an increase in endoplasmic reticulum (ER) inducing ER stress and apoptosis [26].

A central role for NETs in coronary artery disease (CAD) has been proposed and main studies investigating this relationship are summarized in Table 1. For example, NETs were retrieved at a higher extent in older thrombi showing lytic changes compared to fresh ones, but never in organized thrombi, thus suggesting that NET formation occurs early in the thrombus dissolution process [27]. In another study, coronary thrombi were confirmed to contain a large amount of NETs, which are deemed as a scaffold for platelets, red blood cells, and fibrin [28].

Table 1. Main studies investigating NETs in coronary artery disease.

Author	Year	Patients	Biomarkers	Results
Borissoff et al. [29]	2013	282 patients with suspected CAD undergoing coronary CTA, grouped based on the presence and severity of CAD	dsDNA, nucleosomes, citH4, and MPO-DNA complexes	dsDNA, nucleosome, and MPO-DNA complex levels were higher in patients with severe CAD ($p < 0.05$ for all) compared to healthy controls and correlated with the severity of luminal stenosis and the number of diseased coronary artery vessels ($p \leq 0.001$ for all). Baseline higher-than-median values of dsDNA (OR 3.12, $p = 0.013$), nucleosome (OR 2.59, $p = 0.030$), and MPO–DNA complexes (OR 3.53, $p = 0.009$) were significantly associated with the occurrence of MACEs.
Cui et al. [30]	2013	137 ACS patients (51 UA, 37 NSTEMI, and 49 STEMI), 13 stable AP patients, and 60 healthy controls	dsDNA	ACS patients showed higher dsDNA levels compared to stable AP patients and control group ($p < 0.05$ for both). Significant differences in dsDNA concentrations were observed among UA, NSTEMI, and STEMI sub-groups ($p < 0.05$ for all).
Mangold et al. [28]	2015	111 patients with STEMI undergoing PCI (TIMI flow 0–1)	Nucleosomes and dsDNA	NE, MPO, nucleosome, and dsDNA concentrations were increased at the CLS compared to the femoral site ($p < 0.001$ for all). Nucleosome and dsDNA levels positively correlated with coronary thrombus NET burden ($p < 0.05$ for both), the latter being positively correlated with ST resolution and both enzymatic (CK-MB AUC) and CMR-assessed infarct size ($p < 0.01$ for all).
Helseth et al. [31]	2016	30 patients with CAD undergoing PCI (20 with STEMI and 10 with stable AP)	Nucleosomes and dsDNA	dsDNA and nucleosome levels were higher in patients with STEMI compared to those with AP ($p < 0.05$ for both). dsDNA significantly correlated with peak TnT and CK-MB at day 5 ($p = 0.03$ for both) and with CMR-assessed infarct size at days 5 and 7 ($p < 0.05$ for both), while only nucleosomes correlated with infarct size at day 5 ($p = 0.02$).
Hofbauer et al. [32]	2019	50 patients with STEMI undergoing PCI (TIMI flow 0)	dsDNA and citH3	dsDNA and citH3 levels were significantly increased at the CLS than at the femoral artery ($p < 0.01$ for both). This trend was confirmed only for dsDNA when compared to healthy controls ($p < 0.0001$). Both dsDNA and citH3 were positively correlated with enzymatic infarct size ($p < 0.05$ for both). dsDNA measured at the CLS at the time of PCI was positively correlated with WMSI at the 24 ± 8-month follow-up ($p = 0.039$).

Table 1. *Cont.*

Author	Year	Patients	Biomarkers	Results
Liu et al. [33]	2019	83 patients with STEMI undergoing PCI (TIMI 0)	dsDNA and MPO-DNA complexes	A larger number of NETting neutrophils from IRA was found compared to peripheral arteries and healthy controls ($p < 0.05$ for both). Higher concentrations of dsDNA and MPO-DNA complexes were retrieved within IRA compared to peripheral arteries ($p < 0.05$ for both). Baseline levels of coronary dsDNA were higher in patients experiencing a MACE (0.70 vs. 0.46 µg/mL, $p = 0.002$). Additionally, dsDNA was found to independently predict in-hospital MACEs (OR 46.26, $p = 0.001$). A cutoff of 0.39 µg/mL for dsDNA was reported as a better prognostic marker compared to TnT and CK-MB (sensitivity 78%, specificity 53%).
Helseth et al. [34]	2019	224 patients with STEMI undergoing PCI followed for 3 months	dsDNA and MPO-DNA complexes	dsDNA and MPO-DNA levels were correlated to leukocyte count at admission ($p < 0.01$ for both) and to each other only in the acute phase ($p < 0.001$), but not after 3 months. dsDNA weakly correlated with glucose in the acute phase and after 3 months ($p < 0.05$ for both), while MPO-DNA did not.
Mangold et al. [35]	2019	91 patients with STEMI receiving thrombectomy during PCI	dsDNA and citH3	dsDNA and citH3 were significantly elevated at the CLS compared to femoral plasma ($p < 0.0001$ for both) and correlated with enzymatic infarct size (CK-MB AUC, $p < 0.001$ and $p < 0.01$, respectively). High CLS dsDNA correlated with low, non-classical (anti-inflammatory) monocyte percentage at the culprit site ($p < 0.05$). Low CX3CR1 expression of non-classical monocytes (i.e., anti-inflammatory) negatively correlated with high CLS dsDNA and citH3 levels ($p < 0.05$ for both).
Liberale et al. [36]	2019	66 patients undergoing PCI	MPO-DNA and TF-DNA complexes	MPO-DNA complexes were higher in the high- compared to the low-CRP group ($p < 0.01$). Patients with high CRP levels showed increased levels of TF-DNA complexes than patients with low CRP levels ($p < 0.01$). A positive correlation with NETosis markers (MPO-DNA and TF-DNA complexes) was recorded ($p < 0.0001$).

ACS: acute coronary syndrome. AMI: acute myocardial infarction. AP: angina pectoris. AUC: area under the curve. citH3: citrullinated histone H3. citH4: citrullinated histone H4. CAD: coronary artery disease. CK: creatine-phosphokinase. CK-MB: creatine-phosphokinase isoform muscle and brain. CLS: culprit lesion site. CMR: cardiac magnetic resonance. CRP: C-reactive protein. CTA: computed tomography angiography. CX3CR1: C-X3-C motif chemokine receptor 1. dsDNA: double-stranded deoxyribonucleic acid. IRA: infarct-related artery. MACEs: major cardiovascular events. MPO/DNA: myeloperoxidase/deoxyribonucleic acid. NET: neutrophil extracellular trap. NSTEMI: non ST elevation myocardial infarction. OR: odds ratio. PCI: percutaneous coronary intervention. STEMI: ST elevation myocardial infarction. TF: tissue factor. TIMI: Thrombolysis In Myocardial Infarction. TnT: troponin T. UA: unstable angina. WMSI: wall motion score index.

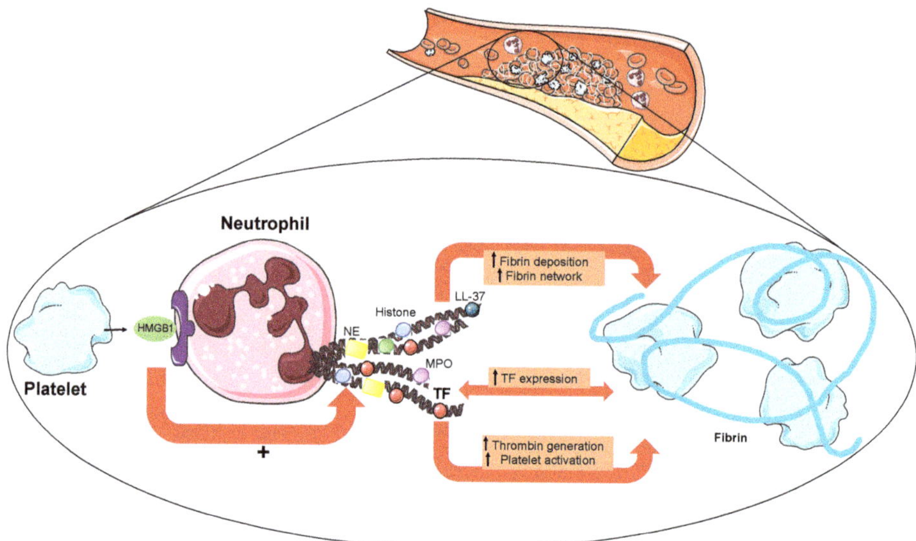

Figure 2. The interplay between NETs and platelets. NETs promote thrombosis by favoring fibrin deposition. Recently, a notion has been added by showing that NETs can express tissue factor further triggering thrombin generation and platelet activation and finally increasing the thrombogenic potential of NETs. This was reported especially at the site of plaque rupture during acute myocardial infarction when platelets and neutrophils interact with each other. In this view, activated platelets present HMGB1 to neutrophils and stimulate them to form NETs. Legend. HMGB1: high-mobility group box 1. NE: neutrophil elastase. MPO: myeloperoxidase. TF: tissue factor.

Nucleosomes (DNA-histone complexes) and double-stranded DNA (dsDNA)—key components of NETs proposed as sensitive biomarkers for CV events—were found at increased levels at the culprit site and correlated with the coronary thrombus NET burden. Interestingly, the latter negatively correlated with ST resolution, but was positively associated with the infarct size expressed both as area under the curve of creatine phosphokinase isoform muscle brain (CK-MB) and through cardiac magnetic resonance (CMR) assessment [28]. These data underline the detrimental role played by NETs at the culprit site through the stimulation of thrombosis and inflammation into the infarcted myocardium. Additionally, the activity of DNase at the culprit site was negatively correlated with the coronary NET burden, the area at risk, ST resolution, and infarct size measured through CMR [28]. Hence, the balance between NET burden and endogenous DNase activity might be responsible for different outcomes and eventually represent a field of research for targeted therapies. This is also true for other surrogate markers of NET burden (dsDNA and citrullinated histone H3 [citH3]), whose concentration was increased at the culprit site [32]. Interestingly, in patients evaluated through transthoracic echocardiography after 24 ± 8 months from AMI, dsDNA at the culprit site positively correlated with the wall motion score index (the higher the index, the worse the left ventricular function) [32]. Another study pointed out the prognostic role of NETs. In a cohort of patients with recent STEMI, higher levels of coronary dsDNA were found to independently predict in-hospital major adverse CV events (MACEs) [33]. These results, however, confirmed those previously reported by Borissoff et al., who in 2013 described for the first time a positive association between high levels of circulating dsDNA, nucleosomes, and MPO-DNA complexes and the occurrence of MACEs [29].

Some studies followed the time course of NETs at different time points. In a cohort of 30 patients with STEMI and stable angina undergoing successful PCI [31], a progressive decrease of dsDNA in all patients following PCI was reported across 14 days, although STEMI patients exhibited higher levels throughout the observation time. Differently, nucleosomes were found to peak after 12 h from PCI in STEMI patients and then to progressively reduce until day 7 with a slight increase at day 14, remaining higher in patients with stable angina [31]. In another study, both dsDNA and MPO-DNA concentrations were higher in the acute phase than after three months and correlated with the total leukocyte count at the time of the admission and to each other only in the acute phase. Interestingly, the acute glucose load provided by the oral glucose tolerance test performed three months after the STEMI resulted in an increased gene expression of peptidylarginine deiminase 4 (PAD4), but it was not paralleled by an increase in dsDNA and/or MPO-DNA levels [34]. Based on the available literature [37], the authors concluded that this may be probably due to a delayed release of NETs or to the fact that NETosis might be triggered by acute changes in plasma glucose in the stable setting (i.e., three months) following an AMI.

NETs are likely to behave in a similar manner also in stable CAD. In a large study including >1000 patients previously enrolled in the ASCET (ASpirin non-responsiveness and Clinical Endpoints Trial) [38], dsDNA and MPO-DNA significantly correlated with neutrophil count, but only dsDNA levels were strongly associated with prothrombin fragment 1 and 2 and D-dimer, two in vivo markers of thrombin generation and fibrin turnover hypercoagulability. These findings further underpinned how NETs exert a negative impact beyond their prothrombotic potential [38] and confirmed previous findings by Borissoff et al. [29]. When analyzing the outcomes (including a composite of unstable angina, non-hemorrhagic stroke, AMI, or all-cause mortality), patients experiencing an event presented with significantly higher dsDNA levels as compared to patients without events. A trend toward an increased number of endpoints across quartiles was found, especially for quartiles from 2nd to 4th. Additionally, increased dsDNA levels in 2nd–4th quartiles were associated with a 2-fold increased risk of experiencing a composite of unstable angina, non-hemorrhagic stroke, AMI, or all-cause mortality, independently of treatment allocation and markers of hypercoagulability [38].

4. NETs in Diabetes

Diabetes is characterized by a low-grade inflammation [39] explaining the typical complications of the disease through endothelial dysfunction, hyperreactivity of platelets, and elevated levels of pro-coagulant mediators [40,41]. Hyperglycemic conditions were reported to limit lipopolysaccharide (LPS)-induced neutrophil degranulation and the following release of granular proteins, i.e., MPO and NE [42,43]. In recent years, a progressive number of evidences shed light on the role played by neutrophils in the pathophysiology of diabetes (both type 1 diabetes [T1D] and type 2 diabetes [T2D]) [44–47]. Additionally, the expression of PAD4 in neutrophils is elevated in patients with T1D and T2D, thus explaining their special attitude to produce NETs [48].

Neutrophils were recognized to infiltrate the pancreas of subjects with T1D [49] and to have a role in the onset and the progression of T1D [50]. Neutrophils might accumulate at all disease stages, including pre-symptomatic subjects with positive autoantibodies [51]. Through the colocalization between dsDNA and MPO, it emerged that pancreas-residing neutrophils were able to form NETs, as confirmed by the decoration of decondensed DNA with citrullinated histones [51]. Indeed, a reduction in the neutrophil count in patients with T1D at onset was paralleled by a marked increase in NE and proteinase 3 (PR3) levels and activity, that in turn were associated with an increased NETosis [49,50,52,53]. It is then likely that the reduced number of circulating neutrophils might be due to an increased NET production, which is also responsible for the augmented levels of NE and PR3 in the bloodstream.

Additional studies are available describing the role played by NETs in T2D, but they appear controversial. Although high glucose levels were described to induce NETosis and NET-related products both in vitro and in vivo in a dose-dependent fashion [54], both spontaneously and when induced by phorbol 12-myristate 13-acetate (PMA) [55], a deeper investigation provided somewhat different results. In fact, Joshi et al. reported that in vitro NET formation was impaired at progressively increasing glucose concentrations, being delayed and resulting in short-lived and unstable NETs [56]. This was later confirmed when neutrophils from T2D subjects were stimulated for 3 h with LPS.

In patients with T2D, a pre-activated condition was observed, i.e., NETting neutrophils without any external stimulus, only in presence of normal glucose concentration (5.5 mM). This was probably due to the incapacity of neutrophils to respond to other stimuli (e.g., PMA) when already exposed to hyperglycemia [56]. An explanation for these different results in pretty similar conditions may be the different time of incubation (4 h vs. 24 h, respectively) affecting the process of NET formation. Hence, diabetes represents a trigger for the constitutive NET activation, but the continuous stimulus provided by higher glucose concentrations is likely to detrimentally impact on the ability of neutrophils to produce fully working NETs. This aspect, therefore, deserves further investigation in the future in order to better clarify these mechanisms.

Neutrophils from T2D patients were shown to produce a large amount of IL-6, which in turn induced NET formation in an autocrine fashion at the same extent of LPS, except when neutrophils were cultured under high glucose conditions (30 mM) [56]. This latter finding was confirmed in a small cohort of T2D patients followed for one year from the time of the diagnosis and treated with metformin 500–2500 mg/daily [57]. Indeed, neutrophils from T2D patients produced a larger amount of NETs compared to healthy controls, but not when stimulated with PMA [57]. Additionally, NET formation, nucleosome, and NE-dsDNA complexes were still present in the plasma of patients after 6 months of metformin treatment, while all neutrophil functional responses returned to normal values after 12 months with no change in neutrophil count across this period [57]. This finding about metformin was later investigated by Menegazzo et al. confirming that metformin reduced NE, PR3, histones, and dsDNA levels [58]. Indeed, metformin blocked in vitro pathologic changes in nuclear dynamics and DNA release provoking a blunted NETosis in response to classical NET stimuli [58]. As NET formation is likely to be associated with glucose-stimulated reactive oxygen species (ROS) production, it is possible that ROS have a direct effect on NET production. In fact, diphenyleneiodonium and apocynin, two inhibitors of NADPH oxidase, reduce NET formation in neutrophils exposed to high glucose stimulation [59]. Accordingly, the inhibition of NADPH oxidase markedly decreased the release of extracellular DNA compared to high glucose condition, thus suggesting that glucose-induced NET production might be dependent on NADPH oxidase [59].

NETs were described to be implicated in diabetic complications. Indeed, a poor outcome for diabetic wounds in subjects with T1D and T2D was recorded [48,60]. In a case-control association study, dsDNA-histone complex and NE levels were significantly increased in patients with diabetic retinopathy compared with those without [55]. As a further proof of it, Wang et al. reported that an increased NET formation was observed in the serum of T2D patients with diabetic retinopathy irrespective of the stage of the disease, with NE driving this trend [59].

5. NETs in Obesity

Obesity is considered an inflammatory disease since adipose tissue dysfunction is responsible for an impairment in adipocytokine production [61]. In addition, inflammatory cells can infiltrate the adipose tissue [62] and release pro-inflammatory mediators [63,64]. NETs were shown to have a role in the obesity-related inflammation both in pre-clinical and clinical studies.

In an experimental mouse model of high-fat, high-sucrose diet, the immunostaining for cathelicidin-related antimicrobial peptide (CRAMP), a surrogate marker of NETting neutrophils, was markedly more positive compared to control lean mice and reduced after treatment with Cl-amidine, a PAD4 inhibitor, or DNase [65]. Additionally, the effect of NETs in mediating endothelial dysfunction in obese mice was studied with Cl-amidine administered for 2 weeks or DNase for 8 days, after 8 and 9 weeks of high fat, respectively. Blocking NETs is beneficial for the recovery from the endothelial dysfunction provoked by the high-fat diet [65]. The main explanation of the role of NETs in obesity-induced endothelial dysfunction might be an abnormal production of MPO. MPO, in fact, increases the production of ROS, which in turn oxidize the endothelial-derived nitric oxide production. Different results were reported by Braster et al. in another model of high-fat diet, in which the presence of NETting neutrophils in the adipose tissue was confirmed at a higher extent in obese than in lean mice [66]. Despite the administration of Cl-amidine for 10 weeks since the beginning of the high-fat diet, no beneficial effect in terms of improved metabolic parameters was found [66]. This is likely to suggest that an early blockade of NETs might not be effective in blunting NET-related effects probably due to the presence of a kind of 'escape' mechanism.

Recently, in a cohort of patients with morbid obesity who underwent sleeve gastrectomy, a higher amount of MPO-DNA complexes compared to healthy controls was found [67]. Levels of MPO-DNA complexes positively correlated with body weight, body mass index, waist and hip circumference, and glyco-metabolic profile. One year after the surgical intervention, MPO-DNA complexes did not show any absolute change compared to baseline. In some patients, however, MPO-DNA complexes were reduced, whereas in some others increased [67], thus suggesting that the mere weight loss may not modify neutrophil activation. Interestingly, the sub-group with reduced MPO-DNA complexes after sleeve gastrectomy presented with a reduced body weight and BMI and an improved glycemic status. On the contrary, those with persisting high levels of MPO-DNA complexes after surgery had a history of stroke and thromboembolism and therefore may represent a high CV risk population [67].

6. NETs and the Inflammasome

Depending on different sensor components, various inflammasomes can oligomerize [68,69] and the activation of the caspase-1 takes place [70]. The common, final stage of this process is the proteolytic cleavage of pro-IL-1β and pro-IL-18 to their active forms. The NACHT, LRR, and PYD domain-containing protein 3 (NLRP3) inflammasome was largely studied in the CV field, as confirmed by their role in atherosclerosis, acute myocardial infarction, heart failure, and pericarditis [71–76]. Of note, the role of the NLRP3 inflammasome and IL-1β is well established in many rheumatic diseases, too [77].

Cathelicidin LL-37 is an antimicrobial peptide released within NETs and was previously recognized to induce IL-1β from monocytes following the activation of the P2X purinoreceptor 7 (P2X7R) [78], that mediates the potassium efflux during inflammasome activation (Figure 3). Kahlenberg et al. reported some interesting findings on the role played by NETs in triggering the NLRP3 inflammasome activation in macrophages of patients with systemic lupus erythematosus (SLE) [79]. Indeed, they found a positive correlation between the concentration of LL-37 within NETs and their ability to activate the NLRP3 inflammasome and release IL-1β and IL-18 through caspase-1. As well, LL-37 played a major role in potassium efflux through the P2X7R activation. A central role for IL-18 was shown, which effectively stimulated NET release at the same extent of other known NETosis stimuli (i.e., PMA and LPS) [79]. Additionally, IL-18-stimulated NET release significantly increased caspase-1 activation in primed macrophages compared to IL-18 alone. This might suggest a feed-forward loop through which NETs increase the synthesis of IL-1β and IL-18 in macrophages, that in turn can stimulate NET formation in neutrophils (Figure 3). Similarly to what happens in SLE, the pivotal role of NETs was demonstrated in acute gout, too [80]. As well, patients with adult-onset Still's disease (AOSD) presented with higher levels of circulating NETs compared to controls, which contributed to the NLRP3 inflammasome and macrophage activation, finally increasing the release of pro-inflammatory cytokines [81]. An interplay between NETs and the inflammasome has been described also in severe asthma [82]. Among patients included in the Severe Asthma Research Program (SARP)-3, increased caspase-1 concentrations were measured in patients with high levels of NETs, thus suggesting the inflammasome activation. This may suggest that patients with severe asthma have a marked neutrophil activation in their airways, as proved by the increased concentrations of NETs, the latter being able to further trigger the inflammasome in monocytes or macrophages and release IL-1β [82,83].

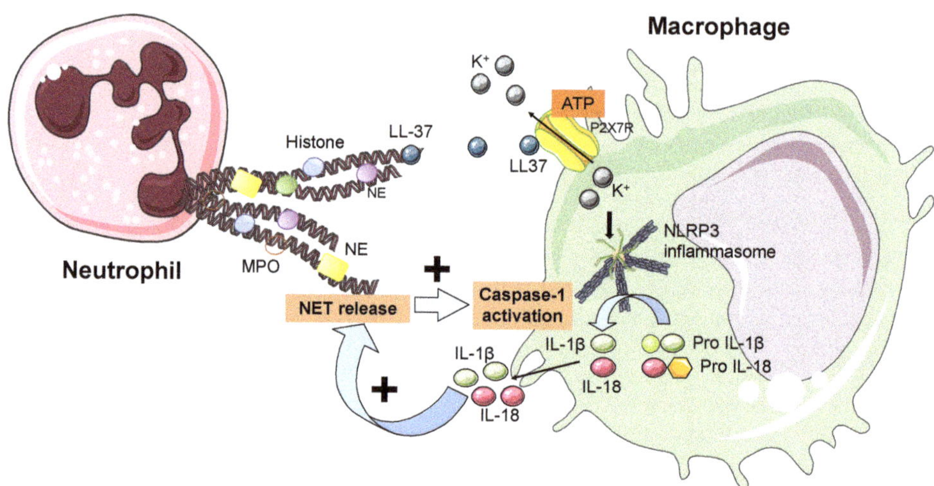

Figure 3. Interactions between neutrophils and macrophages. The NLRP3 inflammasome is an intracellular macromolecular structure recognizing danger signals and activating an inflammatory response, especially by the release of IL-1β and IL-18. In recent works, NETs have been described to play a central role in activating the NLRP3 inflammasome in macrophages. This happens through LL-37 triggering potassium efflux from the cell via the activation of the P2X7R. Additionally, IL-18 may stimulate NET release and increase caspase-1 activation in macrophages in a feed-forward loop. Accordingly, NETs trigger IL-1β and IL-18 synthesis in macrophages, that promote NET formation in neutrophils. Legend. IL: interleukin. MPO: myeloperoxidase. NET: neutrophil extracellular trap. NLRP3: NACHT, LRR, and PYD domain-containing protein 3. P2X7R: P2X purinoreceptor 7.

Caspases are important in pyroptosis, a regulated cellular death depending on the activation of the inflammasome [84,85]. Typical substrates are IL-1β and IL-18. Recently, gasdermin D (GSDMD) has been identified as an important pyroptotic effector activated by caspase-11 and less often by caspase-1 [86,87]. Caspases are responsible for the cleavage of the Asp275 and Asp276 residues on GSDMD, that generates an N-terminal GSDMD product, namely GSDMD-NT or GSDMD-p30. GSDMD-NT is responsible for the pores through the cytoplasmic membrane [88,89] leading to osmotic swelling and membrane rupture. Pyroptosis can, however, be also activated in a non-canonical fashion through caspase-11 (caspase-4/5 in human cells) activity following LPS stimulation [87].

Recently, Sollberger et al. investigated the role of GSDMD as a common effector of both pyroptosis and NETosis [90]. In an in vitro experiment, GSDMD was cleaved during NET formation and localized to the plasma membrane of neutrophils. Additionally, some neutrophil proteases (NE, PR3, and cathepsin G) were found to induce GSDMD cleavage at different sites leading to lysis-inducing fragments. The authors then concluded that GSDMD may represent a key player in pro-inflammatory cell death through two functions [90]. First of all, NE and GSDMD look like to be involved in a feed-forward loop, in which GSDMD and NE help each other for their own activation. Once GSDMD activates, it is able to form pores in the membrane of granules favoring NE release into the cytoplasm toward the nucleus, where it gets processed with histones and increases nuclear expansion [91]. As a second function, following NET formation, GSDMD forms pores in the cell membrane allowing NET release. Along with these interesting findings and the knowledge that neutrophils appear to be resistant to caspase-1-dependent pyroptosis, neutrophils were recently described to release NETs in a GSDMD-dependent manner following the non-canonical inflammasome signaling [92]. Indeed, pyroptosis was previously described to depend on the proteolytic cleavage of GSDMD by caspase 11 in neutrophils [86,87].

The role of the NLRP3 inflammasome in AMI was largely investigated in recent years [93–95]. Actually, we now know that the NLRP3 inflammasome activation is important in the determination of the infarct size (mainly through pyroptosis) [96,97] and in the so-called "wavefront of reperfusion injury," through which the infarct size expands in the 3–6 h after reperfusion through an increasing activation of the NLRP3 inflammasome [94]. For a more in-depth discussion on the role of the NLRP3 inflammasome, readers are referred elsewhere [13,75,95]. Therefore, the link between NETs and the NLRP3 inflammasome in the pathophysiology of AMI is still under investigation and not completely understood yet. Cholesterol crystals are recognized as important drivers in atherosclerosis [98], as supported by studies in mice with defective cholesterol efflux [99,100]. Additionally, the excess of cholesterol crystals is uptaken by lysosomes, whose membrane may be damaged and then activate the NLRP3 inflammasomes [99]. Besides, cholesterol crystals were found to prime the NLRP3 inflammasome through the production of NETs [101].

With regard to diabetes, very few data are available evaluating the relationship between NETs and the inflammasome, although data from the CANTOS (Canakinumab Anti-Inflammatory Thrombosis Outcomes Study) trial did not show any effectiveness of IL-1β blocking in reducing incident diabetes [102]. Future studies unraveling this interplay may be beneficial in developing targeted therapies for patients developing diabetes.

7. Conclusions and Future Perspectives

NETs primarily represent an essential barrier in response to inflammatory stimuli provided by a wealth of pathogens. An excessive production of NETs may, however, end in chronic inflammation, as occurs in CV diseases, where NETs play an important role. Additionally, NETs can trigger other cells, such as monocytes and macrophages, to release IL-1β through the NLRP3 inflammasome, which in turn is responsible for the persistence of a pro-inflammatory milieu. In vitro studies reported that proteases on NETs can adjust cytokine levels either by destroying or activating them, thus blunting or favoring inflammation [103–105]. Therefore, NETs are likely to behave as a double-edged sword in the innate immune system. An exaggerated NET formation is responsible for different diseases, both infectious and non-infectious. NETs can bind to platelets and red blood cells and impair the coagulation cascade by increasing the efficiency of fibrin aggregation and the risk of thrombotic events. Recently, new information emerged showing that multiple receptors and various redundant signaling pathways are involved in NETosis, suggesting that a fine tuning is strictly required to address different biological effects [106]. Further studies, however, are warranted to thoroughly understand all the different functions of NETs and their importance in the clinical setting.

In light of the pathophysiological relevance of NETs, the development of therapies blocking NETs is ongoing [107]. For example, the inhibition of PAD4 was proved effective in different conditions, such as AMI, stroke, and diabetes [108]. Besides, Janus Kinase (JAK)1/2 inhibitor, that lowers NET formation in mice and humans, was found to experimentally reduce thrombosis [109]. The negative side of these potential therapeutic pathways relies on the non-uniqueness of the targets acting also in processes other than NETosis, hence this research field needs to be further deepened. Along with pharmacological inhibition, some cells (i.e., macrophages) as well as plasma own a system for NET degradation to directly digest extracellular DNA and dampen inflammation, as witnessed by the decreased clearance of NETs occurring in or causing SLE and rheumatoid arthritis [110].

Although the discovery of NETs has revolutionized the understanding of the pathophysiology and the natural history of some human diseases, additional efforts are needed to understand the real impact of NETs and therefore address targeted therapeutic strategies. Finally, a standardized nomenclature and standardized techniques for NET assessment would definitely help to obtain a wealth of comparable data, no matter what the studied disease is [111].

Author Contributions: A.B. conceived the structure of the review. A.B. and A.V. wrote the first manuscript draft. A.V. designed the figures and Table 1. A.A. and F.M. critically revised the manuscript and gave suggestions to improve it. All authors have read and agreed to the published version of the manuscript.

Funding: This research was funded by a grant from the Italian Ministry of Health (Italian Cardiovascular Network, #2754291) to dr. Fabrizio Montecucco. The APC was funded by the same grant.

Acknowledgments: The figures were created using Servier Medical Art templates, which are licensed under a Creative Commons Attribution 3.0 Unported License; https://smart.servier.com.

Conflicts of Interest: Dr. Abbate has served as a consultant for Astra Zeneca, Janssen, Merck, Novartis, Olatec, and Serpin pharma. All other authors declare no conflicts of interest.

References

1. Borregaard, N. Neutrophils, from marrow to microbes. *Immunity* **2010**, *33*, 657–670. [CrossRef] [PubMed]
2. Bonaventura, A.; Montecucco, F.; Dallegri, F.; Carbone, F.; Luscher, T.F.; Camici, G.G.; Liberale, L. Novel findings in neutrophil biology and their impact on cardiovascular disease. *Cardiovasc. Res.* **2019**, *115*, 1266–1285. [CrossRef] [PubMed]
3. Cowland, J.B.; Borregaard, N. Granulopoiesis and granules of human neutrophils. *Immunol. Rev.* **2016**, *273*, 11–28. [CrossRef] [PubMed]
4. Papayannopoulos, V. Neutrophil extracellular traps in immunity and disease. *Nat. Rev. Immunol.* **2018**, *18*, 134–147. [CrossRef] [PubMed]
5. Sorensen, O.E.; Borregaard, N. Neutrophil extracellular traps—The dark side of neutrophils. *J. Clin. Investig.* **2016**, *126*, 1612–1620. [CrossRef] [PubMed]
6. Bonaventura, A.; Liberale, L.; Carbone, F.; Vecchie, A.; Diaz-Canestro, C.; Camici, G.G.; Montecucco, F.; Dallegri, F. The Pathophysiological Role of Neutrophil Extracellular Traps in Inflammatory Diseases. *Thromb. Haemost.* **2018**, *118*, 6–27. [CrossRef]
7. Mohanan, S.; Cherrington, B.D.; Horibata, S.; McElwee, J.L.; Thompson, P.R.; Coonrod, S.A. Potential role of peptidylarginine deiminase enzymes and protein citrullination in cancer pathogenesis. *Biochem. Res. Int.* **2012**, *2012*, 895343. [CrossRef]
8. Papayannopoulos, V.; Metzler, K.D.; Hakkim, A.; Zychlinsky, A. Neutrophil elastase and myeloperoxidase regulate the formation of neutrophil extracellular traps. *J. Cell Biol.* **2010**, *191*, 677–691. [CrossRef]
9. Metzler, K.D.; Fuchs, T.A.; Nauseef, W.M.; Reumaux, D.; Roesler, J.; Schulze, I.; Wahn, V.; Papayannopoulos, V.; Zychlinsky, A. Myeloperoxidase is required for neutrophil extracellular trap formation: Implications for innate immunity. *Blood* **2011**, *117*, 953–959. [CrossRef]
10. Belaaouaj, A.; McCarthy, R.; Baumann, M.; Gao, Z.; Ley, T.J.; Abraham, S.N.; Shapiro, S.D. Mice lacking neutrophil elastase reveal impaired host defense against gram negative bacterial sepsis. *Nat. Med.* **1998**, *4*, 615–618. [CrossRef]
11. Doring, Y.; Soehnlein, O.; Weber, C. Neutrophils cast NETs in atherosclerosis: Employing peptidylarginine deiminase as a therapeutic target. *Circ. Res.* **2014**, *114*, 931–934. [CrossRef] [PubMed]
12. Castanheira, F.V.S.; Kubes, P. Neutrophils and NETs in modulating acute and chronic inflammation. *Blood* **2019**, *133*, 2178–2185. [CrossRef]
13. Toldo, S.; Abbate, A. The NLRP3 inflammasome in acute myocardial infarction. *Nat. Rev. Cardiol.* **2018**, *15*, 203–214. [CrossRef] [PubMed]
14. Jorch, S.K.; Kubes, P. An emerging role for neutrophil extracellular traps in noninfectious disease. *Nat. Med.* **2017**, *23*, 279–287. [CrossRef] [PubMed]
15. Crea, F.; Libby, P. Acute Coronary Syndromes: The Way Forward from Mechanisms to Precision Treatment. *Circulation* **2017**, *136*, 1155–1166. [CrossRef] [PubMed]
16. Bonaventura, A.; Montecucco, F.; Dallegri, F. Cellular recruitment in myocardial ischaemia/reperfusion injury. *Eur. J. Clin. Investig.* **2016**, *46*, 590–601. [CrossRef] [PubMed]
17. Montecucco, F.; Liberale, L.; Bonaventura, A.; Vecchie, A.; Dallegri, F.; Carbone, F. The Role of Inflammation in Cardiovascular Outcome. *Curr. Atheroscler. Rep.* **2017**, *19*, 11. [CrossRef]
18. Distelmaier, K.; Adlbrecht, C.; Jakowitsch, J.; Winkler, S.; Dunkler, D.; Gerner, C.; Wagner, O.; Lang, I.M.; Kubicek, M. Local complement activation triggers neutrophil recruitment to the site of thrombus formation in acute myocardial infarction. *Thromb. Haemost.* **2009**, *102*, 564–572. [CrossRef]
19. Horne, B.D.; Anderson, J.L.; John, J.M.; Weaver, A.; Bair, T.L.; Jensen, K.R.; Renlund, D.G.; Muhlestein, J.B. Which white blood cell subtypes predict increased cardiovascular risk? *J. Am. Coll. Cardiol.* **2005**, *45*, 1638–1643. [CrossRef]

20. Distelmaier, K.; Winter, M.P.; Dragschitz, F.; Redwan, B.; Mangold, A.; Gleiss, A.; Perkmann, T.; Maurer, G.; Adlbrecht, C.; Lang, I.M. Prognostic value of culprit site neutrophils in acute coronary syndrome. *Eur. J. Clin. Investig.* **2014**, *44*, 257–265. [CrossRef]

21. Ge, L.; Zhou, X.; Ji, W.J.; Lu, R.Y.; Zhang, Y.; Zhang, Y.D.; Ma, Y.Q.; Zhao, J.H.; Li, Y.M. Neutrophil extracellular traps in ischemia-reperfusion injury-induced myocardial no-reflow: Therapeutic potential of DNase-based reperfusion strategy. *Am. J. Physiol. Heart Circ. Physiol.* **2015**, *308*, H500–H509. [CrossRef] [PubMed]

22. Fuchs, T.A.; Brill, A.; Duerschmied, D.; Schatzberg, D.; Monestier, M.; Myers, D.D., Jr.; Wrobleski, S.K.; Wakefield, T.W.; Hartwig, J.H.; Wagner, D.D. Extracellular DNA traps promote thrombosis. *Proc. Natl. Acad. Sci. USA* **2010**, *107*, 15880–15885. [CrossRef] [PubMed]

23. Stakos, D.A.; Kambas, K.; Konstantinidis, T.; Mitroulis, I.; Apostolidou, E.; Arelaki, S.; Tsironidou, V.; Giatromanolaki, A.; Skendros, P.; Konstantinides, S.; et al. Expression of functional tissue factor by neutrophil extracellular traps in culprit artery of acute myocardial infarction. *Eur. Heart J.* **2015**, *36*, 1405–1414. [CrossRef] [PubMed]

24. Noubouossie, D.F.; Whelihan, M.F.; Yu, Y.B.; Sparkenbaugh, E.; Pawlinski, R.; Monroe, D.M.; Key, N.S. In vitro activation of coagulation by human neutrophil DNA and histone proteins but not neutrophil extracellular traps. *Blood* **2017**, *129*, 1021–1029. [CrossRef]

25. Maugeri, N.; Campana, L.; Gavina, M.; Covino, C.; De Metrio, M.; Panciroli, C.; Maiuri, L.; Maseri, A.; D'Angelo, A.; Bianchi, M.E.; et al. Activated platelets present high mobility group box 1 to neutrophils, inducing autophagy and promoting the extrusion of neutrophil extracellular traps. *J. Thromb. Haemost.* **2014**, *12*, 2074–2088. [CrossRef]

26. Quillard, T.; Araujo, H.A.; Franck, G.; Shvartz, E.; Sukhova, G.; Libby, P. TLR2 and neutrophils potentiate endothelial stress, apoptosis and detachment: Implications for superficial erosion. *Eur. Heart J.* **2015**, *36*, 1394–1404. [CrossRef]

27. De Boer, O.J.; Li, X.; Teeling, P.; Mackaay, C.; Ploegmakers, H.J.; van der Loos, C.M.; Daemen, M.J.; de Winter, R.J.; van der Wal, A.C. Neutrophils, neutrophil extracellular traps and interleukin-17 associate with the organisation of thrombi in acute myocardial infarction. *Thromb. Haemost.* **2013**, *109*, 290–297.

28. Mangold, A.; Alias, S.; Scherz, T.; Hofbauer, T.; Jakowitsch, J.; Panzenbock, A.; Simon, D.; Laimer, D.; Bangert, C.; Kammerlander, A.; et al. Coronary neutrophil extracellular trap burden and deoxyribonuclease activity in ST-elevation acute coronary syndrome are predictors of ST-segment resolution and infarct size. *Circ. Res.* **2015**, *116*, 1182–1192. [CrossRef]

29. Borissoff, J.I.; Joosen, I.A.; Versteylen, M.O.; Brill, A.; Fuchs, T.A.; Savchenko, A.S.; Gallant, M.; Martinod, K.; Ten Cate, H.; Hofstra, L.; et al. Elevated levels of circulating DNA and chromatin are independently associated with severe coronary atherosclerosis and a prothrombotic state. *Arterioscler. Thromb. Vasc. Biol.* **2013**, *33*, 2032–2040. [CrossRef]

30. Cui, M.; Fan, M.; Jing, R.; Wang, H.; Qin, J.; Sheng, H.; Wang, Y.; Wu, X.; Zhang, L.; Zhu, J.; et al. Cell-Free circulating DNA: A new biomarker for the acute coronary syndrome. *Cardiology* **2013**, *124*, 76–84. [CrossRef]

31. Helseth, R.; Solheim, S.; Arnesen, H.; Seljeflot, I.; Opstad, T.B. The Time Course of Markers of Neutrophil Extracellular Traps in Patients Undergoing Revascularisation for Acute Myocardial Infarction or Stable Angina Pectoris. *Mediat. Inflamm.* **2016**, *2016*, 2182358. [CrossRef] [PubMed]

32. Hofbauer, T.M.; Mangold, A.; Scherz, T.; Seidl, V.; Panzenbock, A.; Ondracek, A.S.; Muller, J.; Schneider, M.; Binder, T.; Hell, L.; et al. Neutrophil extracellular traps and fibrocytes in ST-segment elevation myocardial infarction. *Basic Res. Cardiol.* **2019**, *114*, 33. [CrossRef] [PubMed]

33. Liu, J.; Yang, D.; Wang, X.; Zhu, Z.; Wang, T.; Ma, A.; Liu, P. Neutrophil extracellular traps and dsDNA predict outcomes among patients with ST-elevation myocardial infarction. *Sci. Rep.* **2019**, *9*, 11599. [CrossRef] [PubMed]

34. Helseth, R.; Knudsen, E.C.; Eritsland, J.; Opstad, T.B.; Arnesen, H.; Andersen, G.O.; Seljeflot, I. Glucose associated NETosis in patients with ST-elevation myocardial infarction: An observational study. *BMC Cardiovasc. Disord.* **2019**, *19*, 221. [CrossRef] [PubMed]

35. Mangold, A.; Hofbauer, T.M.; Ondracek, A.S.; Artner, T.; Scherz, T.; Speidl, W.S.; Krychtiuk, K.A.; Sadushi-Kolici, R.; Jakowitsch, J.; Lang, I.M. Neutrophil extracellular traps and monocyte subsets at the culprit lesion site of myocardial infarction patients. *Sci. Rep.* **2019**, *9*, 16304. [CrossRef] [PubMed]

36. Liberale, L.; Holy, E.W.; Akhmedov, A.; Bonetti, N.R.; Nietlispach, F.; Matter, C.M.; Mach, F.; Montecucco, F.; Beer, J.H.; Paneni, F.; et al. Interleukin-1β Mediates Arterial Thrombus Formation via NET-Associated Tissue Factor. *J. Clin. Med.* **2019**, *8*, 2072. [CrossRef]

37. Rodriguez-Espinosa, O.; Rojas-Espinosa, O.; Moreno-Altamirano, M.M.; Lopez-Villegas, E.O.; Sanchez-Garcia, F.J. Metabolic requirements for neutrophil extracellular traps formation. *Immunology* **2015**, *145*, 213–224. [CrossRef]

38. Langseth, M.S.; Opstad, T.B.; Bratseth, V.; Solheim, S.; Arnesen, H.; Pettersen, A.A.; Seljeflot, I.; Helseth, R. Markers of neutrophil extracellular traps are associated with adverse clinical outcome in stable coronary artery disease. *Eur. J. Prev. Cardiol.* **2018**, *25*, 762–769. [CrossRef]

39. Wellen, K.E.; Hotamisligil, G.S. Inflammation, stress, and diabetes. *J. Clin. Investig.* **2005**, *115*, 1111–1119. [CrossRef]

40. Bonaventura, A.; Liberale, L.; Montecucco, F. Aspirin in primary prevention for patients with diabetes: Still a matter of debate. *Eur. J. Clin. Investig.* **2018**, *48*, e13001. [CrossRef]

41. Vecchie, A.; Montecucco, F.; Vecchie, F.; Dallegri, F.; Bonaventura, A. Diabetes and Vascular Disease: Is it all about Glycemia? *Curr. Pharm. Des.* **2019**, *25*, 3112–3127. [CrossRef] [PubMed]

42. Stegenga, M.E.; van der Crabben, S.N.; Blumer, R.M.; Levi, M.; Meijers, J.C.; Serlie, M.J.; Tanck, M.W.; Sauerwein, H.P.; van der Poll, T. Hyperglycemia enhances coagulation and reduces neutrophil degranulation, whereas hyperinsulinemia inhibits fibrinolysis during human endotoxemia. *Blood* **2008**, *112*, 82–89. [CrossRef] [PubMed]

43. De Souza Ferreira, C.; Araujo, T.H.; Angelo, M.L.; Pennacchi, P.C.; Okada, S.S.; de Araujo Paula, F.B.; Migliorini, S.; Rodrigues, M.R. Neutrophil dysfunction induced by hyperglycemia: Modulation of myeloperoxidase activity. *Cell Biochem. Funct.* **2012**, *30*, 604–610. [CrossRef] [PubMed]

44. Battaglia, M. Neutrophils and type 1 autoimmune diabetes. *Curr. Opin. Hematol.* **2014**, *21*, 8–15. [CrossRef] [PubMed]

45. Zhang, H.; Yang, Z.; Zhang, W.; Niu, Y.; Li, X.; Qin, L.; Su, Q. White blood cell subtypes and risk of type 2 diabetes. *J. Diabetes Complicat.* **2017**, *31*, 31–37. [CrossRef] [PubMed]

46. Bonaventura, A.; Liberale, L.; Carbone, F.; Vecchie, A.; Bonomi, A.; Scopinaro, N.; Camerini, G.B.; Papadia, F.S.; Maggi, D.; Cordera, R.; et al. Baseline neutrophil-to-lymphocyte ratio is associated with long-term T2D remission after metabolic surgery. *Acta Diabetol.* **2019**, *56*, 741–748. [CrossRef]

47. Milosevic, D.; Panin, V.L. Relationship Between Hematological Parameters and Glycemic Control in Type 2 Diabetes Mellitus Patients. *J. Med. Biochem.* **2019**, *38*, 164–171. [CrossRef]

48. Wong, S.L.; Demers, M.; Martinod, K.; Gallant, M.; Wang, Y.; Goldfine, A.B.; Kahn, C.R.; Wagner, D.D. Diabetes primes neutrophils to undergo NETosis, which impairs wound healing. *Nat. Med.* **2015**, *21*, 815–819. [CrossRef]

49. Valle, A.; Giamporcaro, G.M.; Scavini, M.; Stabilini, A.; Grogan, P.; Bianconi, E.; Sebastiani, G.; Masini, M.; Maugeri, N.; Porretti, L.; et al. Reduction of circulating neutrophils precedes and accompanies type 1 diabetes. *Diabetes* **2013**, *62*, 2072–2077. [CrossRef]

50. Harsunen, M.H.; Puff, R.; D'Orlando, O.; Giannopoulou, E.; Lachmann, L.; Beyerlein, A.; von Meyer, A.; Ziegler, A.G. Reduced blood leukocyte and neutrophil numbers in the pathogenesis of type 1 diabetes. *Horm. Metab. Res.* **2013**, *45*, 467–470. [CrossRef]

51. Vecchio, F.; Lo Buono, N.; Stabilini, A.; Nigi, L.; Dufort, M.J.; Geyer, S.; Rancoita, P.M.; Cugnata, F.; Mandelli, A.; Valle, A.; et al. Abnormal neutrophil signature in the blood and pancreas of presymptomatic and symptomatic type 1 diabetes. *JCI Insight* **2018**, *3*. [CrossRef]

52. Wang, Y.; Xiao, Y.; Zhong, L.; Ye, D.; Zhang, J.; Tu, Y.; Bornstein, S.R.; Zhou, Z.; Lam, K.S.; Xu, A. Increased neutrophil elastase and proteinase 3 and augmented NETosis are closely associated with beta-cell autoimmunity in patients with type 1 diabetes. *Diabetes* **2014**, *63*, 4239–4248. [CrossRef] [PubMed]

53. Qin, J.; Fu, S.; Speake, C.; Greenbaum, C.J.; Odegard, J.M. NETosis-associated serum biomarkers are reduced in type 1 diabetes in association with neutrophil count. *Clin. Exp. Immunol.* **2016**, *184*, 318–322. [CrossRef] [PubMed]

54. Menegazzo, L.; Ciciliot, S.; Poncina, N.; Mazzucato, M.; Persano, M.; Bonora, B.; Albiero, M.; Vigili de Kreutzenberg, S.; Avogaro, A.; Fadini, G.P. NETosis is induced by high glucose and associated with type 2 diabetes. *Acta Diabetol.* **2015**, *52*, 497–503. [CrossRef] [PubMed]

55. Park, J.H.; Kim, J.E.; Gu, J.Y.; Yoo, H.J.; Park, S.H.; Kim, Y.I.; Nam-Goong, I.S.; Kim, E.S.; Kim, H.K. Evaluation of Circulating Markers of Neutrophil Extracellular Trap (NET) Formation as Risk Factors for Diabetic Retinopathy in a Case-Control Association Study. *Exp. Clin. Endocrinol. Diabetes* **2016**, *124*, 557–561. [CrossRef] [PubMed]

56. Joshi, M.B.; Lad, A.; Bharath Prasad, A.S.; Balakrishnan, A.; Ramachandra, L.; Satyamoorthy, K. High glucose modulates IL-6 mediated immune homeostasis through impeding neutrophil extracellular trap formation. *FEBS Lett.* **2013**, *587*, 2241–2246. [CrossRef] [PubMed]

57. Carestia, A.; Frechtel, G.; Cerrone, G.; Linari, M.A.; Gonzalez, C.D.; Casais, P.; Schattner, M. NETosis before and after Hyperglycemic Control in Type 2 Diabetes Mellitus Patients. *PLoS ONE* **2016**, *11*, e0168647. [CrossRef]

58. Menegazzo, L.; Scattolini, V.; Cappellari, R.; Bonora, B.M.; Albiero, M.; Bortolozzi, M.; Romanato, F.; Ceolotto, G.; Vigili de Kreutzeberg, S.; Avogaro, A.; et al. The antidiabetic drug metformin blunts NETosis in vitro and reduces circulating NETosis biomarkers in vivo. *Acta Diabetol.* **2018**, *55*, 593–601. [CrossRef]

59. Wang, L.; Zhou, X.; Yin, Y.; Mai, Y.; Wang, D.; Zhang, X. Hyperglycemia Induces Neutrophil Extracellular Traps Formation Through an NADPH Oxidase-Dependent Pathway in Diabetic Retinopathy. *Front. Immunol.* **2018**, *9*, 3076. [CrossRef]

60. Fadini, G.P.; Menegazzo, L.; Rigato, M.; Scattolini, V.; Poncina, N.; Bruttocao, A.; Ciciliot, S.; Mammano, F.; Ciubotaru, C.D.; Brocco, E.; et al. NETosis Delays Diabetic Wound Healing in Mice and Humans. *Diabetes* **2016**, *65*, 1061–1071. [CrossRef]

61. Vecchie, A.; Dallegri, F.; Carbone, F.; Bonaventura, A.; Liberale, L.; Portincasa, P.; Fruhbeck, G.; Montecucco, F. Obesity phenotypes and their paradoxical association with cardiovascular diseases. *Eur. J. Intern. Med.* **2018**, *48*, 6–17. [CrossRef] [PubMed]

62. Lee, B.C.; Lee, J. Cellular and molecular players in adipose tissue inflammation in the development of obesity-induced insulin resistance. *Biochim. Biophys. Acta* **2014**, *1842*, 446–462. [CrossRef] [PubMed]

63. Liberale, L.; Bertolotto, M.; Carbone, F.; Contini, P.; Wust, P.; Spinella, G.; Pane, B.; Palombo, D.; Bonaventura, A.; Pende, A.; et al. Resistin exerts a beneficial role in atherosclerotic plaque inflammation by inhibiting neutrophil migration. *Int. J. Cardiol.* **2018**, *272*, 13–19. [CrossRef] [PubMed]

64. Liberale, L.; Bonaventura, A.; Carbone, F.; Bertolotto, M.; Contini, P.; Scopinaro, N.; Camerini, G.B.; Papadia, F.S.; Cordera, R.; Camici, G.G.; et al. Early reduction of matrix metalloproteinase-8 serum levels is associated with leptin drop and predicts diabetes remission after bariatric surgery. *Int. J. Cardiol.* **2017**, *245*, 257–262. [CrossRef] [PubMed]

65. Wang, H.; Wang, Q.; Venugopal, J.; Wang, J.; Kleiman, K.; Guo, C.; Eitzman, D.T. Obesity-induced Endothelial Dysfunction is Prevented by Neutrophil Extracellular Trap Inhibition. *Sci. Rep.* **2018**, *8*, 4881. [CrossRef] [PubMed]

66. Braster, Q.; Silvestre Roig, C.; Hartwig, H.; Beckers, L.; den Toom, M.; Doring, Y.; Daemen, M.J.; Lutgens, E.; Soehnlein, O. Inhibition of NET Release Fails to Reduce Adipose Tissue Inflammation in Mice. *PLoS ONE* **2016**, *11*, e0163922. [CrossRef]

67. D'Abbondanza, M.; Martorelli, E.E.; Ricci, M.A.; De Vuono, S.; Migliola, E.N.; Godino, C.; Corradetti, S.; Siepi, D.; Paganelli, M.T.; Maugeri, N.; et al. Increased plasmatic NETs by-products in patients in severe obesity. *Sci. Rep.* **2019**, *9*, 14678. [CrossRef]

68. Toldo, S.; Mezzaroma, E.; Mauro, A.G.; Salloum, F.; Van Tassell, B.W.; Abbate, A. The inflammasome in myocardial injury and cardiac remodeling. *Antioxid. Redox Signal.* **2015**, *22*, 1146–1161. [CrossRef]

69. Schroder, K.; Tschopp, J. The inflammasomes. *Cell* **2010**, *140*, 821–832. [CrossRef]

70. Franchi, L.; Eigenbrod, T.; Munoz-Planillo, R.; Nunez, G. The inflammasome: A caspase-1-activation platform that regulates immune responses and disease pathogenesis. *Nat. Immunol.* **2009**, *10*, 241–247. [CrossRef]

71. Jin, Y.; Fu, J. Novel Insights into the NLRP 3 Inflammasome in Atherosclerosis. *J. Am. Heart Assoc.* **2019**, *8*, e012219. [CrossRef] [PubMed]

72. Abbate, A.; Van Tassell, B.W.; Biondi-Zoccai, G.G. Blocking interleukin-1 as a novel therapeutic strategy for secondary prevention of cardiovascular events. *BioDrugs* **2012**, *26*, 217–233. [CrossRef] [PubMed]

73. Zuurbier, C.J.; Abbate, A.; Cabrera-Fuentes, H.A.; Cohen, M.V.; Collino, M.; De Kleijn, D.P.V.; Downey, J.M.; Pagliaro, P.; Preissner, K.T.; Takahashi, M.; et al. Innate immunity as a target for acute cardioprotection. *Cardiovasc. Res.* **2019**, *115*, 1131–1142. [CrossRef] [PubMed]

74. Bonaventura, A.; Montecucco, F. Inflammation and pericarditis: Are neutrophils actors behind the scenes? *J. Cell. Physiol.* **2019**, *234*, 5390–5398. [CrossRef] [PubMed]

75. Mauro, A.G.; Bonaventura, A.; Mezzaroma, E.; Quader, M.; Toldo, S. NLRP3 Inflammasome in Acute Myocardial Infarction. *J. Cardiovasc. Pharmacol.* **2019**, *74*, 175–187. [CrossRef] [PubMed]

76. Bonaventura, A.; Cannata, A.; Mezzaroma, E.; Sinagra, G.; Bussani, R.; Toldo, S.; Gandhi, R.; Kim, M.; Paolini, J.; Montecucco, F.; et al. Abstract 13363: Intensification of the Inflammasome Formation in the Pericardium of Patients with Chronic Severe Pericarditis. *Circulation* **2019**, *140* (Suppl. 1), A13363.

77. Dinarello, C.A. The IL-1 family of cytokines and receptors in rheumatic diseases. *Nat. Rev. Rheumatol.* **2019**, *15*, 612–632. [CrossRef]

78. Elssner, A.; Duncan, M.; Gavrilin, M.; Wewers, M.D. A novel P2X7 receptor activator, the human cathelicidin-derived peptide LL37, induces IL-1 beta processing and release. *J. Immunol.* **2004**, *172*, 4987–4994. [CrossRef]

79. Kahlenberg, J.M.; Carmona-Rivera, C.; Smith, C.K.; Kaplan, M.J. Neutrophil extracellular trap-associated protein activation of the NLRP3 inflammasome is enhanced in lupus macrophages. *J. Immunol.* **2013**, *190*, 1217–1226. [CrossRef]

80. Mitroulis, I.; Kambas, K.; Chrysanthopoulou, A.; Skendros, P.; Apostolidou, E.; Kourtzelis, I.; Drosos, G.I.; Boumpas, D.T.; Ritis, K. Neutrophil extracellular trap formation is associated with IL-1beta and autophagy-related signaling in gout. *PLoS ONE* **2011**, *6*, e29318. [CrossRef]

81. Hu, Q.; Shi, H.; Zeng, T.; Liu, H.; Su, Y.; Cheng, X.; Ye, J.; Yin, Y.; Liu, M.; Zheng, H.; et al. Increased neutrophil extracellular traps activate NLRP3 and inflammatory macrophages in adult-onset Still's disease. *Arthritis Res. Ther.* **2019**, *21*, 9. [CrossRef] [PubMed]

82. Lachowicz-Scroggins, M.E.; Dunican, E.M.; Charbit, A.R.; Raymond, W.; Looney, M.R.; Peters, M.C.; Gordon, E.D.; Woodruff, P.G.; Lefrancais, E.; Phillips, B.R.; et al. Extracellular DNA, Neutrophil Extracellular Traps, and Inflammasome Activation in Severe Asthma. *Am. J. Respir. Crit. Care Med.* **2019**, *199*, 1076–1085. [CrossRef] [PubMed]

83. Awad, F.; Assrawi, E.; Jumeau, C.; Georgin-Lavialle, S.; Cobret, L.; Duquesnoy, P.; Piterboth, W.; Thomas, L.; Stankovic-Stojanovic, K.; Louvrier, C.; et al. Impact of human monocyte and macrophage polarization on NLR expression and NLRP3 inflammasome activation. *PLoS ONE* **2017**, *12*, e0175336. [CrossRef] [PubMed]

84. Stephenson, H.N.; Herzig, A.; Zychlinsky, A. Beyond the grave: When is cell death critical for immunity to infection? *Curr. Opin. Immunol.* **2016**, *38*, 59–66. [CrossRef] [PubMed]

85. Mishra, P.K.; Adameova, A.; Hill, J.A.; Baines, C.P.; Kang, P.M.; Downey, J.M.; Narula, J.; Takahashi, M.; Abbate, A.; Piristine, H.C.; et al. Guidelines for evaluating myocardial cell death. *Am. J. Physiol. Heart Circ. Physiol.* **2019**, *317*, H891–H922. [CrossRef] [PubMed]

86. Kayagaki, N.; Stowe, I.B.; Lee, B.L.; O'Rourke, K.; Anderson, K.; Warming, S.; Cuellar, T.; Haley, B.; Roose-Girma, M.; Phung, Q.T.; et al. Caspase-11 cleaves gasdermin D for non-canonical inflammasome signalling. *Nature* **2015**, *526*, 666–671. [CrossRef] [PubMed]

87. Shi, J.; Zhao, Y.; Wang, K.; Shi, X.; Wang, Y.; Huang, H.; Zhuang, Y.; Cai, T.; Wang, F.; Shao, F. Cleavage of GSDMD by inflammatory caspases determines pyroptotic cell death. *Nature* **2015**, *526*, 660–665. [CrossRef]

88. Liu, X.; Zhang, Z.; Ruan, J.; Pan, Y.; Magupalli, V.G.; Wu, H.; Lieberman, J. Inflammasome-activated gasdermin D causes pyroptosis by forming membrane pores. *Nature* **2016**, *535*, 153–158. [CrossRef]

89. Shi, J.; Gao, W.; Shao, F. Pyroptosis: Gasdermin-Mediated Programmed Necrotic Cell Death. *Trends Biochem. Sci.* **2017**, *42*, 245–254. [CrossRef]

90. Sollberger, G.; Choidas, A.; Burn, G.L.; Habenberger, P.; Di Lucrezia, R.; Kordes, S.; Menninger, S.; Eickhoff, J.; Nussbaumer, P.; Klebl, B.; et al. Gasdermin D plays a vital role in the generation of neutrophil extracellular traps. *Sci. Immunol.* **2018**, *3*. [CrossRef]

91. Metzler, K.D.; Goosmann, C.; Lubojemska, A.; Zychlinsky, A.; Papayannopoulos, V. A myeloperoxidase-containing complex regulates neutrophil elastase release and actin dynamics during NETosis. *Cell Rep.* **2014**, *8*, 883–896. [CrossRef]

92. Chen, K.W.; Monteleone, M.; Boucher, D.; Sollberger, G.; Ramnath, D.; Condon, N.D.; von Pein, J.B.; Broz, P.; Sweet, M.J.; Schroder, K. Noncanonical inflammasome signaling elicits gasdermin D-dependent neutrophil extracellular traps. *Sci. Immunol.* **2018**, *3*, eaar6676. [CrossRef] [PubMed]

93. Toldo, S.; Mezzaroma, E.; McGeough, M.D.; Pena, C.A.; Marchetti, C.; Sonnino, C.; Van Tassell, B.W.; Salloum, F.N.; Voelkel, N.F.; Hoffman, H.M.; et al. Independent roles of the priming and the triggering of the NLRP3 inflammasome in the heart. *Cardiovasc. Res.* **2015**, *105*, 203–212. [CrossRef] [PubMed]

94. Toldo, S.; Marchetti, C.; Mauro, A.G.; Chojnacki, J.; Mezzaroma, E.; Carbone, S.; Zhang, S.; Van Tassell, B.; Salloum, F.N.; Abbate, A. Inhibition of the NLRP3 inflammasome limits the inflammatory injury following myocardial ischemia-reperfusion in the mouse. *Int. J. Cardiol.* **2016**, *209*, 215–220. [CrossRef] [PubMed]

95. Toldo, S.; Mauro, A.G.; Cutter, Z.; Abbate, A. Inflammasome, pyroptosis, and cytokines in myocardial ischemia-reperfusion injury. *Am. J. Physiol. Heart Circ. Physiol.* **2018**, *315*, H1553–H1568. [CrossRef]

96. Kawaguchi, M.; Takahashi, M.; Hata, T.; Kashima, Y.; Usui, F.; Morimoto, H.; Izawa, A.; Takahashi, Y.; Masumoto, J.; Koyama, J.; et al. Inflammasome activation of cardiac fibroblasts is essential for myocardial ischemia/reperfusion injury. *Circulation* **2011**, *123*, 594–604. [CrossRef]

97. Mezzaroma, E.; Toldo, S.; Farkas, D.; Seropian, I.M.; Van Tassell, B.W.; Salloum, F.N.; Kannan, H.R.; Menna, A.C.; Voelkel, N.F.; Abbate, A. The inflammasome promotes adverse cardiac remodeling following acute myocardial infarction in the mouse. *Proc. Natl. Acad. Sci. USA* **2011**, *108*, 19725–19730. [CrossRef]

98. Duewell, P.; Kono, H.; Rayner, K.J.; Sirois, C.M.; Vladimer, G.; Bauernfeind, F.G.; Abela, G.S.; Franchi, L.; Nunez, G.; Schnurr, M.; et al. NLRP3 inflammasomes are required for atherogenesis and activated by cholesterol crystals. *Nature* **2010**, *464*, 1357–1361. [CrossRef]

99. Tall, A.R.; Westerterp, M. Inflammasomes, neutrophil extracellular traps, and cholesterol. *J. Lipid Res.* **2019**, *60*, 721–727. [CrossRef]

100. Westerterp, M.; Fotakis, P.; Ouimet, M.; Bochem, A.E.; Zhang, H.; Molusky, M.M.; Wang, W.; Abramowicz, S.; la Bastide-van Gemert, S.; Wang, N. Cholesterol Efflux Pathways Suppress Inflammasome Activation, NETosis, and Atherogenesis. *Circulation* **2018**, *138*, 898–912. [CrossRef]

101. Warnatsch, A.; Ioannou, M.; Wang, Q.; Papayannopoulos, V. Inflammation. Neutrophil extracellular traps license macrophages for cytokine production in atherosclerosis. *Science* **2015**, *349*, 316–320. [CrossRef] [PubMed]

102. Everett, B.M.; Donath, M.Y.; Pradhan, A.D.; Thuren, T.; Pais, P.; Nicolau, J.C.; Glynn, R.J.; Libby, P.; Ridker, P.M. Anti-Inflammatory Therapy with Canakinumab for the Prevention and Management of Diabetes. *J. Am. Coll. Cardiol.* **2018**, *71*, 2392–2401. [CrossRef] [PubMed]

103. Hahn, J.; Schauer, C.; Czegley, C.; Kling, L.; Petru, L.; Schmid, B.; Weidner, D.; Reinwald, C.; Biermann, M.H.C.; Blunder, S.; et al. Aggregated neutrophil extracellular traps resolve inflammation by proteolysis of cytokines and chemokines and protection from antiproteases. *FASEB J.* **2019**, *33*, 1401–1414. [CrossRef] [PubMed]

104. Schauer, C.; Janko, C.; Munoz, L.E.; Zhao, Y.; Kienhofer, D.; Frey, B.; Lell, M.; Manger, B.; Rech, J.; Naschberger, E.; et al. Aggregated neutrophil extracellular traps limit inflammation by degrading cytokines and chemokines. *Nat. Med.* **2014**, *20*, 511–517. [CrossRef]

105. Clancy, D.M.; Henry, C.M.; Sullivan, G.P.; Martin, S.J. Neutrophil extracellular traps can serve as platforms for processing and activation of IL-1 family cytokines. *FEBS J.* **2017**, *284*, 1712–1725. [CrossRef]

106. Petretto, A.; Bruschi, M.; Pratesi, F.; Croia, C.; Candiano, G.; Ghiggeri, G.; Migliorini, P. Neutrophil extracellular traps (NET) induced by different stimuli: A comparative proteomic analysis. *PLoS ONE* **2019**, *14*, e0218946. [CrossRef]

107. Sorvillo, N.; Cherpokova, D.; Martinod, K.; Wagner, D.D. Extracellular DNA NET-Works with Dire Consequences for Health. *Circ. Res.* **2019**, *125*, 470–488. [CrossRef]

108. Wong, S.L.; Wagner, D.D. Peptidylarginine deiminase 4: A nuclear button triggering neutrophil extracellular traps in inflammatory diseases and aging. *FASEB J.* **2018**, *32*, 6358–6370. [CrossRef]

109. Wolach, O.; Sellar, R.S.; Martinod, K.; Cherpokova, D.; McConkey, M.; Chappell, R.J.; Silver, A.J.; Adams, D.; Castellano, C.A.; Schneider, R.K.; et al. Increased neutrophil extracellular trap formation promotes thrombosis in myeloproliferative neoplasms. *Sci. Transl. Med.* **2018**, *10*, eaan8292. [CrossRef]

110. Keyel, P.A. Dnases in health and disease. *Dev. Biol.* **2017**, *429*, 1–11. [CrossRef]

111. Boeltz, S.; Amini, P.; Anders, H.J.; Andrade, F.; Bilyy, R.; Chatfield, S.; Cichon, I.; Clancy, D.M.; Desai, J.; Dumych, T.; et al. To NET or not to NET:current opinions and state of the science regarding the formation of neutrophil extracellular traps. *Cell Death Differ.* **2019**, *26*, 395–408. [CrossRef] [PubMed]

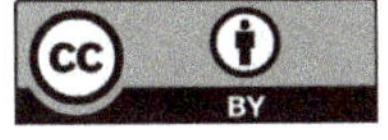

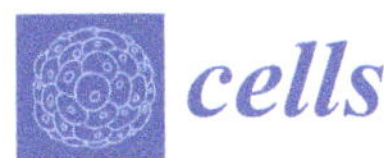 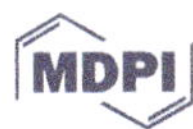

Article

Neutrophil Chemotaxis and NETosis in Murine Chronic Liver Injury via Cannabinoid Receptor 1/G$\alpha_{i/o}$/ROS/p38 MAPK Signaling Pathway

Xuan Zhou [†], Le Yang [†], Xiaoting Fan [†], Xinhao Zhao, Na Chang, Lin Yang and Liying Li *

Department of Cell Biology, Municipal Laboratory for Liver Protection and Regulation of Regeneration, Capital Medical University, Beijing 100069, China; zhouxuanyee@126.com (X.Z.); yangle@ccmu.edu.cn (L.Y.); 18210564428@163.com (X.F.); xinhaozhao0010@163.com (X.Z.); changna@ccmu.edu.cn (N.C.); yang_lin@ccmu.edu.cn (L.Y.)
* Correspondence: liliying@ccmu.edu.cn
† These authors contributed equally.

Received: 22 January 2020; Accepted: 3 February 2020; Published: 5 February 2020

Abstract: Neutrophils play an essential role in the control of inflammatory diseases. However, whether cannabinoid receptors (CBs) play a role in neutrophil chemotaxis and NETosis in sterile liver inflammation remains unknown. The expression of marker genes on neutrophils was characterized by FACS, immunofluorescence, qRT-PCR, and Western blot. The amount of neutrophils was significantly elevated from 7 days and reached the peak at 2 weeks in carbon tetrachloride (CCl$_4$)-treated mouse liver. The mRNA expression of neutrophil marker Ly6G had positive correlation with CB1 and CB2 expression in injured liver. In vitro CBs were abundantly expressed in isolated neutrophils and CB1 agonist ACEA promoted the chemotaxis and cytoskeletal remodeling, which can be suppressed by CB1 antagonist AM281. Moreover, ACEA induced NETosis, myeloperoxidase release from lysosome and ROS burst, indicating neutrophil activation, via G$\alpha_{i/o}$. Conversely, CB2 agonist JWH133 had no effect on neutrophil function. ROS and p38 MAPK signaling pathways were involved in CB1-mediated neutrophil function, and ROS was upstream of p38 MAPK. CB1 blockade in vivo significantly attenuated neutrophil infiltration and liver inflammation in CCl$_4$-treated mice. Taken together, CB1 mediates neutrophil chemotaxis and NETosis via G$\alpha_{i/o}$/ROS/p38 MAPK signaling pathway in liver inflammation, which represents an effective therapeutic strategy for liver diseases.

Keywords: liver injury; neutrophil extracellular trap; myeloperoxidase; carbon tetrachloride

1. Introduction

Neutrophils are the most abundant white blood cells and among the first cells recruited to an inflammatory site, thus mediating the early responses to tissue injury [1]. Neutrophil activation is characterized by neutrophil extracellular trap (NET) formation (NETosis) [2,3], granule enzymes myeloperoxidase (MPO) release from lysosome (azurophilic granules) [4] and ROS burst [5], further contributes to inflammation-associated damage in injured tissue. NETosis was first described in 2004 as highly decondensed chromatin structures, which was associated with citrullination of histone H3 [6,7]. NETosis has been found in response to various stimuli such as LPS, damage-associated molecular patterns (DAMPs), and PMA [6,8]. Recent studies have implicated that neutrophils play an essential role in the control of sterile inflammatory diseases, which are also characterized by a sustained influx of neutrophils and persistent NET release, and contribute to various injury processes [9,10]. For instance, in chronic obstructive pulmonary disease and cystic fibrosis, neutrophils and NETs contribute to chronic inflammatory and lung tissue damage [11,12]. Peptidylarginine deiminase (PAD) inhibition reduces NETosis and protects against lupus-related vasculature, kidney and skin injury in various lupus models [13]. In pyogenic arthritis, pyoderma gangrenosum and acne syndrome, an imbalance of NET formation and degradation are detected that enhances the half-life of these structures in vivo and promotes inflammation [14]. Especially, the important role of neutrophils has been identified in acute liver injury. In liver ischemia/reperfusion, interleukin-33, which is released from liver sinusoidal endothelial cells, promotes NETosis of infiltrating neutrophils and exacerbates inflammatory injury [15]. Disruption of the miR-223 gene exacerbates acetaminophen-induced hepatic neutrophil infiltration, oxidative stress, and injury, and enhances TLR9 ligand-mediated activation of pro-inflammatory mediators in neutrophils [16]. However, it remains unknown about the mediator and underlying molecular mechanism of regulating neutrophil recruitment and activation during chronic liver injury.

The endocannabinoid system (ECS) comprises cannabinoid receptors (CBs; CB1 and CB2), endocannabinoids and their synthesis and degradation enzymes [17]. CB1 is highly expressed in central nervous system and is also found in the periphery, including immune system and liver at a lower level, while CB2 is mainly expressed in immune cells [18]. ECS has been proven to be involved in the regulation of multiple physiological processes, such as appetite control, energy balance, pain perception, and immune response [19–21]. Notably CBs have been identified as pivotal regulators of acute and chronic liver injury, especially in inflammation-related liver injury [22]. For examples, a potential impact of CB1 on the inflammatory response associated with NASH has been suggested by experiments in obese rats, showing that CB1 antagonist rimonabant plays a hepatoprotective role in the treatment of obesity-associated liver diseases and related features of metabolic syndrome [23,24]. Moreover, CB1 and CB2 participate in the resveratrol-induced anti-NASH effect by maintaining the gut barrier integrity and inhibiting gut inflammation in high-fat diet-induced NASH rat models [25]. Our previous studies have also found that CB1 promotes the infiltration and activation of bone marrow (BM)-derived monocytes/macrophages in carbon tetrachloride (CCl_4)-induced liver injury mouse model, which could be inhibited by the blockade of CB1 [26,27]. However, the knowledge of whether CBs are involved in neutrophil function during sterile liver inflammation remains limited.

Here we investigate the effects of CBs on neutrophil chemotaxis and activation in isolated neutrophils and CCl_4-induced murine models. Our findings suggest that CB1 but not CB2 mediates neutrophil chemotaxis and NETosis in vitro, which are dependent of ROS and MAPK signaling pathways. Furthermore, blockade of CB1 in vivo reduces the infiltration and activation of neutrophils and attenuates liver injury in CCl_4-treated mice, which may represent an effective therapeutic strategy for liver diseases.

2. Materials and Methods

2.1. Materials

RPMI Medium 1640 was from GIBCO/Invitrogen (Grand Island, NY, USA). PCR reagents were from Applied Biosystems. ACEA (special CB1 agonists), AM281 (CB1 antagonist), JWH133 (CB2 antagonist), SB203580 (p38 inhibitor) were from TOCRIS/R&D (Minneapolis, MN, USA). NAC and PTX were from Sigma-Aldrich (St. Louis, MO, USA). Fibronectin was from Calbiochem (Germany). YM254890 was from Adipogen Corp. (San Diego, CA, USA). SYTOX Green Nucleic Acid Stain was from Molecular Probes, Inc. (Eugene, OR, USA).

2.2. Mouse Models of Liver Fibrosis

A CCl_4 (1 μL/g BW)/OO mixture (1:9 v/v) was injected into abdominal cavity of mice twice per week. Mice were sacrificed at 1, 2, and 3 days and 1, 2, and 4 weeks. The liver tissues were harvested. The intraperitoneal injection of AM281 (2.5 mg/kg BW) or DNAase I (11284932001, 50 μg/mouse, Roche, Swiss) was performed at 4 or 24 h before CCl_4 administration. All animal work was conformed to the Ethics Committee of Capital Medical University and in accordance with the approved guidelines (approval number: AEEI-2014-131).

2.3. BM Transplantation

ICR male mice aged 6 weeks received lethal irradiation (8 Grays) and immediately received transplantation by a tail vein injection of 1.5×10^7 whole BM cells obtained from 3-week-old EGFP transgenic mice. Four weeks later, mice of BM-rebuild were subjected to CCl_4-induced liver injury. After another 2 weeks, mice were sacrificed and liver tissues were harvested.

2.4. FACS

Non-parenchymal cells of mouse liver were isolated as described previously [28]. APC-Ly6G (BD Biosciences, Franklin Lakes, NJ, USA) and its isotype-matched negative control were added to the non-parenchymal cell suspension, respectively. After 15 min incubation in the dark, the cells were washed with PBS and subjected to FACS, which was performed on a FACSAria and analyzed with FACS Diva 4.1 (BD, Biosciences).

2.5. Isolation of Mouse BM Neutrophils

ICR mice aged 6 weeks were sacrificed by cervical dislocation at the time of neutrophils harvest. Tibias and femurs were removed and stripped of their muscles. The BM was flushed using PBS, and cell aggregates were disrupted via filtration through 70-μm cell strainer (BD Bioscience) and washed with PBS. Cell suspension was layered in a ratio of 1 to 3 on top of Histopaque 1077 (Sigma Aldrich), after centrifugation, precipitate was resuspended the with PBS. The cell suspension was layered in a ratio of 1 to 2 on top of Histopaque 1119 (Sigma Aldrich), after centrifugation, neutrophils were recovered on the top of Histopaque 1119. Neutrophils were washed with PBS and then resuspended in RPMI Medium 1640. The purity of neutrophils was determined by immunofluorescence staining for Ly6G (almost 100% cells were positive for Ly6G). Neutrophil viability was analyzed using Cell Counting Kit-8 (CCK-8) (Dojindo, Kumamoto, Japan) according to the manufacturer's procedure.

2.6. Neutrophils Chemotaxis Assay

Isolated bone marrow neutrophils were incubated with Calcein-AM (Life Technologies, CA, USA) to label cells and treated with AM281 (10 μM), NAC (5 mM), PTX (5 ng/mL), YM254890 (10 μM) or SB203580 (10 μM) for 20 min, then seeded to the upper chambers of a 3 μm-transwell (Corning). Then cells were allowed to migrate for another 2 h in the presence of ACEA (1 μM) or JWH133 (1 μM) in the lower chambers. The chambers were incubated at 37 °C in 5% CO_2. Subsequently, chemotaxis of neutrophils was determined by the fluorescence value of Calcein-AM in the lower chambers, using a fluorescent plate reader EnVision 2104-0010 (Perkinelmer, MA, USA).

2.7. Western Blot Analysis

Proteins were extracted from cells (50 μg) or liver tissue (100 μg) using RIPA Lysis Buffer (R0010, Solarbio, China) added with Complete Protease Inhibitor Cocktail Tablets (04693116001, Roche, Swiss). The components of RIPA Lysis Buffer were as follows: 50 mM Tris (pH 7.4), 150 mM NaCl, 1%TritonX-100, 1% sodium deoxycholate, 0.1% SDS, 2 mM sodium pyrophosphate, 25 mM b-glycerophosphate, 1 mM EDTA, 1mM Na_3VO_4, 0.5 mg/mL leupeptin. Then the extract was separated by SDS-PAGE and subjected to Western blot analysis. Membranes were incubated overnight using the following antibodies: rabbit anti-citrullinated-histone H3 (CitH3) polyclonal antibody (ab5103, 1:200, Abcam, Cambridge, United Kingdom), rabbit anti-ERK1/2 monoclonal antibody (4695) and rabbit anti-phorspho-ERK1/2 monoclonal antibody (4376, 1:1000, Cell Signaling, Beverly, MA, USA); rabbit anti-p38 polyclonal antibody (9212) and rabbit anti-phorspho-p38 polyclonal antibody (9211, 1:1000, Cell Signaling); rabbit anti-JNK polyclonal antibody (9252) and rabbit anti-phospho-JNK monoclonal antibody (4668, 1:1000, Cell Signaling); mouse anti-β-tubulin (HC101, 1:1000, TransGen Biotech, China) and anti-β-actin monoclonal antibodies (HC201, 1:1000, TransGen Biotech, China). IRDye 800CW Goat anti-Mouse IgG (H + L) Secondary Antibody (92632210), IRDye 800CW Goat anti-Rabbit IgG (H + L)

Secondary Antibody (92632211, 1:10000, LI-COR, NE, USA) were used. The bands were displayed using ODYSSEY and quantified by Odyssey v3.0 software. β-tubulin or β-actin were as references.

2.8. Immunofluorescence Staining

Isolated BM neutrophils were plated to adhere in fibronectin-coated 96-well plates (Corning) or Nunc glass base dishes (Thermo Fisher Scientific, MA, USA) and pretreated with vehicle, AM281 (10 μM), NAC (5 mM), PTX (5 ng/mL), YM254890 (10 μM) or SB203580 (10 μM) for 20 min, respectively, and stimulated for 2 h with ACEA or JWH133. Neutrophils were fixed by 4% paraformaldehyde for 30 min, after blocked with 2% BSA (Roche, Switzerland), they were incubated with the specific primary antibodies for CitH3 (1:200), MPO (1:200) or Ly-6G (Clone 1A8, 551459, 1:100, BD pharmingen), CB1 (10006590, 1:200, Cayman Chemical, Ann Arbor, MI, USA), CB2 (1:200, 101550, Cayman Chemical) or Rabbit IgG Isotype Control (1:100, 10500C, Invitrogen, CA, USA). Cy3-conjugate affinipure goat-anti-rabbit IgG (111165003, 1:100) or Cy5-conjugate affinipure goat-anti-rat IgG (112175143, 1:100, Jackson Immunoresearch, PA, USA) were as secondary antibodies. For F-actin, neutrophils were fixed by 4% paraformaldehyde for 30 min, penetrated by 0.5% Triton X-100 for 15 min and after blocked with 2% BSA, FITC-conjugated phalloidin (A12379, 1:100, Molecular Probes, OR, USA) was incubated for 20 min. Nuclei were stained with DAPI and SYTOX Green. The sample was observed under confocal microscope (LSM510, Carl Zeiss MicroImaging GmbH, Germany). For high content analysis, the plates were imaged on Thermo Scientific CellInsight personal cell imaging platform (Thermo Fisher Scientific). Fluorescence intensity of each well was analyzed by Cellomics Cell Health Profiling BioApplication software.

2.9. RT-qPCR

Total RNA was extracted from liver frozen specimens with or without treatments using an RNeasy kit (Qiagen, Germany). RT-qPCR was performed in an ABI Prism 7300 sequence detecting system (Applied Biosystems, CA, USA). Primers were as follows: 18s rRNA: Sense, 5′-GTA ACC CGT TGA ACC CCA TT-3′; Antisense, 5′-CCA TCC AAT CGG TAG TAG CG-3′. Ly6G: Sense, 5′-AGA AGC AAA GTC AAG AGC AAT CTC T-3′; Antisense, 5′-TGA CAG CAT TAC CAG TGA TCT CAG T-3′. CB1: Sense, 5′-GGC GGT GGC CGA TCT C-3′; Antisense, 5′-CGG TAA CCC CAC CCA GTT T-3′. CB2: Sense, 5′-AGC GCC CTG GAG AAC ATG-3′; Antisense, AGC TGC TGA TGA ACA GGT ACG A-3′. MCP-1: Sense, 5′-TCT GGG CCT GCT GTT CAC A-3′; Antisense, 5′-GGA TCA TCT TGC TGG TGA ATG A-3′. IL-1β: Sense, 5′-GCA ACT GTT CCT GAA CTC AAC T-3′; Antisense, 5′-ATC TTT TGG GGT CCG TCA ACT-3′. IL-6: Sense, 5′-TAG TCC TTC CTA CCC CAA TTT CC-3′; Antisense, 5′-TTG GTC CTT AGC CAC TCC TTC-3′. CD86: Sense, 5′-TCC AAG TTT TTG GGC AAT GTC-3′; Antisense, 5′-CCT ATG AGT GTG CAC TGA GTT AAA CA-3′.

2.10. ROS Production

2′,7′-Dichlorofluorescin diacetate (DCFHDA) (Sigma Aldrich) is a cell-permeable non-fluorescent probe, which is de-esterified intracellularly and turns to highly fluorescent 2′,7′-dichlorofluorescein upon oxidation. Isolated neutrophils were incubated with DCFHDA for 20 min and after seeded to 96-well plate, they were treated with different stimulators. The plate was then transferred onto a fluorescent plate reader, EnVision 2104-0010 (Perkinelmer, MA, USA), and detected the fluorescent value or Thermo Scientific CellInsight personal cell imaging platform to acquire ROS immunofluorescence images.

2.11. Liver Damage Assessment

Serum ALT and AST levels were detected by BS-200 Chemistry Analyzer (MINDARY, China).

2.12. Histology Analysis

Liver tissues were fixed in 4% paraformaldehyde. Liver tissue sections (5 μm) were stained with H&E for assessment of liver inflammation and injury. The inflammatory response was quantified by calculating inflammatory area using Image J software. Fifteen randomly selected areas per sample were measured as the mean value of the expressed percentage of inflammatory area.

2.13. Statistical Analysis

The results are expressed as mean ± standard error of the mean (SEM). Statistical significance was assessed by Student's t-test or one-way ANOVA for analysis of variance when appropriate. Correlation coefficients were calculated by Pearson test. $p < 0.05$ was considered to be significant. All results were verified in at least three independent experiments.

3. Results

3.1. Numerous Neutrophils Are Recruited and Activated in the Liver of CCl4-Treated Mice

To investigate the dynamic change of neutrophil signatures in sterile liver inflammation, we examined the mRNA expression of neutrophil marker Ly6G in the liver treated by CCl_4 for different time points. Our results showed that Ly6G mRNA expression up-regulated from 7 days of CCl_4 administration and reached the peak at 2 weeks, whereas the expression evidently decreased at 4 weeks compared with 2 weeks (Figure 1A), indicating that numerous neutrophils were recruited to injured liver during the early stage of chronic liver injury. Further, FACS analysis revealed that percentage of Ly6G$^+$ neutrophils was much higher in CCl_4-treated mice for 2 weeks compared with that in olive oil (OO)-treated mice (Figure 1B,C).

To clarify the origin of neutrophils recruited to the injured liver, we performed a genetic EGFP-labeled BM cell transplantation to the mice that had been lethally irradiated. Then the chimeric mice received intraperitoneal injection of CCl_4 for 2 weeks to induce liver injury. We isolated hepatic non-parenchymal cells from liver tissue and detected Ly6G$^+$ cells by FACS. The percentage of Ly6G$^+$EGFP$^+$ neutrophils (BM origin, OO group: 1.81%; CCl_4 group: 12.00%) was much higher than Ly6G$^+$EGFP$^-$ neutrophils (non-BM origin, OO group: 0.07%; CCl_4 group: 0.13%) in both OO and CCl_4 groups (Figure 1D,E). Moreover, Ly6G$^+$EGFP$^+$ neutrophils were significantly increased after CCl_4 administration compared with that in OO group (Figure 1D,E), indicating the recruited neutrophils in injured liver were mostly derived from BM. Then we performed immunofluorescent staining to examine CitH3 expression in the neutrophils of injured liver (Figure 1F). Further, increased hepatic level of citrullinated histone H3 (CitH3, specific marker of NETosis) was detected in CCl_4-treated mice (Figure 1G,H), suggesting the activation of these infiltrating neutrophils in the injured liver. Correlation analysis showed a positive correlation between CitH3 protein levels and Ly6G mRNA expression in liver tissue (Figure 1I). Altogether these results demonstrate that large numbers of BM-derived neutrophils are recruited and activated in the early stage of chronic liver injury.

3.2. CB Expression Positively Correlates with Neutrophil Signatures in CCl4-Treated Mice, and CBs Are Abundantly Expressed in Isolated Neutrophils

Our previous study had showed that CB1 and CB2 expression were increased in CCl_4-induced liver injury [27]. Here we undertook correlation analysis of mRNA expression levels between CB1 or CB2 and Ly6G. Each dot represented one liver sample from all mice (including OO and CCl_4-treated groups). Correlation coefficients were calculated using relative mRNA expression levels of CB1/CB2 and Ly6G from the same sample by Pearson correlation test (Figure 2A). Although both CB1 and CB2 were positively correlated with Ly6G ($p < 0.05$), CB1 represented a particularly higher correlation coefficient (Figure 2A). Based on the prevailing amount of BM-derived neutrophils in injured liver, we used mouse neutrophils isolated from BM in subsequent cellular experiments. The expression of CB1 and CB2 in mouse BM derived-neutrophils were detected at mRNA level (Figure 2B), and protein level by immunofluorscence (Figure 2C). These results demonstrated the positive correlation between the expression of CB1 and neutrophil signatures in CCl$_4$-treated mice and the abundant expression of CB1 in isolated neutrophils, suggesting that CB1 might play an important role in the recruitment and activation of neutrophils during sterile liver injury.

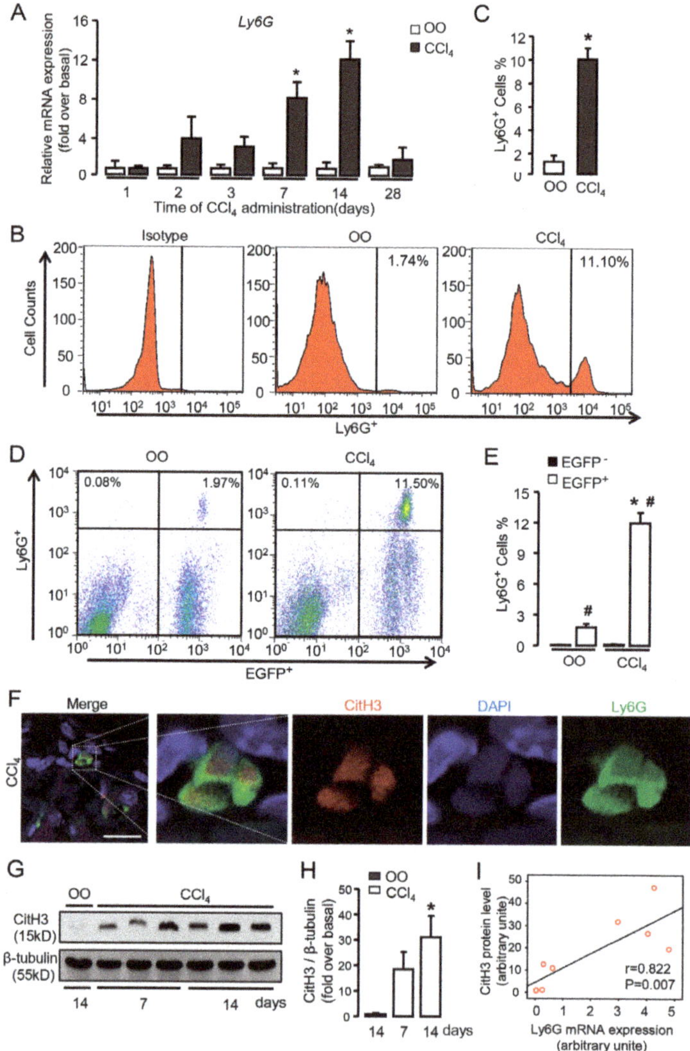

Figure 1. Numerous neutrophils are recruited and activated in the liver of carbon tetrachloride (CCl$_4$)-treated mice. (**A**) The mRNA expression of neutrophil marker Ly6G was examined by qRT-PCR in the injured liver of CCl$_4$ mice. (**B,C**) Representative FACS plots and quantification for total neutrophils (Ly6G$^+$). (**D,E**) Representative FACS plots and quantification for neutrophils of BM origin (Ly6G$^+$EGFP$^+$) and non-BM origin (Ly6G$^+$EGFP$^-$). (**F**) Immunofluorescent staining for CitH3 in the liver of CCl$_4$-treated mice. Scale bars, 20 μm. (**G,H**) CitH3 expression in the injured liver was examined by Western blot. (**I**) The correlation between CitH3 protein levels and Ly6G mRNA expression in liver tissue. Data are presented as the mean ± SEM. N = 6 per group. * $p < 0.05$ vs. control. # $p < 0.05$ vs. EGFP$^-$ neutrophils with the same treatment.

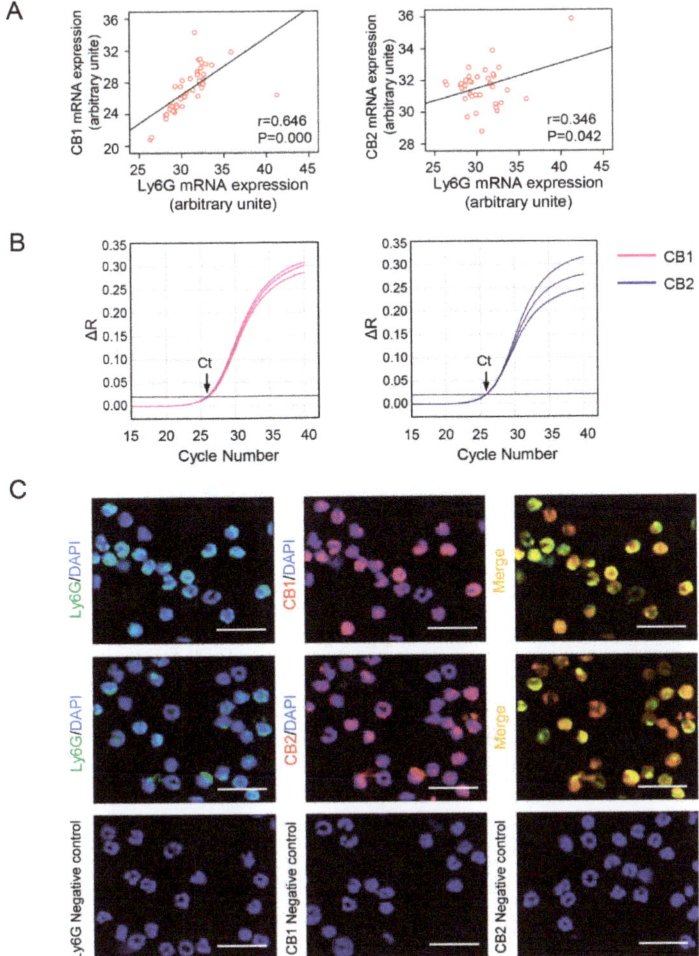

Figure 2. Cannabinoid receptor (CB) expression positively correlates with neutrophil signatures in CCl$_4$-treated mice, and CBs are abundantly expressed in isolated neutrophils. (**A**) The correlation between Ly6G and CB1 or CB2 in liver tissue. (**B**) The amplification plots of CB1 and CB2 expression in neutrophils by RT-qPCR. (**C**) Representative images of immunofluorescent staining for Ly6G (green) and CB1 or CB2 (red) in neutrophils. The nuclei were stained with DAPI (blue). Scale bars, 20 μm. N = 6 per group.

3.3. CB1 Rather than CB2 Mediates the Chemotaxis and Cytoskeletal Remodeling of Neutrophils In Vitro

Transwell assay was performed to explore whether CBs were involved in the chemotaxis of neutrophils in vitro. Treatment with ACEA (CB1 agonist) significantly increased the migration capacity of neutrophils in a dose-dependent manner, while JWH133 (CB2 agonist) had no such effect (Figure 3A). Due to the weak affinity between ACEA and CB2, we pretreated neutrophils with CB1 antagonist AM281 (1 and 10 μM) in ACEA-stimulated cells and showed declined chemotaxis of neutrophils with AM281 pretreatment (Figure 3B), further proving that CB1 mediated the chemotaxis of neutrophils.

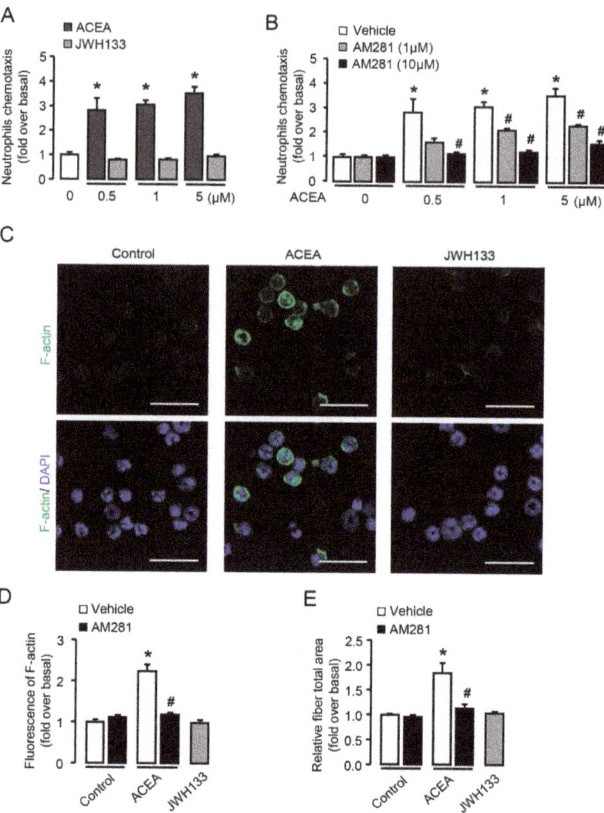

Figure 3. CB1 rather than CB2 mediates the chemotaxis and cytoskeletal remodeling of neutrophils in vitro. Chemotaxis assays were performed by transwell chambers. (**A**) Neutrophil chemotaxis with ACEA (CB1 agonist) or JWH133 (CB2 agonist) treatment for 2 h. (**B**) Effect of AM281 (CB1 antagonist) on neutrophil chemotaxis. (**C**) Representative images of F-actin remodeling with ACEA (1 μM, 2 h) and JWH 133 (1 μM, 2 h) treatment in neutrophils. Scale bars, 20 μm. (**D**) Quantification of F-actin with or without AM281 (10 μM) in ACEA-treated neutrophils. (**E**) The total fiber area was qualified by high content analysis in ACEA-treated neutrophils with or without AM281 pretreatment. Data are presented as the mean ± SEM. N = 5 per group. * $p < 0.05$ vs. control. # $p < 0.05$ vs. ACEA-treated alone.

Cytoskeletal remodeling is a prerequisite for cell chemotaxis and migration [29]. To evaluate the involvement of CB1 in cytoskeletal remodeling, neutrophils were stimulated with ACEA or JWH133 and then stained with FITC-conjugated phalloidin. Our findings indicated that ACEA-treated neutrophils were able to form a well-defined F-actin-rich leading edge (Figure 3C) and induced an increase in F-actin content (Figure 3D), whereas JWH133-treated neutrophils did not show obvious polymerized F-actin (Figure 3C,D). Consistent with the chemotaxis results above, AM281 could significantly reduce the increase of F-actin content induced by ACEA (Figure 3D). Moreover, the amount and distribution of actin fibers in neutrophils were determined by high content analysis. Treatment with ACEA showed significant increases in the total fiber area, which can be reversed by AM281 (Figure 3E). These results support that CB1 rather than CB2 plays an important role in neutrophil chemotaxis and cytoskeletal remodeling.

3.4. CB1 but not CB2 is Involved in the Activation of Neutrophils In Vitro

Next we sought to determine whether CBs played a role in the activation of neutrophils, including NETosis, MPO release from lysosome and ROS burst. Neutrophils stimulated with ACEA exhibited increased CitH3 fluorescence compared with untreated cells and represented manifest web-like chromatin release, in which chromatin and CitH3 (red) had good co-localization in neutrophils (Ly6G$^+$, violet) (Figure 4A,B), and can be suppressed by AM281 (Figure 4B). Western blot results showed the same effect of ACEA on CitH3 expression (Figure 4C). In contrast, JWH133-treated neutrophils did not exhibit increased level of CitH3 or web-like chromatin release (Figure 4A–C). We performed CCK-8 assay to measure neutrophil viability under the treatment of ACEA, the condition to induce NETosis. Our results showed that ACEA decreased the cell viability of neutrophils, while CB2 agonist JWH133 had no such effect, which was in accordance with the results of NETosis (Figure 4D).

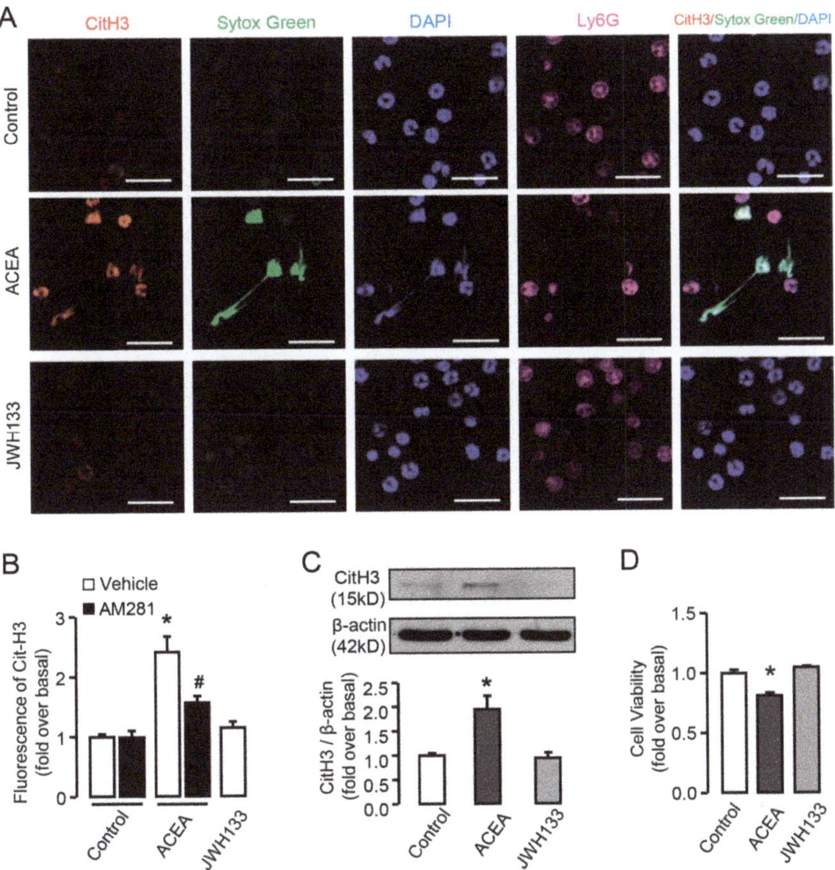

Figure 4. CB1 but not CB2 is involved in CitH3 expression and NETosis in vitro. (**A**) Representative confocal images of CitH3 (red) and Ly6G (violet) immunofluorescent staining and NETosis in ACEA or JWH133-treated neutrophils. The nuclei were stained with SYTOX® Green (green) and DAPI (blue). Scale bars, 20 μm. (**B**) Quantification of CitH3 and NETosis in ACEA or JWH133-treated neutrophils. (**C**) CitH3 protein level in ACEA or JWH133-stimulated neutrophils was examined by Western blot. (**D**) Cell viability of neutrophils treated by ACEA or JWH-133 by CCK-8 assay. Data are presented as the mean ± SEM. N = 4 per group. * $p < 0.05$ vs. control. # $p < 0.05$ vs. ACEA-treated alone.

Normally, MPO exists in lysosome and is undetectable by antibodies, when stimulated MPO is released from lysosome becoming detectable [30]. Further we detected the release of MPO in neutrophils by immunofluorescence. ACEA treatment resulted in more MPO release of neutrophils compared with control, while JWH133 treatment had no such effect (Figure 5A,B). Similar to the results of CitH3, AM281 also blocked ACEA-induced MPO release in neutrophils (Figure 5B). We then measured ROS burst in neutrophils with ACEA treatment. In response to ACEA stimulation, neutrophils showed a significant increase of ROS burst at 10 min, and this increase could be significantly prevented by pre-incubation with NAC which is the scavenger of ROS (Figure 5C). In addition, pretreatment with AM281 repressed ACEA-induced ROS burst, and JWH133 could not induce ROS burst in neutrophils (Figure 5D). ROS immunofluorescence images also displayed the increase of ROS burst by ACEA treatment (Figure 5E). Altogether these results display that CB1 but not CB2 mediates the activation of neutrophils.

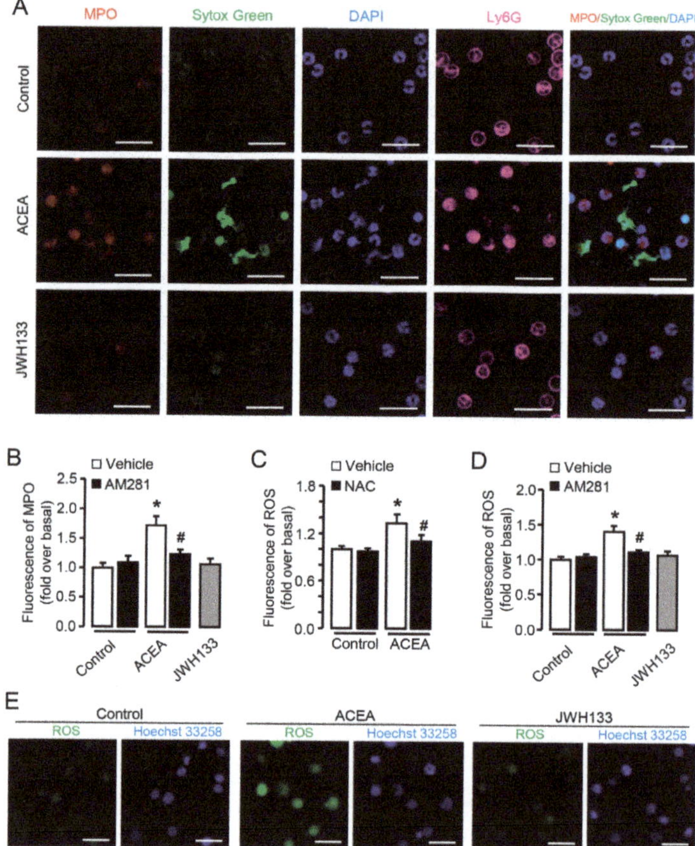

Figure 5. CB1 but not CB2 mediates MPO release and ROS burst in vitro. (**A**) Representative confocal images myeloperoxidase (MPO) (red) and Ly6G (violet) immunofluorescent staining in ACEA or JWH133-stimulated neutrophils. The nuclei were stained with SYTOX® Green (green) and DAPI (blue). Scale bars, 20μm. (**B**) Quantification of MPO in ACEA or JWH133-treated neutrophils. (**C**) ROS burst in ACEA-treated neutrophils with or without NAC. (**D**) ROS burst in ACEA-treated neutrophils with or without AM281. (**E**) ROS immunofluorescence images in ACEA- or JWH-133-treated neutrophils. Data are presented as the mean ± SEM. N = 4 per group. * $p < 0.05$ vs. control. # $p < 0.05$ vs. ACEA-treated alone.

3.5. Blockade of CB1 Significantly Attenuates Neutrophil Infiltration and Liver Inflammation in CCl₄-Treated Mice

The effects of CB1 blockade on neutrophil function and liver inflammation were further verified in vivo in mice treated with CCl_4 for 2 weeks, when the hepatic levels of neutrophil signatures were highest. CB1 blockade by the administration of AM281 restrained the mRNA levels of Ly6G in injured livers (Figure 6A). In line with this, FACS analysis showed decreased neutrophils infiltration after AM281 administration in CCl_4-treated mice compared with CCl_4-treated alone (Figure 6B,C). Similarly, the down-regulated expression of CitH3 (Figure 6D,E) was observed in CCl_4-treated mice with the administration of AM281, indicating less formation of NETs. Representative H&E-stained images showed a significant decrease of infiltrated inflammatory cells (Figure 6F) and the inflammatory area was quantified by digital image analysis (Figure 6G). Besides, AM281 administration protected liver against CCl_4-induced injury with lower levels of alanine aminotransferase (ALT) and aspartate aminotransferase (AST) in mouse serum (Figure 6H). To elucidate the significance of NETs formation in liver inflamamtion, DNase I was administrated in CCl_4-treated mice. Our results showed that DNase I significantly reduced mRNA expression of markers for liver inflammation (MCP1, IL-1β, IL-6) and macrophage activation (CD86) in the liver of CCl_4-treated mice (Figure 6I). Altogether these results demonstrate that blockade of CB1 inhibits the recruitment and activation of neutrophils in the early stage of chronic liver injury and significantly attenuates liver injury.

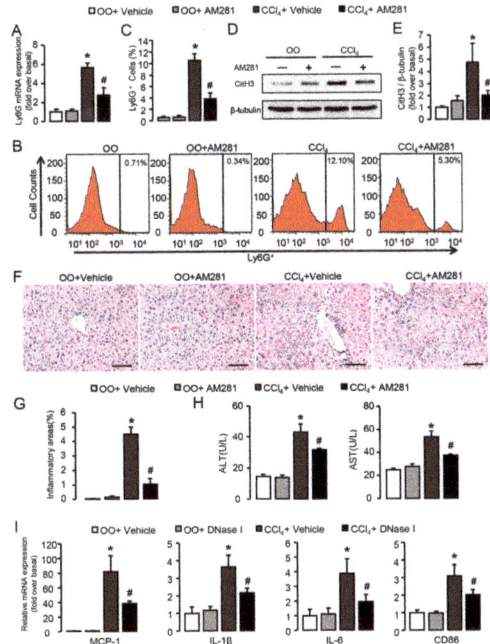

Figure 6. Blockade of CB1 significantly attenuates neutrophil infiltration and liver inflammation in CCl_4-treated mice. (**A**) Ly6G mRNA expression in CCl_4- or olive oil (OO)-treated liver with or without the administration of AM281. (**B,C**) Representative FACS plots and quantification for neutrophils in liver. (**D,E**) CitH3 protein levels in liver. (**F**) Representative H&E staining images of liver sections. Scale bars, 100 μm. (**G**) Quantitative analysis of liver inflammation areas. (**H**) Alanine aminotransferase (ALT) and aspartate aminotransferase (AST) levels were detected by chemistry analyzer. (**I**) mRNA expression of MCP-1, IL-1β, IL-6, and CD86 in CCl_4- or OO-treated liver with or without the administration of DNase I. Data are presented as the mean ± SEM. N = 6 per group. * $p < 0.05$ vs. OO. # $p < 0.05$ vs. CCl_4-treated alone.

3.6. $G\alpha_{i/o}$ Signal Is Involved in CB1-Mediated Chemotaxis and NETosis In Vitro

CB1 is a G-protein-coupled receptor which can transduce corresponding G protein-related signaling. To determine the distinct G-protein subtype involved in neutrophil chemotaxis and NETosis, we pre-treated cells with pertussis toxin (PTX) ($G\alpha_{i/o}$ inhibitor) or YM254890 ($G\alpha_q$ inhibitor). PTX prevented ACEA-induced neutrophil chemotaxis, while YM254890 exhibited no effect on it (Figure 7A). In line with this, the up-regulation of Cit-H3 protein induced by ACEA can be reversed by PTX, not YM254890 (Figure 7B–D). Moreover, less MPO release of neutrophils was observed after the pre-incubation of PTX in ACEA-stimulated cells compared with control, while YM254890 treatment had no such effect (Figure 7E). Markedly, PTX pretreatment inhibited ACEA-induced ROS burst, while YM254890 could not reduce ROS burst in neutrophils (Figure 7F). Taken together, these results indicate that $G\alpha_{i/o}$, not $G\alpha_q$ signal is involved in CB1-mediated chemotaxis and NETosis.

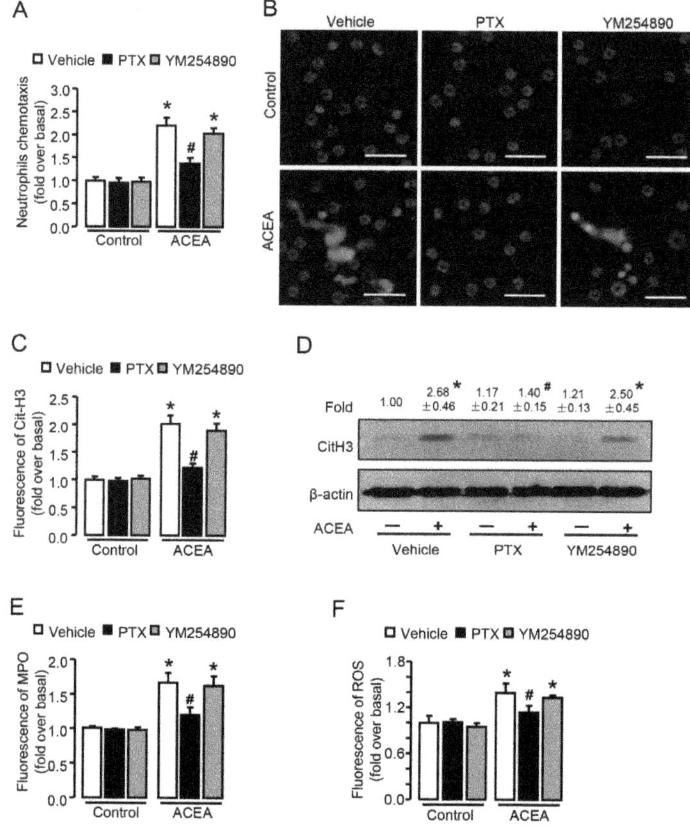

Figure 7. $G\alpha_{i/o}$ signal is involved in CB1-mediated chemotaxis and NETosis in vitro. (**A**) ACEA-induced neutrophil chemotaxis pretreated with $G\alpha_{i/o}$ inhibitor PTX or $G\alpha_q$ inhibitor YM254890. (**B,C**) Representative images and quantification of CitH3 immunofluorescent staining (green) and NETosis in ACEA-treated neutrophils pretreated with PTX or YM254890. The nuclei were stained with DAPI (blue). Scale bars, 20 μm. (**D**) CitH3 protein level with PTX or YM254890 pretreatment was examined by Western blot. (**E**) Quantification of myeloperoxidase (MPO) immunofluorescence with pertussis toxin (PTX) or YM254890 pretreatment. (**F**) ROS burst in ACEA-treated neutrophils with or without PTX or YM254890 pretreatment. Data are presented as the mean ± SEM. N = 4 per group. * $p < 0.05$ vs. control. # $p < 0.05$ vs. ACEA-treated alone.

3.7. ROS Is Required for CB1-Mediated Neutrophil Chemotaxis and NETosis In Vitro

Since ROS burst was markedly induced by ACEA, we then explored whether ROS was involved in CB1-mediated neutrophil chemotaxis and NETosis. Transwell assay showed that CB1-mediated chemotaxis in neutrophils was suppressed by NAC (Figure 8A), suggesting that ROS acted as a signaling molecule in CB1-mediated neutrophil chemotaxis. As NETosis can either be ROS-dependent or ROS-independent [31,32], we pre-treated neutrophils with NAC before stimulation with ACEA and detected CitH3 expression and MPO release, to investigate whether CB1-induced NETosis required ROS in vitro. NAC significantly blocked ACEA-induced increase of CitH3 detected by immunofluorescence (Figure 8B,C) and Western blot (Figure 8D). Similarly, lower MPO fluorescence was observed in neutrophils pre-incubated with NAC before ACEA stimulation compared with that without NAC (Figure 8E). Collectively, elimination of ROS suppresses CB1-mediated chemotaxis and NETosis in neutrophils, suggesting that ROS acts as an important signaling molecule in CB1-mediated neutrophil function.

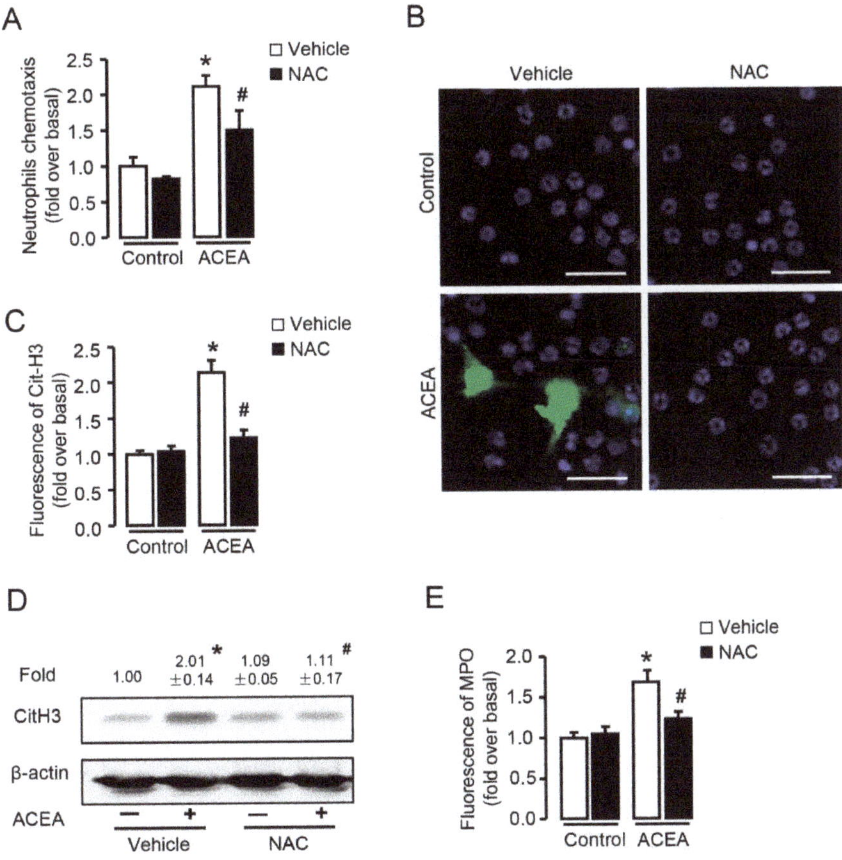

Figure 8. ROS is required in CB1-mediated chemotaxis and NETosis in vitro. (**A**) ACEA-induced neutrophil chemotaxis pretreated with or without NAC (5 mM). (**B,C**) Representative images and quantification of CitH3 immunofluorescent staining (green) and NETosis in ACEA-treated neutrophils pretreated with or without NAC. The nuclei were stained with DAPI (blue). Scale bars, 20 μm. (**D**) CitH3 protein level with or without NAC pretreatment was examined by Western blot. (**E**) Quantification of MPO immunofluorescence with or without NAC pretreatment. Data are presented as the mean ± SEM. N = 4 per group. * $p < 0.05$ vs. control. # $p < 0.05$ vs. ACEA-treated alone.

3.8. p38 MAPK Signaling Pathway, Located In the Downstream of ROS, Is Involved in CB1-Mediated Neutrophil Chemotaxis and NETosis

CB1 is a G-protein-coupled receptor whose biological function depends on multiple signaling pathways, such as AMPK and MAPK signaling pathways [33]. To identify which pathway controls the chemotaxis and NETosis of neutrophils, we first detected the phosphorylation of p38, JNK and ERK after ACEA treatment. Stimulation with ACEA led to a significant increase in the protein level of phosphor-p38 (Figure 9A,B), but failed to activate JNK (Figure 9C,D) and ERK (Figure 9E,F) in neutrophils. Based on these, we focused on the key role of p38 in neutrophil function in the following experiments.

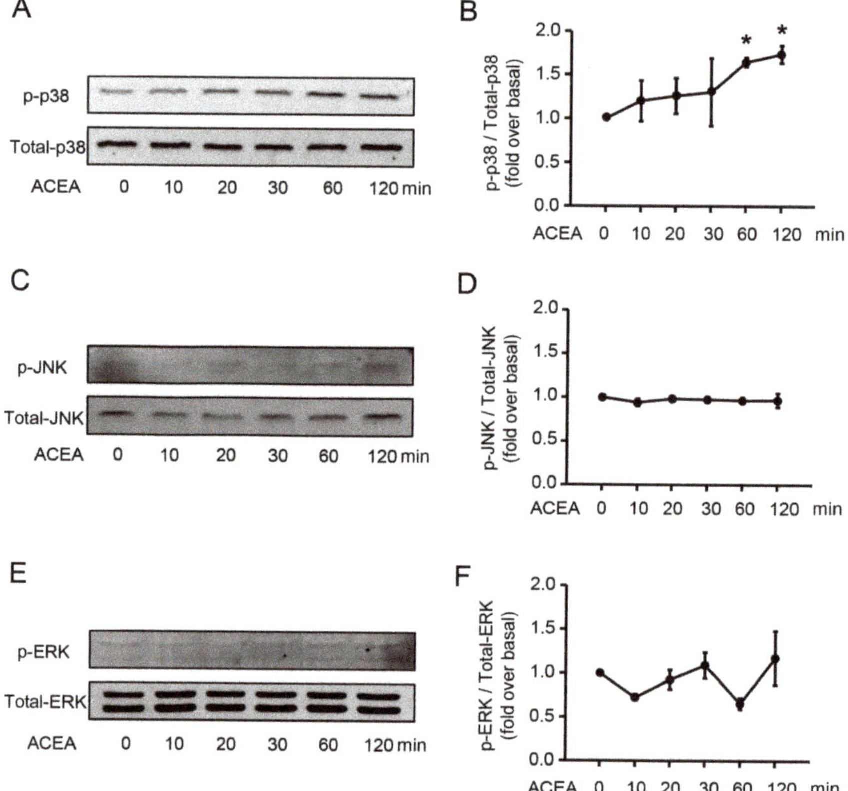

Figure 9. ACEA increases the protein level of phosphor-p38 in neutrophils. (**A,B**) Phosphor-p38 and total p38 expression after ACEA treatment was measured by Western blot. (**C,D**) Phosphor-JNK and total JNK expression. (**E,F**) Phosphor-ERK and total ERK expression. Data are presented as the mean ± SEM. N = 3 per group. * $p < 0.05$ vs. control.

Moreover, ACEA-induced neutrophil chemotaxis was significantly suppressed by p38 inhibitor SB203580 (Figure 10A), indicating the key role of p38 in neutrophil chemotaxis. In case of CB1-mediated NETosis, p38 inhibition restrained CitH3 expression detected by both fluorescence (Figure 10B,C) and Western blot (Figure 10D). Similarly, lower MPO fluorescence was observed in neutrophils pre-incubated with p38 inhibitor before ACEA stimulation (Figure 10E). These results indicate that CB1-mediated p38 phosphorylation is involved in neutrophil chemotaxis and NETosis. Furthermore, inhibition of p38 had no effect on the production of ROS (Figure 10F), whereas elimination of ROS inhibited CB1-mediated phosphorylation of p38 (Figure 10G), suggesting that ROS was upstream of p38. Combining the above results, p38 MAPK signaling pathway is required for CB1-mediated neutrophil chemotaxis and NETosis, and locates in the downstream of ROS (Figure 10H).

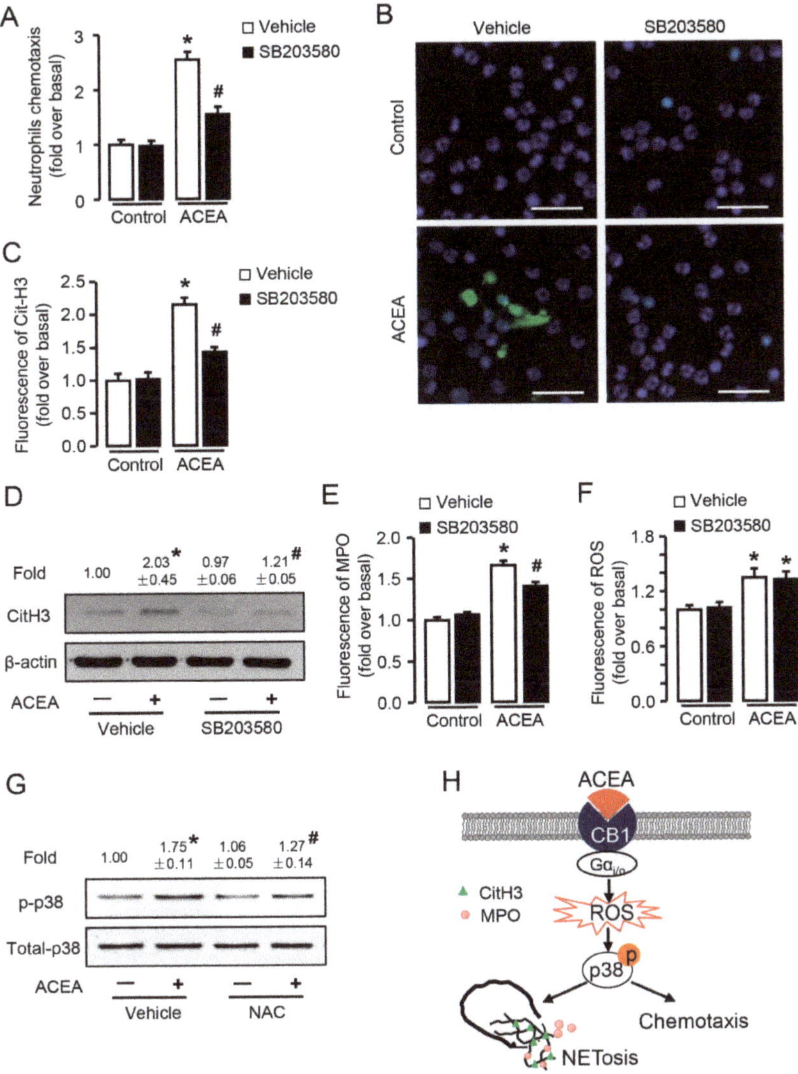

Figure 10. p38 MAPK signaling pathway is involved in CB1-mediated neutrophil chemotaxis and NETosis, and located in the downstream of ROS. (**A**) ACEA-induced neutrophil chemotaxis with or without p38 inhibitor SB203580 (10 µM). (**B,C**) Quantification of CitH3 immunofluorescence with or without SB203580. Scale bars, 20 µm. (**D**) CitH3 protein level with or without SB203580 was examined by Western blot. (**E**) Quantification of MPO immunofluorescence with or without SB203580. (**F**) ROS burst in ACEA-treated neutrophils with or without SB203580. (**G**) Phosphor-p38 and total p38 expression was measured by Western blot with or without NAC. (**H**) Schema graph of CB1 in neutrophil chemotaxis and NETosis. Data are presented as the mean ± SEM. N = 4 per group. * $p < 0.05$ vs. control. # $p < 0.05$ vs. ACEA-treated alone.

4. Discussion

In summary, this study demonstrates for the first time that CB1 mediates neutrophil chemotaxis and activation in a ROS- and p38 MAPK-dependent manner in sterile liver inflammation. Our work provides several new findings as follows: 1. Numerous bone marrow-derived neutrophils are recruited and activated in the liver of CCl$_4$-treated mice; 2. CBs positively correlate with neutrophil signatures in CCl$_4$-treated mice, and are abundantly expressed in isolated neutrophils; 3. In vitro CB1 rather than CB2 mediates neutrophil chemotaxis, NETosis, MPO release and ROS burst via G$\alpha_{i/o}$ signal; 4. ROS and p38 MAPK signaling pathway are both required for CB1-mediated neutrophil chemotaxis and NETosis, and p38 MAPK signaling pathway locates in the downstream of ROS; 5. Blockade of CB1 significantly attenuates neutrophil infiltration and liver inflammation in CCl$_4$-treated mice.

Neutrophils act as the first responders of the innate immune system and their crucial role in fighting invading pathogens during bacterial inflammation has been well established by published literature [34,35]. Recently more and more studies have been focusing on the prevailing role of neutrophils in sterile inflammation, and overexuberant neutrophil recruitment is associated with collateral tissue damage, defective healing, and chronic inflammation [36,37]. In the current study, we show that numerous BM-derived neutrophils are recruited to the site of liver injury shortly. The hepatic levels of neutrophil marker Ly6G begin to rise from 7 days of CCl$_4$ administration and peek at 2 weeks, which is the early stage of chronic liver injury. This is in agreement with published studies demonstrating that neutrophil depletion by injection of Ly6G antibody markedly reduces chronic-binge ethanol feeding-induced liver injury and liver transplantation ischemia–reperfusion injury [8,38,39]. However, there are studies identifying the dual role for neutrophils in acetaminophen-induced acute liver injury, with neutrophil-mediated injury amplification early on, but exerting protective effects during the repair phase as depletion of neutrophils increases liver damage [40,41]. Also neutrophils contribute to spontaneous resolution of liver inflammation and fibrosis via microRNA-223 in CCl$_4$-induced chronic liver injury [41]. More studies will be needed to figure out the mechanism underlying differential role of neutrophils in different models of liver inflammation and fibrosis.

ECS is implicated in the pathogenesis of numerous diseases, including cancer, cardiovascular disease, and liver disease [42,43]. Especially CB1 has emerged as a pivotal mediator in liver and exerts profibrogenic effects in chronic liver diseases including hepatic fibrosis, liver cirrhosis alcoholic fatty liver and nonalcoholic fatty liver [44]. Our previous studies have also demonstrated the vital role of CB1 in the migration and activation of BM-derived mesenchymal stromal cells and monocytes/macrophages in CCl$_4$-induced chronic liver injury [26,27,45,46]. However, the effect of CBs on neutrophil function during sterile liver inflammation is unclear up to now and is first documented in the present study. Our data display that CB1 rather than CB2 mediates the chemotaxis of neutrophils and NETosis, and CB1 blockade with AM281 reduces the infiltration and NETosis of neutrophils and attenuates liver injury in vivo, which can be used as a novel target for the treatment of liver fibrosis.

NETs, DNA webs released into the extracellular environment by activated neutrophils, are thought to play a key role in the function of neutrophils [47,48]. Unlike nuclear chromatin, NETs are highly decondensed chromatin structures, and PAD4 has been reported to be essential in chromatin decondensation to form NETs by catalyzing histone citrullination [49]. The partial PAD4-deficiency (Pad4$^{+/-}$) reduced acute lung injury induced by bacteria and improved survival, while complete NET inhibition by PAD4 deficiency (Pad4$^{-/-}$) reduced lung injury [50]. Further studies will be needed to investigate PAD4 expression and the effect of PAD4 on NETosis in our CCl$_4$-treated mice and ACEA-treated neutrophils.

NETosis was initially found dependent on the ROS by NADPH [32], and was subsequently found also to be independent of ROS [31]. In the present study, ACEA-mediated neutrophil chemotaxis and NETosis can be significantly suppressed by ROS scavenger NAC, indicating that CB1 induces the chemotaxis and NETosis of neutrophils in a ROS-dependent manner. Since ROS could activate MAPK pathway and then mediate PMA-induced NETosis [51], here we detect the activation of p38, JNK, and ERK after ACEA stimulation, showing that only p38 MAPK pathway is activated and involved in

CB1-mediated neutrophil chemotaxis and NETosis. Further we identify the upstream and downstream relationship of ROS and p38 MAPK signaling pathways by the fact that p38 inhibition has no effect on the production of ROS, whereas ROS elimination inhibits CB1-mediated phosphorylation of p38, suggesting that ROS acts as an upstream signaling molecule of p38 MAPK in neutrophil chemotaxis and NETosis.

In conclusion, we identify the critical role of CB1 in neutrophil chemotaxis and NETosis during sterile liver inflammation and explore the underlying mechanism associated with $G\alpha_{i/o}$/ROS/p38 MAPK signaling pathway, which may open new perspectives for pharmacological treatment of liver disease.

Author Contributions: Conceptualization, L.L. (Lin Yang); Methodology, X.Z. (Xuan Zhou), X.F. and X.Z. (Xinhao Zhao); Formal Analysis, X.Z. (Xuan Zhou), L.Y. (Le Yang) and N.C.; Investigation, X.Z. (Xuan Zhou), X.F. and X.Z. (Xinhao Zhao); Writing—Original Draft Preparation, X.Z. (Xuan Zhou) and L.Y. (Le Yang); Writing—Review and Editing, L.L. (Lin Yang); Project Administration, L.Y. (Lin Yang); Funding Acquisition, L.L. (Lin Yang). All authors have read and agree to the published version of the manuscript.

Funding: This research was funded by National Natural and Science Foundation of China (81670550, 81430013), Beijing Natural Science Foundation (7172019).

Conflicts of Interest: The authors declare no conflict of interest.

References

1. Bardoel, B.W.; Kenny, E.F.; Sollberger, G.; Zychlinsky, A. The balancing act of neutrophils. *Cell Host Microbe* **2014**, *15*, 526–536. [CrossRef]
2. Jorch, S.K.; Kubes, P. An emerging role for neutrophil extracellular traps in noninfectious disease. *Nat. Med.* **2017**, *23*, 279–287. [CrossRef]
3. Cools-Lartigue, J.; Spicer, J.; Najmeh, S.; Ferri, L. Neutrophil extracellular traps in cancer progression. *Cell. Mol. Life Sci.* **2014**, *71*, 4179–4194. [CrossRef] [PubMed]
4. Metzler, K.D.; Goosmann, C.; Lubojemska, A.; Zychlinsky, A.; Papayannopoulos, V. A myeloperoxidase-containing complex regulates neutrophil elastase release and actin dynamics during NETosis. *Cell Rep.* **2014**, *8*, 883–896. [CrossRef] [PubMed]
5. Sun, L.; Wu, Q.; Nie, Y.; Cheng, N.; Wang, R.; Wang, G.; Zhang, D.; He, H.; Ye, R.D.; Qian, F. A Role for MK2 in Enhancing Neutrophil-Derived ROS Production and Aggravating Liver Ischemia/Reperfusion Injury. *Front. Immunol.* **2018**, *9*, 2610. [CrossRef] [PubMed]
6. de Bont, C.M.; Koopman, W.; Boelens, W.C.; Pruijn, G. Stimulus-dependent chromatin dynamics, citrullination, calcium signalling and ROS production during NET formation. *Biochim. Biophys. Acta Mol. Cell Res.* **2018**, *1865*, 1621–1629. [CrossRef]
7. Brinkmann, V.; Reichard, U.; Goosmann, C.; Fauler, B.; Uhlemann, Y.; Weiss, D.S.; Weinrauch, Y.; Zychlinsky, A. Neutrophil extracellular traps kill bacteria. *Science* **2004**, *303*, 1532–1535. [CrossRef] [PubMed]
8. Huang, H.; Tohme, S.; Al-Khafaji, A.B.; Tai, S.; Loughran, P.; Chen, L.; Wang, S.; Kim, J.; Billiar, T.; Wang, Y.; et al. Damage-associated molecular pattern-activated neutrophil extracellular trap exacerbates sterile inflammatory liver injury. *Hepatology* **2015**, *62*, 600–614. [CrossRef]
9. Sollberger, G.; Tilley, D.O.; Zychlinsky, A. Neutrophil Extracellular Traps: The Biology of Chromatin Externalization. *Dev. Cell* **2018**, *44*, 542–553. [CrossRef]
10. Hisada, Y.; Grover, S.P.; Maqsood, A.; Houston, R.; Ay, C.; Nconuossie, D.F.; Cooley, B.C.; Wallen, H.; Key, N.S.; Thalin, C.; et al. Neutrophils and neutrophil extracellular traps enhance venous thrombosis in mice bearing human pancreatic tumors. *Haematologica* **2019**. [CrossRef]
11. Castanheira, F.; Kubes, P. Neutrophils and NETs in modulating acute and chronic inflammation. *Blood* **2019**, *133*, 2178–2185. [CrossRef] [PubMed]
12. Grabcanovic-Musija, F.; Obermayer, A.; Stoiber, W.; Krautgartner, W.D.; Steinbacher, P.; Winterberg, N.; Bathke, A.C.; Klappacher, M.; Studnicka, M. Neutrophil extracellular trap (NET) formation characterises stable and exacerbated COPD and correlates with airflow limitation. *Respir. Res.* **2015**, *16*, 59. [CrossRef] [PubMed]

13. Knight, J.S.; Subramanian, V.; O'Dell, A.A.; Yalavarthi, S.; Zhao, W.; Smith, C.K.; Hodgin, J.B.; Thompson, P.R.; Kaplan, M.J. Peptidylarginine deiminase inhibition disrupts NET formation and protects against kidney, skin and vascular disease in lupus-prone MRL/lpr mice. *Ann. Rheum. Dis.* **2015**, *74*, 2199–2206. [CrossRef] [PubMed]

14. Mistry, P.; Carmona-Rivera, C.; Ombrello, A.K.; Hoffmann, P.; Seto, N.L.; Jones, A.; Stone, D.L.; Naz, F.; Carlucci, P.; Dell'Orso, S.; et al. Dysregulated neutrophil responses and neutrophil extracellular trap formation and degradation in PAPA syndrome. *Ann. Rheum. Dis.* **2018**, *77*, 1825–1833. [CrossRef]

15. Yazdani, H.O.; Chen, H.W.; Tohme, S.; Tai, S.; van der Windt, D.J.; Loughran, P.; Rosborough, B.R.; Sud, V.; Beer-Stolz, D.; Turnquist, H.R.; et al. IL-33 exacerbates liver sterile inflammation by amplifying neutrophil extracellular trap formation. *J. Hepatol.* **2017**. [CrossRef] [PubMed]

16. He, Y.; Feng, D.; Li, M.; Gao, Y.; Ramirez, T.; Cao, H.; Kim, S.J.; Yang, Y.; Cai, Y.; Ju, C.; et al. Hepatic mitochondrial DNA/Toll-like receptor 9/MicroRNA-223 forms a negative feedback loop to limit neutrophil overactivation and acetaminophen hepatotoxicity in mice. *Hepatology* **2017**, *66*, 220–234. [CrossRef]

17. Mallat, A.; Lotersztajn, S. Targeting cannabinoid receptors in hepatocellular carcinoma? *Gut* **2016**, *65*, 1582–1583. [CrossRef]

18. Fonseca, B.M.; Costa, M.A.; Almada, M.; Correia-da-Silva, G.; Teixeira, N.A. Endogenous cannabinoids revisited: A biochemistry perspective. *Prostag. Other Lipid Med.* **2013**, *102–103*, 13–30. [CrossRef]

19. Rossi, F.; Tortora, C.; Punzo, F.; Bellini, G.; Argenziano, M.; Di Paola, A.; Torella, M.; Perrotta, S. The Endocannabinoid/Endovanilloid System in Bone: From Osteoporosis to Osteosarcoma. *Int. J. Mol. Sci.* **2019**, *20*, 1919. [CrossRef]

20. Rossi, F.; Punzo, F.; Umano, G.R.; Argenziano, M.; Miraglia, D.G.E. Role of Cannabinoids in Obesity. *Int. J. Mol. Sci.* **2018**, *19*, 2690. [CrossRef]

21. Starowicz, K.; Przewlocka, B. Modulation of neuropathic-pain-related behaviour by the spinal endocannabinoid/endovanilloid system. *Philos. Trans. R. Soc. Lond. B Biol. Sci.* **2012**, *367*, 3286–3299. [CrossRef] [PubMed]

22. Mallat, A.; Teixeira-Clerc, F.; Lotersztajn, S. Cannabinoid signaling and liver therapeutics. *J. Hepatol.* **2013**, *59*, 891–896. [CrossRef] [PubMed]

23. Tam, J.; Vemuri, V.K.; Liu, J.; Batkai, S.; Mukhopadhyay, B.; Godlewski, G.; Osei-Hyiaman, D.; Ohnuma, S.; Ambudkar, S.V.; Pickel, J.; et al. Peripheral CB1 cannabinoid receptor blockade improves cardiometabolic risk in mouse models of obesity. *J. Clin. Investig.* **2010**, *120*, 2953–2966. [CrossRef] [PubMed]

24. Gary-Bobo, M.; Elachouri, G.; Gallas, J.F.; Janiak, P.; Marini, P.; Ravinet-Trillou, C.; Chabbert, M.; Cruccioli, N.; Pfersdorff, C.; Roque, C.; et al. Rimonabant reduces obesity-associated hepatic steatosis and features of metabolic syndrome in obese Zucker fa/fa rats. *Hepatology* **2007**, *46*, 122–129. [CrossRef] [PubMed]

25. Chen, M.; Hou, P.; Zhou, M.; Ren, Q.; Wang, X.; Huang, L.; Hui, S.; Yi, L.; Mi, M. Resveratrol attenuates high-fat diet-induced non-alcoholic steatohepatitis by maintaining gut barrier integrity and inhibiting gut inflammation through regulation of the endocannabinoid system. *Clin. Nutr.* **2019**. [CrossRef]

26. Tian, L.; Li, W.; Yang, L.; Chang, N.; Fan, X.; Ji, X.; Xie, J.; Yang, L.; Li, L. Cannabinoid Receptor 1 Participates in Liver Inflammation by Promoting M1 Macrophage Polarization via RhoA/NF-kappaB p65 and ERK1/2 Pathways, Respectively, in Mouse Liver Fibrogenesis. *Front. Immunol.* **2017**, *8*, 1214. [CrossRef]

27. Mai, P.; Yang, L.; Tian, L.; Wang, L.; Jia, S.; Zhang, Y.; Liu, X.; Yang, L.; Li, L. Endocannabinoid System Contributes to Liver Injury and Inflammation by Activation of Bone Marrow-Derived Monocytes/Macrophages in a CB1-Dependent Manner. *J. Immunol.* **2015**, *195*, 3390–3401. [CrossRef]

28. Han, Z.; Zhu, T.; Liu, X.; Li, C.; Yue, S.; Liu, X.; Yang, L.; Yang, L.; Li, L. 15-deoxy-Delta12,14 -prostaglandin J2 reduces recruitment of bone marrow-derived monocyte/macrophages in chronic liver injury in mice. *Hepatology* **2012**, *56*, 350–360. [CrossRef]

29. Malinova, T.S.; Huveneers, S. Sensing of Cytoskeletal Forces by Asymmetric Adherens Junctions. *Trends Cell Biol.* **2018**, *28*, 328–341. [CrossRef]

30. Papayannopoulos, V.; Metzler, K.D.; Hakkim, A.; Zychlinsky, A. Neutrophil elastase and myeloperoxidase regulate the formation of neutrophil extracellular traps. *J. Cell Biol.* **2010**, *191*, 677–691. [CrossRef]

31. Pilsczek, F.H.; Salina, D.; Poon, K.K.; Fahey, C.; Yipp, B.G.; Sibley, C.D.; Robbins, S.M.; Green, F.H.; Surette, M.G.; Sugai, M.; et al. A novel mechanism of rapid nuclear neutrophil extracellular trap formation in response to Staphylococcus aureus. *J. Immunol.* **2010**, *185*, 7413–7425. [CrossRef] [PubMed]

32. Fuchs, T.A.; Abed, U.; Goosmann, C.; Hurwitz, R.; Schulze, I.; Wahn, V.; Weinrauch, Y.; Brinkmann, V.; Zychlinsky, A. Novel cell death program leads to neutrophil extracellular traps. *J. Cell Biol.* **2007**, *176*, 231–241. [CrossRef] [PubMed]

33. Turu, G.; Hunyady, L. Signal transduction of the CB1 cannabinoid receptor. *J. Mol. Endocrinol.* **2010**, *44*, 75–85. [CrossRef]

34. Kolaczkowska, E.; Kubes, P. Neutrophil recruitment and function in health and inflammation. *Nat. Rev. Immunol.* **2013**, *13*, 159–175. [CrossRef] [PubMed]

35. Meyer, E.; Beyersmann, J.; Bertz, H.; Wenzler-Rottele, S.; Babikir, R.; Schumacher, M.; Daschner, F.D.; Ruden, H.; Dettenkofer, M. Risk factor analysis of blood stream infection and pneumonia in neutropenic patients after peripheral blood stem-cell transplantation. *Bone Marrow Transpl.* **2007**, *39*, 173–178. [CrossRef] [PubMed]

36. Peiseler, M.; Kubes, P. More friend than foe: The emerging role of neutrophils in tissue repair. *J. Clin. Investig.* **2019**, *130*, 2629–2639. [CrossRef]

37. Phillipson, M.; Kubes, P. The neutrophil in vascular inflammation. *Nat. Med.* **2011**, *17*, 1381–1390. [CrossRef]

38. Bertola, A.; Park, O.; Gao, B. Chronic plus binge ethanol feeding synergistically induces neutrophil infiltration and liver injury in mice: A critical role for E-selectin. *Hepatology* **2013**, *58*, 1814–1823. [CrossRef]

39. Klune, J.R.; Bartels, C.; Luo, J.; Yokota, S.; Du, Q.; Geller, D.A. IL-23 mediates murine liver transplantation ischemia-reperfusion injury via IFN-gamma/IRF-1 pathway. *Am. J. Physiol. Gastrointest. Liver Physiol.* **2018**, *315*, G991–G1002. [CrossRef]

40. Alvarenga, D.M.; Mattos, M.S.; Lopes, M.E.; Marchesi, S.C.; Araujo, A.M.; Nakagaki, B.N.; Santos, M.M.; David, B.A.; De Souza, V.A.; Carvalho, E.; et al. Paradoxical Role of Matrix Metalloproteinases in Liver Injury and Regeneration after Sterile Acute Hepatic Failure. *Cells-Basel* **2018**, *7*, 247. [CrossRef]

41. Calvente, C.J.; Tameda, M.; Johnson, C.D.; Del, P.H.; Lin, Y.C.; Adronikou, N.; De Mollerat, D.J.X.; Llorente, C.; Boyer, J.; Feldstein, A.E. Neutrophils contribute to spontaneous resolution of liver inflammation and fibrosis via microRNA-223. *J. Clin. Investig.* **2019**, *130*, 4091–4109. [CrossRef] [PubMed]

42. Basu, P.P.; Aloysius, M.M.; Shah, N.J.; Brown, R.J. Review article: The endocannabinoid system in liver disease, a potential therapeutic target. *Aliment. Pharmacol. Ther.* **2014**, *39*, 790–801. [CrossRef] [PubMed]

43. Miller, L.K.; Devi, L.A. The highs and lows of cannabinoid receptor expression in disease: Mechanisms and their therapeutic implications. *Pharmacol. Rev.* **2011**, *63*, 461–470. [CrossRef] [PubMed]

44. Mahmoud, M.F.; Swefy, S.E.; Hasan, R.A.; Ibrahim, A. Role of cannabinoid receptors in hepatic fibrosis and apoptosis associated with bile duct ligation in rats. *Eur. J. Pharmacol.* **2014**, *742*, 118–124. [CrossRef] [PubMed]

45. Wang, L.; Yang, L.; Tian, L.; Mai, P.; Jia, S.; Yang, L.; Li, L. Cannabinoid Receptor 1 Mediates Homing of Bone Marrow-Derived Mesenchymal Stem Cells Triggered by Chronic Liver Injury. *J. Cell. Physiol.* **2017**, *232*, 110–121. [CrossRef] [PubMed]

46. Mai, P.; Tian, L.; Yang, L.; Wang, L.; Yang, L.; Li, L. Cannabinoid receptor 1 but not 2 mediates macrophage phagocytosis by G(alpha)i/o /RhoA/ROCK signaling pathway. *J. Cell. Physiol.* **2015**, *230*, 1640–1650. [CrossRef] [PubMed]

47. Liew, P.X.; Kubes, P. The Neutrophil's Role During Health and Disease. *Physiol. Rev.* **2019**, *99*, 1223–1248. [CrossRef]

48. Pfeiler, S.; Stark, K.; Massberg, S.; Engelmann, B. Propagation of thrombosis by neutrophils and extracellular nucleosome networks. *Haematologica* **2017**, *102*, 206–213. [CrossRef]

49. Li, P.; Li, M.; Lindberg, M.R.; Kennett, M.J.; Xiong, N.; Wang, Y. PAD4 is essential for antibacterial innate immunity mediated by neutrophil extracellular traps. *J. Exp. Med.* **2010**, *207*, 1853–1862. [CrossRef]

50. Lefrancais, E.; Mallavia, B.; Zhuo, H.; Calfee, C.S.; Looney, M.R. Maladaptive role of neutrophil extracellular traps in pathogen-induced lung injury. *JCI Insight* **2018**, *3*. [CrossRef]

51. Keshari, R.S.; Verma, A.; Barthwal, M.K.; Dikshit, M. Reactive oxygen species-induced activation of ERK and p38 MAPK mediates PMA-induced NETs release from human neutrophils. *J. Cell. Biochem.* **2013**, *114*, 532–540. [CrossRef] [PubMed]

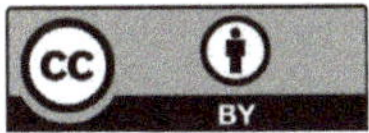

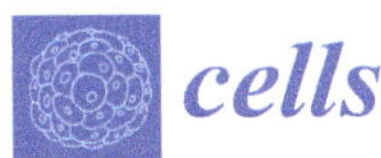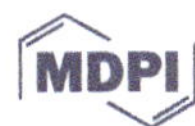

Article

Prognostic Role of Blood NETosis in the Progression of Head and Neck Cancer

Anna Sophie Decker [1], Ekaterina Pylaeva [1], Alexandra Brenzel [2], Ilona Spyra [1], Freya Droege [1], Timon Hussain [1], Stephan Lang [1] and Jadwiga Jablonska [1,*]

[1] Translational Oncology, Department of Otorhinolaryngology, University Hospital Essen, 45147 Essen, Germany
[2] Imaging Center Essen (IMCES), University Hospital Essen, 45147 Essen, Germany
* Correspondence: jadwiga.jablonska@uk-essen.de; Tel.: +49-201-723-3190

Received: 1 January 1970; Accepted: 19 August 2019; Published: 21 August 2019

Abstract: Neutrophil extracellular traps (NETs) represent web-like structures consisting of externalized DNA decorated with granule proteins that are responsible for trapping and killing bacteria. However, undesirable effects of NET formation during carcinogenesis, such as metastasis support, have been described. In the present study, we evaluated the correlation between NETosis and disease progression in head and neck cancer (HNC) patients in order to establish a valid biomarker for an early detection and monitoring of HNC progression. Moreover, factors influencing NET release in HNC patients were revealed. We showed a significantly elevated vital NETosis in neutrophils isolated from early T1–T2 and N0–N2 stage patients, as compared to healthy controls. Additionally, in our experimental setting, we confirmed the involvement of tumor cells in the stimulation of NET formation. Interestingly, in advanced cancer stages (T3–4, N3) NETosis was reduced. This also correlated with the levels of granulocyte colony-stimulating factor (G-CSF) in plasma and tumor tissue. Altogether, we suggest that the elevated NETosis in blood can be used as a biomarker to detect early HNC and to predict patients at risk to develop tumor metastasis. Therapeutic disruption of NET formation may offer new roads for successful treatment of HNC patients in order to prevent metastasis.

Keywords: head-and-neck cancer; metastasis; neutrophils; NETs; NETosis; innate immunity; G-CSF

1. Introduction

Head and neck cancer (HNC) is one of the most common tumor entities worldwide with an incidence of around 680,000 new cases per year [1]. The majority of HNC is histologically diagnosed as squamous cell carcinomas. At the time of diagnosis most HNC are locally advanced, which, despite multimodal treatment, often leads to disease progression or recurrence [2]. Recurrent HNC is often no longer accessible to curative therapy, turning HNC into the ninth deadliest cancer disease [1]. Although some risk factors associated with bad prognosis are well known, it still remains unclear which patients will suffer from recurrent HNC. Thus, this field is lacking a noninvasive diagnostic tool for early HNC diagnosis and for monitoring recurrent HNC progression.

Neutrophils play an important role in innate immunity, as they are the first line of defense during acute infection. Neutrophils show various strategies to protect the body from intruding microbes, fungi, and other pathogens [3]. Besides the well-known mechanisms like phagocytosis, degranulation, or production of reactive oxygen species (ROS), another antimicrobial mechanism of neutrophils has been described—neutrophil extracellular trap (NET) formation. NETs are web-like structures composed of externalized DNA decorated with histone and granule proteins. They can be released upon different stimuli, such as bacteria, cytokines, or the protein kinase C activator phorbole-12-myristat-13-acetat (PMA), resulting in pathogen killing [4]. Intensive investigations on NETs over the last decade revealed a potential involvement of the NETs in cancer progression, as it was shown that tumor cells themselves can activate neutrophils and stimulate NET formation via production of different factors like granulocyte colony-stimulating factor (G-CSF) [5]. Moreover, it was observed that released NETs, produced upon stimulation via tumor cells, are able to capture and surround distant metastatic cells and circulating tumor cells and, so, promote metastatic processes [6]. NETs were also shown to support invasion and migration of tumor cells in vitro. Degradation of NETs by DNase treatment prevented metastasis in a murine tumor model [7].

While localized tumors can be easily removed, metastatic disease remains the leading cause of death among cancer patients. Therefore, since NET formation is supposed to facilitate metastasis, we wanted to evaluate if there is a correlation between disease progression in HNC patients and NET formation by blood neutrophils. Moreover, we wanted to reveal factors that are involved in this phenomenon. This should help to reveal useful prognostic biomarkers to identify patients prone to HNC metastasis.

2. Materials and Methods

2.1. Patients

Patients with HNC (group 1, $n = 36$, blood samples for neutrophil isolation; group 2, $n = 17$, whole blood samples for SYTOX staining; group 3, $n = 20$, tumor samples) and healthy volunteers ($n = 10$) were included in the study after written local ethics committee approval; no previous chemotherapy or radiotherapy was performed. Acute inflammatory events (infectious diseases or acute phase of autoimmune disorders) 6 months prior to the enrollment were the exclusion criteria for this study. Clinico-pathological characteristics of HNC patients enrolled in this study are listed in Table 1.

Table 1. Clinico-pathological characteristics of patients enrolled in this study. HNC—head and neck cancer.

	Healthy ($n = 10$)	HNC group 1 ($n = 36$)	HNC group 2 ($n = 17$)	HNC group 3 ($n = 20$)
Age (years)	33 (22–55)	62 (28–85)	67 (52–75)	68 (52–80)
Gender, male (N, %)	5 (50%)	19 (53%)	10 (59%)	15 (75%)
Localization:				
larynx (N, %)		14 (39%)	6 (35.5%)	8 (40%)
oropharynx (N, %)	-	12 (33%)	5 (29%)	4 (20%)
other * (N, %)		10 (28%)	6 (35.5%)	8 (40%)
T Stage:				
1 (N, %)		14 (39%)	3 (17.5%)	2 (10%)
2 (N, %)	-	10 (28%)	4 (24%)	7 (35%)
3 (N, %)		7 (19%)	3 (17.5%)	5 (25%))
4 (N, %)		5 (14%)	7 (41%)	6 (30%)
N stage:				
0 (N, %)		18 (50%)	5 (29%)	6 (30%)
1 (N, %)	-	4 (11%)	3 (18%)	3 (15%)
2 (N, %)		12 (33%)	8 (47%)	11 (55%)
3 (N, %)		2 (6%)	1 (6%)	0 (0%)

* Oral cavity, glands, nasopharynx, hypopharynx.

2.2. Isolation of Blood Neutrophils

Peripheral blood was drawn into 3.8% sodium citrate anticoagulant monovettes and separated by density gradient centrifugation (Biocoll density 1.077 g/mL, Biochrome). The mononuclear cell fraction was discarded, and neutrophils were isolated by sedimentation over 1% polyvinyl alcohol, followed by hypotonic (0.2% NaCl) lysis of erythrocytes. In view of the emerging diversity of circulating neutrophil subtypes in humans, it should be noted that high-density neutrophils were investigated in this study.

The purity of the isolated neutrophils (>95%) was estimated with flow cytometry after staining with anti-CD66b (Beckman Coulter, Krefeld, Germany). Viability Dye eFluor™ 780 (eBioscience, Affymetrix, Santa Clara, CA, USA) or 4′,6-Diamidino-2-Phenylindole, Dilactate (DAPI) (BioLegend, San Diego, CA, USA) were used to determine viable cells. (Supplementary Figure S1A). Data were collected and analyzed with the BD FACS Canto system and BD FACS Diva 6.0 software (BD Biosciences, BD, Franklin Lakes, NJ, USA).

2.3. Bacteria

To stimulate NET release, *Pseudomonas aeruginosa* strain PA14 (wild-type serogroup O10 strain, cytotoxic ExoU+) was used. Bacteria were cultured in Luria–Bertani (LB) broth for 3 h to reach the early exponential phase, washed twice in phosphate buffered saline (PBS), and the optical density of a 100 µL suspension was measured in 96-well flat-bottom cell culture plates (Cellstar, Greiner Bio One International GmbH, Frickenhausen, Germany) at 600 nm using a microplate reader Synergy 2 (BioTek Instruments, Inc., Winooski, VT, USA). OD 0.4 corresponds to a bacterial density of 5×10^9/mL, as determined by serial dilutions and colony-forming unit assays. Bacteria concentration was adjusted to the desired values and verified by further plating on 2% LB agar plates.

2.4. Head and Neck Cancer (HNC) Tumor

Tumor tissue was digested using dispase 0.2 µg/mL, collagenase A 0.2 µg/mL, and DNase I 100 µg/mL (all Sigma-Aldrich/Merck, Darmstadt, Germany) solution in DMEM (Gibco, Life Technologies/Thermo Fisher Scientific, Waltham, MA, USA) containing 10% fetal bovine serum (FCS) and 1% penicillin–streptomycin to exclude the influence of live bacteria on NET formation by neutrophils. Cells were meshed through 50 µm filters (Cell Trics, Partec, Sysmex Europe GmbH, Goerlitz, Germany), and the concentration was measured with a CASY cell counter (Innovatis, Roche Innovatis AG, Bielefeld, Germany).

The percentage of tumor-associated neutrophils from single live cells in tumor tissue was estimated in a single-cell suspension after staining with anti-CD66b (Beckman Coulter) and Viability Dye eFluor™ 780 (eBioscience, Affymetrix).

For tumor supernatant isolation, tumor weight was measured, the tissue was cut into 0.5–1 mm pieces, and the amount of medium (DMEM (Gibco, Life Technologies/Thermo Fisher Scientific) containing 10% FCS and 1% penicillin–streptomycin) was added accordingly by weight (0.6 mL per 0.02 g). The samples were incubated for 4 h at 37 °C, 5% CO_2, and sterile medium was used as a negative control.

2.5. Induction of Neutrophil Extracellular Trap (NET) Formation with Pseudomonas aeruginosa

Isolated neutrophils, 25,000/well, were incubated with *P. aeruginosa* MOI 10 in a glass-bottom 96-well plate (MatTek Corporation, Ashland, MA, USA) precoated with poly-D-lysine 1 mg/mL (Sigma-Aldrich/Merck, Darmstadt, Germany) for 1 or 4 h at 37 °C and 5% CO_2, and sterile medium was used as a negative control. As we did not observe any significant difference in NET formation in control conditions (in the absence of *P. aeruginosa*) between 1 and 4 h (see Supplementary Figure S1B), the control values for 4 h were used for the further analysis.

To study the effect of G-CSF on the capacity of neutrophils to form NETs, neutrophils isolated from the blood of healthy volunteers ($n = 5$) were challenged with *P. aeruginosa* MOI 10 in the absence or presence of human G-CSF (Filgrastim HEXAL, Holzkirchen, Germany) at a concentration 10 ng/mL for 4 h.

2.6. Induction of NET Formation by HNC Cells

The single-cell suspension of HNC tumor tissue was prepared as described above. Cell concentration was adjusted to 25,000 in 100 μL in a glass-bottom 96-welll plate (MatTek Corporation) precoated with poly-D-lysine 1 mg/mL (Sigma-Aldrich/Merck). Neutrophils isolated from peripheral blood of the same patient 25,000/100 uL were added and incubated for 4 h at 37 °C and 5% CO_2.

2.7. Immunofluorescent Staining, Fluorescence Microscopy of NETs, and Analysis

Samples were fixed with paraformaldehyde (Thermo Fisher Scientific) to a final concentration 4%, permeabilized with Triton X-100 (Sigma Aldrich/Merck, Darmstadt, Germany) 0.2% containing buffer, stained with anti-histone-1 antibodies (Merck Millipore, Darmstadt, Germany) and donkey-anti-mouse-AF546 (Invitrogen, Thermo Fisher Scientific, Waltham, MA, USA) secondary antibodies, and mounted with ProLong Gold Antifade Mountant with DAPI (Invitrogen). Decondensed chromatin structures were histone-1-positive [8] and were determined as NETs. Percentage of NET-producing cells, area covered by NETs, and the average size of NETs were estimated microscopically with Zeiss AxioObserver.Z1 Inverted Microscope with ApoTome Optical Sectioning equipped (filters for DAPI and Alexa Fluor 546). Images were processed with ZEN Blue 2012 software (CarlZeiss Microscopy GmbH, Jena, Germany) and analyzed with ImageJ v1.151j8 (public domain). For obtaining binary masks of nuclei and NET structures from the two channel .czi images, the Auto-Threshold (MaxEntropy dark for nuclei and Li dark for NETs) was used. The analyze particles tool was used to quantify the number of nuclei after performing the watershed function. The same was true for the NET structures. NET area quantification was used for further analysis. All images were analyzed in a batch mode, and individual image results were created and controlled for manual correction (see Supplementary Figure S2).

2.8. SYTOX Staining

To identify the major granulocyte subpopulations and exclude eosinophils and basophils, a DuraClone IM Granulocytes Tube set (Beckman Coulter) was used according to the manufacturer's protocol. The SYTOX Orange (Invitrogen) nucleic acid stain was performed with whole blood from the patients within the first 2 h after obtaining, with subsequent lysis of erythrocytes with Whole Blood Lysing Reagents (Beckman Coulter). Neutrophils were gated as CD45$^+$ CD15$^+$ CD294$^-$ as depicted in Figure 6A. SYTOX-positive cells were considered as spontaneously producing NETs. The percentage of SYTOX-positive cells from neutrophils and the mean fluorescence intensity (MFI) of SYTOX were analyzed with the CytoFLEX system (Beckman Coulter).

2.9. ELISA

G-CSF content in plasma and tumor supernatants was analyzed with ELISA (R&D Systems, Minnesota, U.S.) according to the manufacturer's protocols.

2.10. Statistics

Statistical analysis was performed using a Kruskal–Wallis ANOVA for multiple comparisons with Bonferroni correction, a Mann–Whitney U-test for two independent samples, a Wilcoxon matched-pairs signed rank test for dependent samples, and Spearman's R test for correlations. A $p < 0.05$ was considered significant.

2.11. Study Approval

The study was done in accordance to Helsinki declaration. Human studies were approved by the Ethical Committee at Medical Faculty, University Duisburg-Essen, Essen, Germany (Ethik Votum 16-7135-BO, 14.02.2017). Written informed consent was obtained from participants prior to inclusion in the study.

3. Results

3.1. Elevated Neutrophil Extracellular Trap Formation in HNC Patients

During the course of head and neck cancer, the number of neutrophils in blood and tumor progressively increases (Supplementary Figure S1D). This is associated with an adverse prognosis of patients [9]. However, the exact role of these neutrophils in HNC tumor progression is not clear. Therefore, we aimed to address the functionality of blood neutrophils and its changes during tumor progression. As a first approximation, we analyzed the capability of blood neutrophils, isolated from HNC patients versus healthy controls, to release NETs in the presence of bacteria. Here, the common bacteria *P. aeruginosa* was used, which colonizes the oral cavity and upper respiratory tract in pathological conditions [10]. We observed that NET formation was significantly elevated in HNC compared to healthy individuals. (Figure 1).

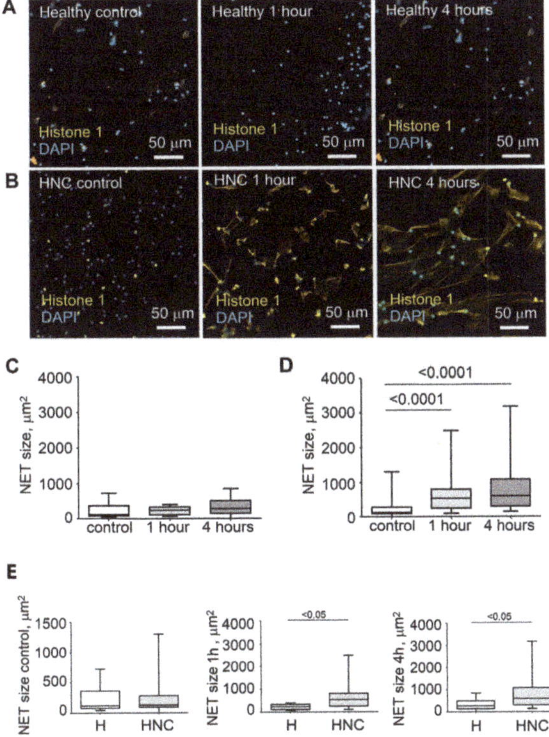

Figure 1. Elevated neutrophil extracellular trap formation in HNC patients. (**A,B**) Representative pictures showing neutrophil extracellular trap (NET) formation by healthy and HNC neutrophils. Isolated neutrophils were incubated with control medium or *Pseudomonas aeruginosa* for 1 and 4 h, fixed, and stained with DAPI (blue) and anti-histone-1 antibodies (orange); scale bar 50 µm. (**C**) Quantification of NET size in healthy individuals. (**D**) Quantification of NET size in HNC patients. (**E**) Comparison of spontaneous, early, and late NET release in healthy and HNC individuals. Blood neutrophils of healthy individuals ($n = 10$) and HNC patients ($n = 36$) were isolated and co-cultured with medium (control) or *P. aeruginosa* for 1 and 4 h. For comparisons of multiple groups, Kruskal–Wallis ANOVA with Bonferroni correction was used; for comparisons of two independent groups, Mann–Whitney U-tests were used; and for comparisons of two dependent groups, a Wilcoxon matched-pairs signed rank test was used. Data are shown as median, interquartile range, and minimal and maximal values.

3.2. Stage of Disease Determines the Ability of Blood Neutrophils to Release NETs

There is increasing evidence that the immune system plays an important role during malignant transformation of cells and the development of cancer. As neutrophils strongly influence tumor progression and metastasis [11–13], we were interested if the capability to produce NETs by these cells correlated with the tumor stage. Therefore, HNC patients were divided into groups concerning their pathologically diagnosed tumor, nodus and metastasis (TNM) stage, blood neutrophils were isolated, and their NET formation capacities were assessed. We could observe that neutrophils isolated from patients in early stages of cancer (T1–T2) already spontaneously produced higher amounts of NET as compared to neutrophils from late-stage cancer patients (Figure 2A,D). After short (1 h) incubation with *Pseudomonas*, NETs were released from early-stage neutrophils at a significantly greater extent as compared to late-stage cancer patients (Figure 2B,D). This difference was gone after longer bacterial stimulation (4 h) (Figure 2C,D), implying that early-stage neutrophils can react faster on the stimulus than late-stage neutrophils. Possibly, neutrophils from early HNC stages are already preactivated in blood, while late-stage HNC neutrophils are not, therefore needing longer activation to release NETs (Supplementary Figure S1C).

Next, we were interested in how NET formation correlated with the stage of lymph node metastasis. Similar to T-stage groups, the early-stage patients (N0–N1) released NETs spontaneously and after only short stimulation with bacteria, while late-stage patient neutrophils needed at least 4 h of stimulation with bacteria to release NETs (Figure 3). Such late/classical NETosis was comparable between early and late stages of HNC (Figure 3C). Here again, spontaneous NETosis was elevated in early stage patients (Figure 3A).

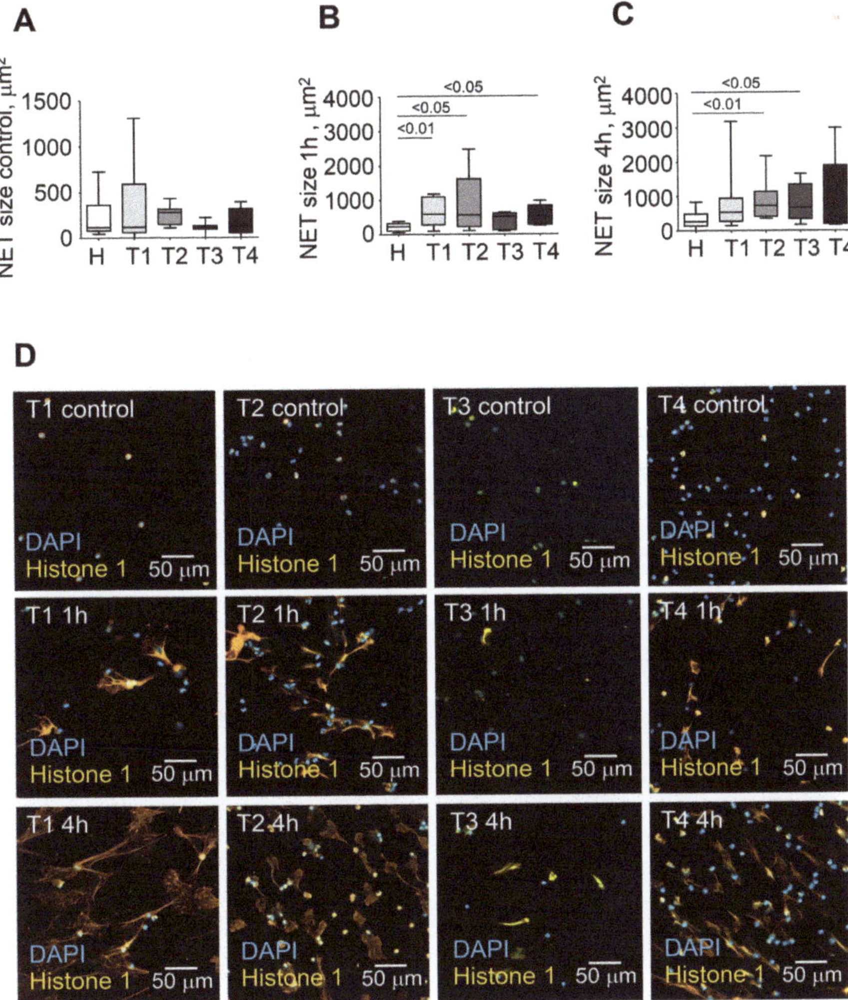

Figure 2. Neutrophils from early T stages of HNC release NETs significantly faster and to a greater extent. (**A**) Quantification of spontaneous NET release in healthy and HNC in different stages of disease. (**B**) Quantification of early NET release in healthy and HNC in different stages. (**C**) Quantification of late NET release in healthy and HNC in different stages. Neutrophils were isolated and stained (control, **A**), or co-cultured with *P. aeruginosa* for 1 (**B**) or for 4 (**C**) h; H—healthy. For comparisons of multiple groups, Kruskal–Wallis ANOVA with Bonferroni correction was used, and for comparisons of two independent groups, Mann–Whitney U-tests were used. Data are shown as median, interquartile range, and minimal and maximal values. (**D**) Exemplified pictures for NET formation in different HNC T stages. Isolated neutrophils were incubated with control medium or *P. aeruginosa* for 1 and 4 h, fixed, and stained with DAPI (blue) and anti-histone-1 antibodies (yellow); scale bar 50 µm.

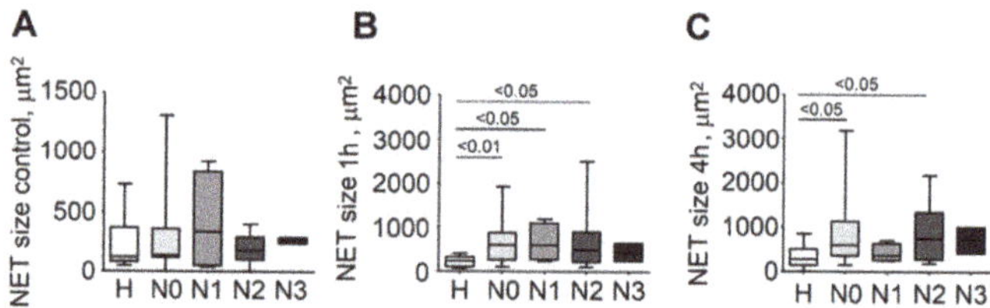

Figure 3. Neutrophils from early N stages of HNC release NETs significantly faster and to a greater extent. (**A**) Quantification of spontaneous NET release by different N stages of HNC neutrophils. (**B**) Quantification of early NET release. (**C**) Quantification of late NET release. Neutrophils were isolated and stained (**A**), or co-cultured with *P. aeruginosa* for 1 h (**B**) and for 4 h (**C**). H—healthy. For comparisons of multiple groups, Kruskal–Wallis ANOVA with Bonferroni correction was used, and for comparisons of two independent groups, Mann–Whitney U-tests were used. Data are shown as median, interquartile range, and minimal and maximal values.

3.3. Formation of NETs Correlates with Serum Levels of G-CSF in HNC Patients

To evaluate the possible mechanism responsible for tumor-mediated activation of NETosis by circulating blood neutrophils, we checked the plasma of HNC patients for tumor-derived factors, and we correlated NET production with the expression of these factors. A significant, positive correlation was observed between serum levels of G-CSF and the percentage of NETs producing neutrophils (Figure 4A).

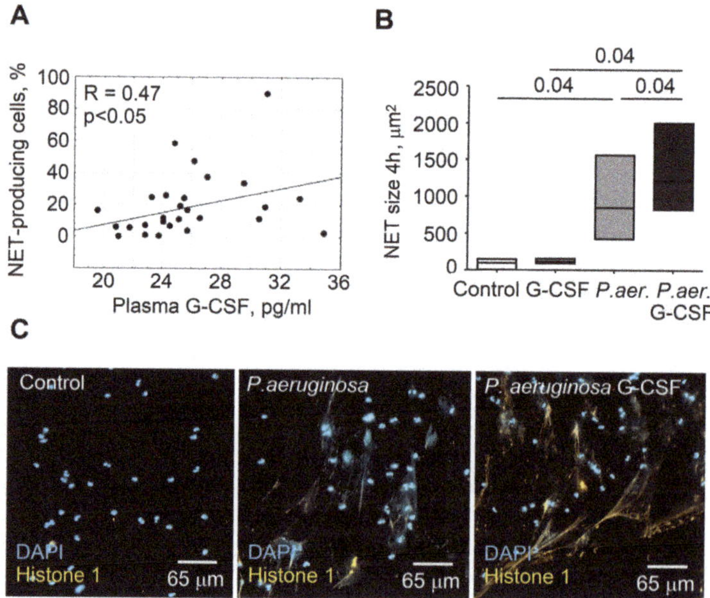

Figure 4. G-CSF stimulates *P. aeruginosa*-induced NET formation. (**A**) Plasma G-CSF levels correlate with the percentage of early (within the first hour of co-incubation with *P. aeruginosa*) NETs. For analysis of correlations, Spearman's R test was used. (**B**) *P. aeruginosa*-induced NET formation of healthy donor ($n = 5$) neutrophils can be stimulated with G-CSF in vitro. Data are shown as median and min/max. For comparisons of two dependent groups, a Wilcoxon matched-pairs signed rank test was used. (**C**) Representative figures illustrating the stimulation of *P. aeruginosa*-induced NET formation by G-CSF. DAPI (blue), histone 1 (orange), scale bar 65 μm.

3.4. G-CSF Stimulates NET Formation in Neutrophils

As the level of NETosis seems to correlate with plasma content of G-CSF in HNC patients, we wanted to confirm if G-CSF can indeed stimulate NET formation by neutrophils in our experimental conditions. We stimulated NET formation in neutrophils, as described above, and treated them additionally with G-CSF. The size of the produced NETs was assessed. We could indeed observe that G-CSF significantly stimulated NET formation (Figure 4B,C).

3.5. Tumor Cells Stimulate NET Release by Blood Neutrophils

Tumor cells produce multiple cytokines and growth factors that may influence neutrophil activation and functions, such as phagocytosis, degranulation, production of reactive oxygen species (ROS), or NETosis. One such factor is G-CSF [10]. To evaluate if tumor cells were able to directly stimulate neutrophil NETosis, we isolated blood neutrophils and tumor cells from the same patient and incubated them at a 1:1 proportion for 4 h in glass-bottom slides. To get single tumor cells, tissue digestion of the patient-derived tumor tissue was performed. After this, we stained DNA and histones to visualize NETs. We could observe that tumor cells indeed strongly stimulated NET release from neutrophils without the need of any additional stimuli (Figure 5).

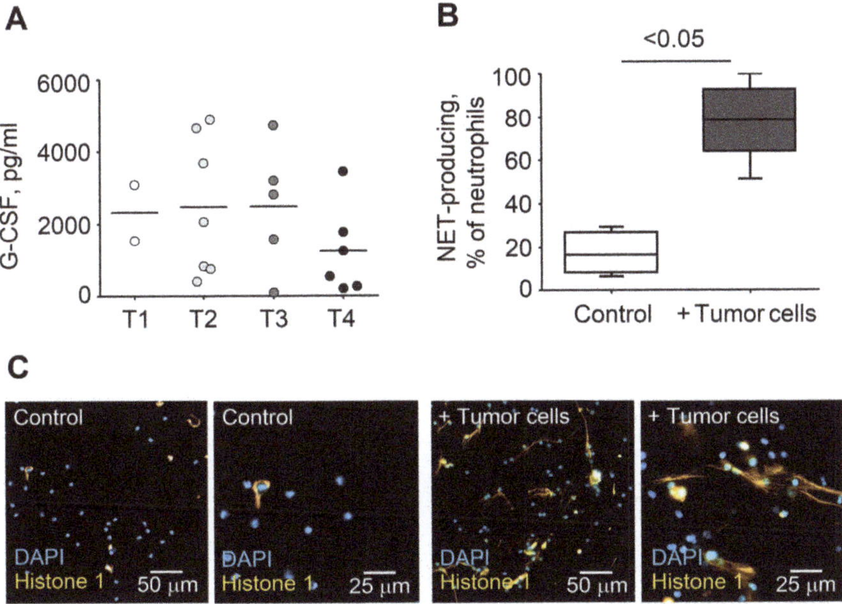

Figure 5. Tumor cells produce high levels of G-CSF and stimulate NETosis of blood neutrophils. (**A**) G-CSF levels in supernatants of cultured tumor tissue (normalized to sample mass). Data are shown as individual values and mean. (**B,C**) Elevated NET production by neutrophils co-incubated with tumor cells. Quantification of NET-positive neutrophils (**B**), and exemplified pictures showing NET release by HNC blood neutrophils (**C**). Isolated neutrophils and tumor cells of HNC patients were co-incubated at a 1:1 proportion for 4 h, fixed, and stained with DAPI (blue) and anti-histone-1 antibodies (orange); scale bars 50 and 25 μm. For comparisons of two independent groups, a Mann–Whitney U-test was used. Data are shown as median, interquartile range, and minimal and maximal values.

3.6. SYTOX Staining of NETs in Blood as a Potential Biomarker that Differentiates Patients Prone to Disease Progression and Metastasis

The ability to release NETs is significantly elevated in patients with an early stage of disease, and late metastatic stages show a NET release comparable to healthy patients. Therefore, we decided to test if simple SYTOX staining of blood neutrophils could provide a useful prognostic tool for HNC patients. We performed SYTOX Orange staining in the DuraClone IM Granulocytes Tube set (Beckman Coulter) and could observe an elevated percentage of SYTOX$^+$ neutrophils in the blood of I–III stage HNC patients, as compared to stage IV (Figure 6B). As the percentage of SYTOX$^+$ neutrophils in the blood of early-stage patients was elevated, we wanted to assess if the amount of released NETs changed in different HNC stages. Indeed, we could observe significantly elevated NET amounts that were released by blood neutrophils from early HNC stages in comparison to late stages (Figure 6C).

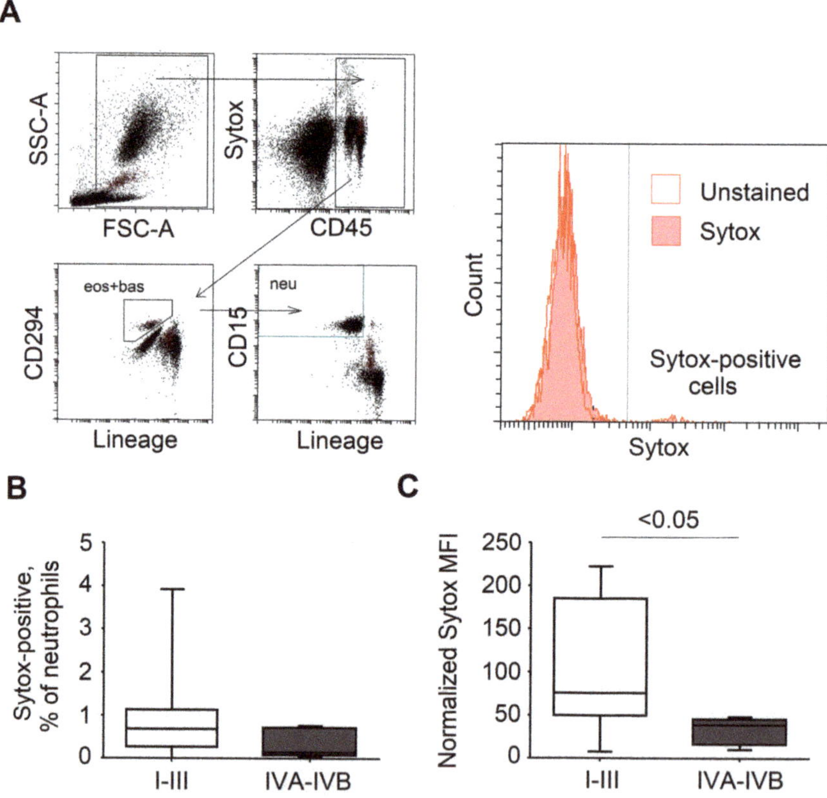

Figure 6. Elevated NET release in early stages of HNC demonstrated in flow cytometry using SYTOX staining. (**A**) Gating strategy for SYTOX expression on blood neutrophils. Neutrophils are gated as CD45$^+$CD15$^+$CD294$^-$cells. NET-releasing neutrophils are determined as SYTOX-positive cells. (**B**) Elevated percentage of SYTOX-positive neutrophils in lower stages of HNC. (**C**) Elevated SYTOX expression on neutrophils (MFI) in lower stages of HNC. For comparisons of two independent groups, a Mann–Whitney U-test was used. Data are shown as median, interquartile range, and minimal and maximal values.

4. Discussion

Neutrophils play a key role in cancer development and progression. This was proven in multiple animal tumor models [12,14,15] and clinical observations [9,16]. While numerous neutrophilic functions are anti-tumoral [17,18], neutrophils can also support tumor development and progression [19–21]. A recently discovered mechanism of anti-bacterial defense, NETosis, was primarily considered to have cytotoxic anti-tumor properties, as NET-derived DNA, histones, and granule proteins are described to be strongly cytotoxic [22,23]. Nevertheless, the ability of such structures to trap tumor cells and attach them to the endothelium, thus supporting their invasion into distant organs, was also demonstrated [6,19].

In this manuscript we focused our attention on the ability of blood neutrophils to form NETs in relation to the stage of HNC disease and to the concentration of plasma G-CSF. The results of the conducted experiments indicate that formation of neutrophil extracellular traps is generally elevated in HNC patients in comparison to healthy individuals. HNC patients showed bigger absolute sizes of NETs after one and after four hours, and spontaneous NET formation in these patients is strongly elevated. This probably is due to the activation of neutrophils with tumor-derived factors, such as G-CSF. Elevated sizes of NETs allow more efficient trapping of circulating tumor cells, thus supporting their spread.

We demonstrated that, particularly in the early stages of disease (T1–2, N0–2), HNC patients showed higher NET formation by blood neutrophils. This was particularly visible for early NET release (one hour of co-incubation with bacteria), implicating significant preactivation of neutrophils by the ongoing disease in early stage patients. Neutrophils isolated from late-stage HNC patients needed longer bacterial stimulation (4 h) in order to produce comparable levels of NETs. This delayed time to react on a stimulus implicates the lack of initial prestimulation in blood in such late-stage patients. The strong spontaneous NET formation in early-stage patients may contribute to their high risk for developing metastases. A similar phenomenon has been described for oral squamous cell carcinoma, when the most prominent NET formation in response to LPS and IL-17 stimuli was detected in the early stages of the disease [24].

Several mechanisms are involved in NET formation. In light of this, classical ROS-dependent and early/rapid ROS-independent ways of NET formation were described [25]. Rapid NET formation is claimed to be "vital" as the phagocytotic and migratory capacity of such neutrophils is preserved. Classic NET release seems to be suicidal, as the neutrophil dies during this process [26]. Here, we observed more rapid NET formation in early stages of HNC and a correlation between early NET release and G-CSF in plasma, while in the late stages of HNC, neutrophils reacted slower and reached high levels of NET formation after four hours of stimulation. The mechanisms responsible for this phenomenon require further investigation, but one can speculate that early-stage HNC neutrophils are more prone to vital NETosis due to the stimulation with tumor-derived factors or circulating tumor cells, while in the late stages the classical 'suicidal' NETosis dominates neutrophil responses. We expect that early vital NETosis can be more supportive for metastatic processes than late suicidal, due to the ability of such neutrophils to remain motile and potentially to migrate into pre-metastatic organs [27,28]. In the present study, the group of HNC patients was significantly older than healthy controls, which may influence NET formation. Nevertheless, literature data has proven that NET release by neutrophils declines with age [29]. Therefore, the observed increase of NET detected in the early stages of HNC is not influenced by the age differences between healthy and HNC individuals.

Because various types of tumors produce several cytokines (IL-6, IL-8, TNFα) and growth factors (G-CSF), which are known to stimulate the activity of neutrophils [30–32], we aimed to investigate the influence of tumor-derived G-CSF on NET formation by the neutrophils isolated from the blood of HNC patients. We observed that the levels of G-CSF positively correlated with the number of NET-producing neutrophils. The increased NET formation in mice bearing G-CSF-producing tumors was reported previously [5]. To confirm that elevated NET release observed in HNC patients is due to G-CSF, we stimulated neutrophils isolated from healthy volunteers with G-CSF in vitro. We could indeed observe a stimulated NET formation in such conditions, while G-CSF alone in the absence of bacterial stimulus did not influence NET formation. Importantly, we could also demonstrate that tumor cells themselves were able to stimulate NET release, possibly due to the high expression of G-CSF.

Monitoring the level of NETs released in the blood of HNC patients could provide a useful, noninvasive biomarker for early diagnosis and monitoring of disease progression. The number of NETs in patient blood can be easily assessed using SYTOX staining of whole blood samples instead of complicated and time-consuming procedures of neutrophil isolation, NET staining, and microscopy [33]. Using this method, we confirmed the results obtained using histological quantification, showing elevated NET release in the early stages of HNC and its decrease in late stages. Nevertheless, further investigations should be performed to increase the specificity of this method [26].

Metastasis of the tumor is the major cause of deaths from cancer, so the prevention of metastases remains one of the most important goals in the therapy of HNC. As NETs are suggested to stimulate this process, the degradation of NETs should provide a possible therapeutic target. In agreement, the treatment with DNase or neutrophil elastase was shown to inhibit adhesion of circulating tumor cells to the endothelium and to reduce development of metastasis in mice [19].

NETs not only take part in killing bacteria or supporting metastasis, but they are also involved in other pathological events like thrombosis. Elevated white blood cells, particularly neutrophils, are strongly associated with an increased risk of deep vein thrombosis and mortality in cancer patients receiving systemic chemotherapy [34]. With their three-dimensional web-like structure, it appears plausible that NETs in the blood stream can bind thrombocytes and participate in forming thrombotic material. Therefore, especially after surgeries when the risk of thromboembolic complication is the highest, NET formation should be therapeutically inhibited.

Clinical observations have proven a worse prognosis of HNC patients treated with G-CSF due to chemo- or radiotherapy-induced neutropenia [35]. At the same time, released G-CSF is associated with increased invasiveness of cancer cells themselves [36] or with diminished anti-tumor effects of chemotherapy. It also promotes re-vascularization and tumor growth [37]. This suggests the prognostic significance of G-CSF levels in patient plasma and suggests re-evaluating its use in cancer patients. Moreover, therapeutic inhibition of G-CSF-signaling pathways in cancer patients prone to metastasis should be considered [12].

5. Conclusions

In sum, we were able to show that NET formation in blood correlates with the progression of HNC disease. Based on this, blood NETosis may serve as a biological marker that can reveal HNC patients with a high risk of cancer progression and metastasis. Early identification of such patients should help to improve disease outcomes via earlier applications of relevant therapies. Moreover, such patients should be included into strict post-treatment observation programs.

Supplementary Materials: The following are available online at http://www.mdpi.com/2073-4409/8/9/946/s1. Figure S1: Gating strategy for determining the purity of isolated blood neutrophils, NET formation, percentage of neutrophils and correlation with tumor-derived factors in different tumor stages; Figure S2: Example analysis of NETs area using ImageJ software.

Author Contributions: A.S.D.: Conceptualization, Methodology, Project Administration, Formal Analysis, Validation, Writing, and Original Draft Preparation; E.P.: Conceptualization, Methodology, Project Administration, Formal Analysis, and Original Draft Preparation; A.B.: Software, Validation; I.S., T.H., and F.D.: Formal Analysis; S.L.: Resources, Writing, and Review & Editing; J.J.: Conceptualization, Project Administration, Supervision, Funding Acquisition, Resources, Writing, and Review & Editing.

Funding: J.J. was supported by Deutsche Forschungsgemeinschaft (DFG/JA 2461/2-1, DFG/JA 2461/5-1) and Deutsche Krebshilfe (No. 70113112).

Acknowledgments: We thank physicians within the Otorhinolaryngology Department at University Hospital Essen for providing subject material and IMCES (University Hospital Essen) for the equipment and support in image analysis. We acknowledge support by the Open Access Publication Fund of the University of Duisburg-Essen.

Conflicts of Interest: The authors declare no conflict of interest.

References

1. Ferlay, J.; Soerjomataram, I.; Dikshit, R.; Eser, S.; Mathers, C.; Rebelo, M.; Parkin, D.M.; Forman, D.; Bray, F. Cancer incidence and mortality worldwide: Sources, methods and major patterns in GLOBOCAN 2012. *Int. J. Cancer* **2015**, *136*, E359–E386. [CrossRef]

2. Leemans, C.R.; Braakhuis, B.J.; Brakenhoff, R.H. The molecular biology of head and neck cancer. *Nat. Rev. Cancer* **2011**, *11*, 9–22. [CrossRef]

3. Borregaard, N. Neutrophils, from marrow to microbes. *Immunity* **2010**, *33*, 657–670. [CrossRef]

4. Brinkmann, V.; Reichard, U.; Goosmann, C.; Fauler, B.; Uhlemann, Y.; Weiss, D.S.; Weinrauch, Y.; Zychlinsky, A. Neutrophil extracellular traps kill bacteria. *Science* **2004**, *303*, 1532–1535. [CrossRef]

5. Demers, M.; Krause, D.S.; Schatzberg, D.; Martinod, K.; Voorhees, J.R.; Fuchs, T.A.; Scadden, D.T.; Wagner, D.D. Cancers predispose neutrophils to release extracellular DNA traps that contribute to cancer-associated thrombosis. *Proc. Natl. Acad. Sci. USA* **2012**, *109*, 13076–13081. [CrossRef]

6. Cools-Lartigue, J.; Spicer, J.; McDonald, B.; Gowing, S.; Chow, S.; Giannias, B.; Bourdeau, F.; Kubes, P.; Ferri, L. Neutrophil extracellular traps sequester circulating tumor cells and promote metastasis. *J. Clin. Investig.* **2013**. [CrossRef]

7. Park, J.; Wysocki, R.W.; Amoozgar, Z.; Maiorino, L.; Fein, M.R.; Jorns, J.; Schott, A.F.; Kinugasa-Katayama, Y.; Lee, Y.; Won, N.H.; et al. Cancer cells induce metastasis-supporting neutrophil extracellular DNA traps. *Sci. Transl. Med.* **2016**, *8*, 361ra138. [CrossRef]

8. Saffarzadeh, M.; Cabrera-Fuentes, H.A.; Veit, F.; Jiang, D.; Scharffetter-Kochanek, K.; Gille, C.; Rooijakkers, S.H.M.; Hartl, D.; Preissner, K.T. Characterization of rapid neutrophil extracellular trap formation and its cooperation with phagocytosis in human neutrophils. *Discoveries* **2014**, *2*, e19. [CrossRef]

9. Dumitru, C.A.; Moses, K.; Trellakis, S.; Lang, S.; Brandau, S. Neutrophils and granulocytic myeloid-derived suppressor cells: Immunophenotyping, cell biology and clinical relevance in human oncology. *Cancer Immunol. Immunother.* **2012**, *61*, 1155–1167. [CrossRef]

10. Lee, W.H.; Chen, H.M.; Yang, S.F.; Liang, C.; Peng, C.Y.; Lin, F.M.; Tsai, L.L.; Wu, B.C.; Hsin, C.H.; Chuang, C.Y.; et al. Bacterial alterations in salivary microbiota and their association in oral cancer. *Sci. Rep.* **2017**, *7*, 16540. [CrossRef]

11. Andzinski, L.; Spanier, J.; Kasnitz, N.; Kroger, A.; Jin, L.; Brinkmann, M.M.; Kalinke, U.; Weiss, S.; Jablonska, J.; Lienenklaus, S. Growing tumors induce a local STING dependent Type I IFN response in dendritic cells. *Int. J. Cancer* **2016**, *139*, 1350–1357. [CrossRef]

12. Pylaeva, E.; Harati, M.D.; Spyra, I.; Bordbari, S.; Strachan, S.; Thakur, B.K.; Hoing, B.; Franklin, C.; Skokowa, J.; Welte, K.; et al. NAMPT signaling is critical for the proangiogenic activity of tumor-associated neutrophils. *Int. J. Cancer* **2019**, *144*, 136–149. [CrossRef]

13. Jablonska, J.; Leschner, S.; Westphal, K.; Lienenklaus, S.; Weiss, S. Neutrophils responsive to endogenous IFN-beta regulate tumor angiogenesis and growth in a mouse tumor model. *J. Clin. Investig.* **2010**, *120*, 1151–1164. [CrossRef]

14. Fridlender, Z.G.; Sun, J.; Kim, S.; Kapoor, V.; Cheng, G.; Ling, L.; Worthen, G.S.; Albelda, S.M. Polarization of tumor-associated neutrophil phenotype by TGF-beta: "N1" versus "N2" TAN. *Cancer Cell* **2009**, *16*, 183–194. [CrossRef]

15. Gershkovitz, M.; Caspi, Y.; Fainsod-Levi, T.; Katz, B.; Michaeli, J.; Khawaled, S.; Lev, S.; Polyansky, L.; Shaul, M.E.; Sionov, R.V.; et al. TRPM2 Mediates Neutrophil Killing of Disseminated Tumor Cells. *Cancer Res.* **2018**, *78*, 2680–2690. [CrossRef]

16. Shaul, M.E.; Fridlender, Z.G. Tumour-associated neutrophils in patients with cancer. *Nat. Rev. Clin. Oncol.* **2019**. [CrossRef]

17. Singhal, S.; Bhojnagarwala, P.S.; O'Brien, S.; Moon, E.K.; Garfall, A.L.; Rao, A.S.; Quatromoni, J.G.; Stephen, T.L.; Litzky, L.; Deshpande, C.; et al. Origin and Role of a Subset of Tumor-Associated Neutrophils with Antigen-Presenting Cell Features in Early-Stage Human Lung Cancer. *Cancer Cell* **2016**, *30*, 120–135. [CrossRef]

18. Eruslanov, E.B.; Bhojnagarwala, P.S.; Quatromoni, J.G.; Stephen, T.L.; Ranganathan, A.; Deshpande, C.; Akimova, T.; Vachani, A.; Litzky, L.; Hancock, W.W.; et al. Tumor-associated neutrophils stimulate T cell responses in early-stage human lung cancer. *J. Clin. Investig.* **2014**, *124*, 5466–5480. [CrossRef]

19. Cools-Lartigue, J.; Spicer, J.; Najmeh, S.; Ferri, L. Neutrophil extracellular traps in cancer progression. *Cell. Mol. Life Sci.* **2014**, *71*, 4179–4194. [CrossRef]

20. Wu, C.F.; Andzinski, L.; Kasnitz, N.; Kroger, A.; Klawonn, F.; Lienenklaus, S.; Weiss, S.; Jablonska, J. The lack of type I interferon induces neutrophil-mediated pre-metastatic niche formation in the mouse lung. *Int. J. Cancer* **2015**, *137*, 837–847. [CrossRef]

21. Negorev, D.; Beier, U.H.; Zhang, T.; Quatromoni, J.G.; Bhojnagarwala, P.; Albelda, S.M.; Singhal, S.; Eruslanov, E.; Lohoff, F.W.; Levine, M.H.; et al. Human neutrophils can mimic myeloid-derived suppressor cells (PMN-MDSC) and suppress microbead or lectin-induced T cell proliferation through artefactual mechanisms. *Sci. Rep.* **2018**, *8*, 3135. [CrossRef]

22. Jablonska, J.; Lang, S.; Sionov, R.V.; Granot, Z. The regulation of pre-metastatic niche formation by neutrophils. *Oncotarget* **2017**, *8*, 112132–112144. [CrossRef]

23. Andzinski, L.; Kasnitz, N.; Stahnke, S.; Wu, C.F.; Gereke, M.; von Kockritz-Blickwede, M.; Schilling, B.; Brandau, S.; Weiss, S.; Jablonska, J. Type I IFNs induce anti-tumor polarization of tumor associated neutrophils in mice and human. *Int. J. Cancer* **2016**, *138*, 1982–1993. [CrossRef]

24. Garley, M.; Dziemianczyk-Pakiela, D.; Grubczak, K.; Surazynski, A.; Dabrowska, D.; Ratajczak-Wrona, W.; Sawicka-Powierza, J.; Borys, J.; Moniuszko, M.; Palka, J.A.; et al. Differences and similarities in the phenomenon of NETs formation in oral inflammation and in oral squamous cell carcinoma. *J. Cancer* **2018**, *9*, 1958–1965. [CrossRef]

25. Rochael, N.C.; Guimaraes-Costa, A.B.; Nascimento, M.T.; DeSouza-Vieira, T.S.; Oliveira, M.P.; Garcia e Souza, L.F.; Oliveira, M.F.; Saraiva, E.M. Classical ROS-dependent and early/rapid ROS-independent release of Neutrophil Extracellular Traps triggered by Leishmania parasites. *Sci. Rep.* **2015**, *5*, 18302. [CrossRef]

26. De Buhr, N.; von Kockritz-Blickwede, M. How Neutrophil Extracellular Traps Become Visible. *J. Immunol. Res.* **2016**, 4604713. [CrossRef]

27. Yipp, B.G.; Kubes, P. NETosis: How vital is it? *Blood* **2013**, *122*, 2784–2794. [CrossRef]

28. Byrd, A.S.; O'Brien, X.M.; Johnson, C.M.; Lavigne, L.M.; Reichner, J.S. An extracellular matrix-based mechanism of rapid neutrophil extracellular trap formation in response to Candida albicans. *J. Immunol.* **2013**, *190*, 4136–4148. [CrossRef]

29. Hazeldine, J.; Harris, P.; Chapple, I.L.; Grant, M.; Greenwood, H.; Livesey, A.; Sapey, E.; Lord, J.M. Impaired neutrophil extracellular trap formation: A novel defect in the innate immune system of aged individuals. *Aging Cell* **2014**, *13*, 690–698. [CrossRef]

30. Kowanetz, M.; Wu, X.; Lee, J.; Tan, M.; Hagenbeek, T.; Qu, X.; Yu, L.; Ross, J.; Korsisaari, N.; Cao, T.; et al. Granulocyte-colony stimulating factor promotes lung metastasis through mobilization of Ly6G+Ly6C+ granulocytes. *Proc. Natl. Acad. Sci. USA* **2010**, *107*, 21248–21255. [CrossRef]

31. Demers, M.; Wagner, D.D. Neutrophil extracellular traps: A new link to cancer-associated thrombosis and potential implications for tumor progression. *Oncoimmunology* **2013**, *2*, e22946. [CrossRef] [PubMed]

32. Kohler, A.; De Filippo, K.; Hasenberg, M.; van den Brandt, C.; Nye, E.; Hosking, M.P.; Lane, T.E.; Mann, L.; Ransohoff, R.M.; Hauser, A.E.; et al. G-CSF-mediated thrombopoietin release triggers neutrophil motility and mobilization from bone marrow via induction of Cxcr2 ligands. *Blood* **2011**, *117*, 4349–4357. [CrossRef] [PubMed]

33. Zharkova, O.; Tay, S.H.; Lee, H.Y.; Shubhita, T.; Ong, W.Y.; Lateef, A.; MacAry, P.A.; Lim, L.H.K.; Connolly, J.E.; Fairhurst, A.M. A Flow Cytometry-Based Assay for High-Throughput Detection and Quantification of Neutrophil Extracellular Traps in Mixed Cell Populations. *Cytom. Part A* **2019**, *95*, 268–278. [CrossRef] [PubMed]

34. Connolly, G.C.; Khorana, A.A.; Kuderer, N.M.; Culakova, E.; Francis, C.W.; Lyman, G.H. Leukocytosis, thrombosis and early mortality in cancer patients initiating chemotherapy. *Thromb. Res.* **2010**, *126*, 113–118. [CrossRef] [PubMed]

35. Staar, S.; Rudat, V.; Stuetzer, H.; Dietz, A.; Volling, P.; Schroeder, M.; Flentje, M.; Eckel, H.E.; Mueller, R.P. Intensified hyperfractionated accelerated radiotherapy limits the additional benefit of simultaneous chemotherapy–results of a multicentric randomized German trial in advanced head-and-neck cancer. *Int. J. Radiat. Oncol. Biol. Phys.* **2001**, *50*, 1161–1171. [CrossRef]

36. Gutschalk, C.M.; Herold-Mende, C.C.; Fusenig, N.E.; Mueller, M.M. Granulocyte colony-stimulating factor and granulocyte-macrophage colony-stimulating factor promote malignant growth of cells from head and neck squamous cell carcinomas in vivo. *Cancer Res.* **2006**, *66*, 8026–8036. [CrossRef] [PubMed]

37. Voloshin, T.; Gingis-Velitski, S.; Bril, R.; Benayoun, L.; Munster, M.; Milsom, C.; Man, S.; Kerbel, R.S.; Shaked, Y. G-CSF supplementation with chemotherapy can promote revascularization and subsequent tumor regrowth: Prevention by a CXCR4 antagonist. *Blood* **2011**, *118*, 3426–3435. [CrossRef] [PubMed]

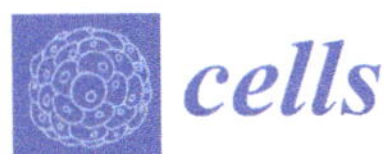 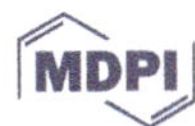

Review

Neutrophil Extracellular Traps (NETs) Take the Central Stage in Driving Autoimmune Responses

Esther Fousert, René Toes and Jyaysi Desai *

Department of Rheumatology, Leiden University Medical Center, 2333 ZA Leiden, The Netherlands; estherfousert@gmail.com (E.F.); R.E.M.Toes@lumc.nl (R.T.)
* Correspondence: j.b.desai@lumc.nl

Received: 16 March 2020; Accepted: 5 April 2020; Published: 8 April 2020

Abstract: Following fifteen years of research, neutrophil extracellular traps (NETs) are widely reported in a large range of inflammatory infectious and non-infectious diseases. Cumulating evidences from in vitro, in vivo and clinical diagnostics suggest that NETs may play a crucial role in inflammation and autoimmunity in a variety of autoimmune diseases, such as rheumatoid arthritis (RA), systemic lupus erythematosus (SLE) and anti-neutrophil cytoplasmic antibodies (ANCA)-associated vasculitis (AAV). Most likely, NETs contribute to breaking self-tolerance in autoimmune diseases in several ways. During this review, we discuss the current knowledge on how NETs could drive autoimmune responses. NETs can break self-tolerance by being a source of autoantigens for autoantibodies found in autoimmune diseases, such as anti-citrullinated protein antibodies (ACPAs) in RA, anti-dsDNA in SLE and anti-myeloperoxidase and anti-protein 3 in AAV. Moreover, NET components could accelerate the inflammatory response by mediating complement activation, acting as danger-associated molecular patterns (DAMPs) and inflammasome activators, for example. NETs also can activate other immune cells, such as B cells, antigen-presenting cells and T cells. Additionally, impaired clearance of NETs in autoimmune diseases prolongs the presence of active NETs and their components and, in this way, accelerate immune responses. NETs have not only been implicated as drivers of inflammation, but also are linked to resolution of inflammation. Therefore, NETs may be central regulators of inflammation and autoimmunity, serve as biomarkers, as well as promising targets for future therapeutics of inflammatory autoimmune diseases.

Keywords: neutrophil extracellular traps (NETs); autoimmunity; autoimmune diseases; inflammation; autoantigens

---

1. Introduction

Known as one of the first responder cells of the innate immune system, neutrophils are described as phagocytes in textbooks that are involved in initial early host-defence responses during infection/injury. However, the discovery of neutrophil extracellular traps (NETs) has shifted the paradigm of our current understanding of neutrophil functions, and their significance during immune responses, quite drastically. Upon interaction with an invading microbe/cytokine, neutrophils release their chromatin material together with a wide range of granular enzymes to form net-like structures known as NETs [1]. NETs cannot only trap the invading pathogen but also degrade them with NET-associated proteolytic enzymes [1]. NETs are involved in numerous infectious/non-infectious diseases and are believed to be crucially involved during inflammation. While NETs are beneficial during infections, they may play a detrimental role in the case of inflammation, autoimmunity and other pathophysiological conditions. NETs accelerate the inflammatory processes by releasing a wide range of active molecules like danger associated molecular patterns (DAMPs), histones, as well as active lytic-enzymes in extracellular space, leading to further immune responses. NETs, therefore, also may serve as a potential source of auto-antigens against which the autoantibodies associated with a wide range of inflammatory autoimmune diseases are directed.

The functions and morphology of neutrophils undergo radical transformation during inflammation, injury and infection. Neutrophils migrate along vesicles by expressing a wide range of migratory protein cascades as well as start to express various pattern recognition receptors and secrete a wide range of cytokines in a process called 'neutrophil activation'. Over the years, it has become clearer that only a fraction of neutrophils can make NETs, indicating the heterogeneity of the neutrophil population, especially during sterile inflammation [2,3] Therefore, it is important to speculate if only a specific subpopulation of neutrophils can undergo NET formation [2,4]. A distinct population of low-density neutrophils, for example, are known to be more vulnerable towards NET formation in systemic lupus erythematosus (SLE) patients [3,5], possibly explaining a link between this disease and NET formation. Interestingly, the composition of NETs may differ based on the stimuli and, therefore, the disease with which it is associated [6]. Furthermore, in certain situations, NETs also might have anti-inflammatory characteristics [7]. It is, therefore, important to characterize NETs in a disease-specific manner to understand their specific involvement during the development of autoimmunity and disease.

2. Composition of Neutrophil Extracellular Traps (NETs)

Neutrophil extracellular traps (NETs) formation can be triggered by a wide range of stimuli in vitro and in vivo during various pathophysiological conditions [6,8]. The protein cargo of NETs induced by different stimuli is heterogenous, making comparing research and drawing conclusions challenging. Due to this, there is an ongoing discussion about the precise mechanisms involved in NET formation, their composition and, thereby, their functional profile specifically their inflammatory/antimicrobial properties [6,9,10]. Recently, there have been new insights about how molecular mechanisms of NET formation may differ in a species specific manner [11,12] but, also based on the location of neutrophils in the blood stream or tissue, as well as local environmental alkaline or oxygen conditions [13]. Therefore, in the context of autoimmune diseases, detailed proteomic analysis of disease-specific NET protein composition (NETome) has the potential to elucidate novel mechanisms of disease onset and progression. The presence of DNase1 inhibitors in SLE)-associated NETs could potentially be demonstrated to lead to impairment of NET degradation [14]. Although disease-specific NETs may have different pathological roles, Chapman et al., recently compared the protein composition of SLE and rheumatoid arthritis (RA) NETs induced by the same stimulant, and showed that only a small number of NET proteins were significantly different between the two diseases [10]. Upon phorbol myristate acetate (PMA) stimulation, RNASE2 was higher in RA NETs, whereas myeloperoxidase (MPO), leukocyte elastase inhibitor and thymidine phosphorylase (TYMP) were higher in SLE NETs. Conversely, NETome comparison between NOX2-dependent (PMA) and NOX2-independent (A23187) showed more distinct protein profiles, irrespective of the disease background of the neutrophils [10]. PMA-induced NETs, for example, were decorated with the annexin proteins azurocidin and histone H3, whereas A23287-induced NETs contained more granule proteins, such as cathelicidin antimicrobial peptides CAMP/LL37 and matrix metalloproteinase-8 (MMP8) [10]. This finding indicates that the in vitro stimulant might be of more influence on the NETome compared to the phenotype of neutrophils. Another study, however, reported the presence of several proteins that varied between PMA–NETs of SLE, lupus nephritis (LN) and healthy neutrophils [15]. LN patient-derived PMA–NETs presented a high expression of α-enolase and annexin A1, compared to SLE PMA–NETs and healthy neutrophils. Accompanying these contradicting findings, however, it is important to take into account that most of these in vitro NETome studies are performed using non-physiological stimuli such as PMA or calcium ionophore A23187 [10,15]. Physiological stimulants might affect protein composition of NETs differently. More research and more critically designed experiments are needed in this direction to understand the role of NETs and the stimuli required to form them during autoimmune responses.

3. Contribution of Neutrophil Extracellular Traps (NETs) to Autoimmunity

Since neutrophils and NETs are present in abundance at the inflammatory sites of various autoimmune diseases, their active involvement in driving autoimmune responses is plausible. Recent evidences from various research groups indeed suggest that (the impaired clearance of) NETs themselves, as well as interactions of NETs with other immune cells could be very crucial for the development of 'autoimmunity' and breaking of self-tolerance (Figure 1). These various aspects associating NETs to autoimmunity are discussed in detail below.

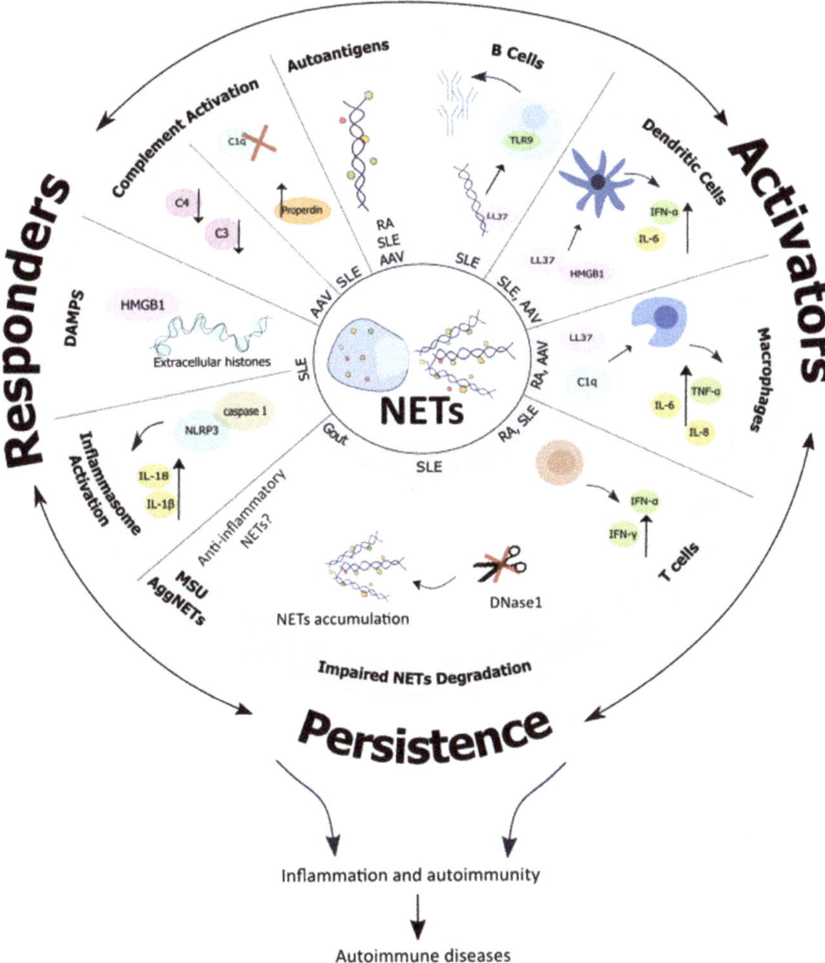

Figure 1. Neutrophil extracellular traps (NETs.) take the central stage in driving autoimmune responses. Abbreviations: AAV: Anti-neutrophil cytoplasmic antibodies associated vasculitis, ANCA: Anti-neutrophil cytoplasmic antibodies, C1q: complement factor 1q, C4: complement factor 3, C4: complement factor 4, DAMPs: damage associated molecular patterns, HMGB1: high mobility group box protein 1, IFN-α: interferon alpha, IFN-γ: interferon gamma, IL: interleukin, LL37: cathelicidin antimicrobial peptides, MSU: monosodium urate crystals, NETs: neutrophil extracellular traps, NLRP3: nucleotide-binding oligomerization domain-like receptor protein 3, RA: rheumatoid arthritis, SLE: systemic lupus erythematosus, TLR9: toll-like receptor 9, TNF-α: tumour necrosis factor alpha.

3.1. Neutrophil Extracellular Traps (NETs) as a Source of Autoantigens

Various neutrophil granular enzymes, together with decondensed chromatin, are present on NETs besides the anti-microbial proteins captured by them. Nonetheless, many of these NET-associated proteins are of "autoantigenic nature" in various rheumatologic diseases (Table 1). Examples include NET-associated MPO and proteinase 3 (PR3) enzymes as major autoantigenic targets of anti-neutrophil cytoplasmic antibody (ANCA)-associated vasculitis (AAV); NET-derived extracellular nucleic acids and dsDNA as the targets of SLE autoantibodies; citrullinated proteins namely citrullinated histones as neoepitopes for anti-citrullinated protein antibodies (ACPA) in RA [16–18]. These NET-associated autoantigens and their contribution are discussed in a disease-specific manner below. It is noteworthy, despite numerous evidences, that the exact mechanisms of how exactly NET autoantigens drive autoimmunity are still in a pre-mature state. There are several missing links and a lack of knowledge so further research is required to define common mechanisms of NET-derived autoimmune responses. Evidences from different in vitro and in vivo studies currently support a theory of what we propose to be a 'vicious loop of inflammation and autoimmunity'. It implies that inflammation-derived NET-components could be a source of autoantigens for autoantibody production. These autoantibodies and associated immune complexes in return may further induce NET formation, leading to a self-amplifying loop of autoimmune-inflammation [19].

Table 1. Neutrophil extracellular traps (NETs)-associated molecules that are known autoantigens in various autoimmune diseases.

Which Autoantigens Are Found on Neutrophil Extracellular Traps (NETs)?		To Which Autoimmune Diseases Are These Autoantigens Associated?	
α-enolase	[10,15]	SLE	[20]
Annexin A1	[10,15]	SLE	[21–23]
		RA	[22]
Apolipoprotein A1	[10]	SLE	[24]
Bb	[25]	AAV	[25]
C1q	[7,26]	SLE	[27]
Catalase	[10]	SLE	[28]
		RA	[28]
Cathelicidin	[10]	SLE	[21]
Citrullinated histones	[7,18,29–32]	RA	[18],
		SLE	[33]
dsDNA		SLE	[33,34]
Histones	[10]	SLE	[35]
HMGB1	[36,37]	SLE	[33,36,37]
LAMP-2	[38]	AAV	[39]
LL37	[5,7,10,40–42]	SLE	[41]
		Psoriasis	[43]
MMP8	[10]	RA	[44]
MMP9	[10,45]	SLE	[45]
MPO	[17,19,46–49]	AAV	[50,51]
PR3	[17,19,48]	AAV	[38]
Properdin	[25]	AAV	[25]
TF	[52,53]	SLE	[53]

Abbreviations: AAV: anti-neutrophil cytoplasmic antibodies (ANCA) vasculitis, Bb: complement factor b, C1q: complement component 1q, HMGB1: high mobility group protein B, LAMP-2: Lysosomal membrane 2 protein, MMP8: matrix metalloproteinases, MMP9: matrix metalloproteinase 9, MPO: myeloperoxidase, PR3: proteinase 3, RA: rheumatoid arthritis, SLE: systemic lupus erythematosus; TF: tissue factor.

3.2. NETs as Complement Activators

Complement activation and consumption is a hallmark of SLE [54]. Lower levels of complement factors C3 and C4, indicating classic complement consumption, was found in sera of a subset of SLE patients with impaired NETs clearance [26]. Seen in AAV, on the other hand, activation of the alternative complement pathway by NETs was demonstrated [25,55]. Tumour necrosis factor alpha (TNF-α)-primed neutrophils stimulated with ANCA lead to C3a, C5a and C5b-9 generation and could be due to granular protein properdin present on NETs [25]. Also, neutrophils stimulated with an anti-MPO antibody generated complement factors C5a and C3d, but not C1q [55]. This indicates that NETs are involved in different complement pathways in specific autoimmune diseases.

3.3. NETs as Damage-Associated Molecular Patterns (DAMPs)

NET-derived products could serve as damage-associated molecular patterns (DAMPs) to initiate further inflammatory response. Particularly, the presence of extracellular histones is perceived as a DAMP [56]. Other DAMPs secreted with NETs are the high-mobility group box 1 (HMGB1) and LL37. NET-derived HMGB1 is associated with SLE [36,37], but not with AAV [36]. Contrarily, HMGB1 contributed to ANCA-induced NET formation [57]. How NET-associated DAMPs may further contribute to tissue injury and inflammation needs to be investigated in detail for autoimmune-inflammatory diseases.

3.4. NETs as Inflammasome Activators

Inflammasomes are key players in the activation of inflammatory responses and NETs can mediate their activation. PMA–NETs activate caspase1 leading to nucleotide-binding oligomerization domain-like receptor protein 3 (NLRP3) inflammasome activation in macrophages of SLE patients [58]. Activation of inflammasome led to secretion of interleukin (IL)-18 and IL-1β. Besides being pro-inflammatory, these cytokines also can induce further NET formation. Adult-onset Still's disease neutrophils, stimulated with PMA, also were found to activate NLRP3 inflammasome through caspase1 [59]. NET formation itself was found to be dependent on noncanonical inflammasome activation, as extrusion of NETs by neutrophils exposed to lipopolysaccharide (LPS) or Gram-negative bacteria relied on activated caspase11 and activated gasdermin D (GSDMD) [60,61]. Together, this implies that NET formation may be both dependent on inflammasome activation and also be able to activate inflammasome.

4. Impaired Clearance of Neutrophil Extracellular Traps (NETs)

NETs contain various active enzymes and DAMPs such as extracellular histones [10]. It is, therefore, important to degrade the NETs by phagocytic cells like macrophages [62]. DNase1 plays an important role to degrade NETs in physiology [14]. After NETs are pre-processed by DNase1, macrophages can ingest NETs for degradation [62]. PMA–NET degradation by macrophages takes place in lysosomes [63]. However, PMA–NET degradation in macrophages also occurs in the cytosol by three prime repair exonuclease (TREX1) enzymes (or DNaseIII), as well as extracellularly by DNase1L3 secreted by dendritic cells (DCs) [62]. PMA–NET clearance by healthy donor macrophages has been described as immunologically silent and without secretion of proinflammatory cytokines [63].

Interestingly, degradation of NETs is found to be impaired in several autoimmune diseases, such as SLE [14,26,64] and AAV [65]. Hakkim et al., reported that reduced DNase1 activity in a subset of SLE patients dysregulated clearance of NETs [14]. Furthermore, SLE-associated NETs activate complement, leading to deposition of C1q on NETs which further inhibits DNase1 activity [26]. A mutation in the DNase1L3 gene also is associated with a familiar form of SLE [66]. Additionally, PMA–NET uptake by monocyte-derived macrophages [67] and LPS–NETs cleared by SLE macrophages [68] led to a pro-inflammatory response, suggesting that clearance of activated NETs in autoimmune diseases also may amplify the inflammatory response. Compromised NET clearance generates the accumulation of active-NETs at inflammatory sites; leading to more inflammation and prolonged presence of

NET autoantigens [69]. This could possibly break self-tolerance and, thereby, intensify the existing autoimmune response.

5. Interplay of Neutrophil Extracellular Traps (NETs) and Other Adaptive Immune Cells

5.1. NET and B Cells

NET formation by splenic neutrophils, but not circulating neutrophils, has been found to induce immunoglobulin class switching, hypermutation and secretion by activating c [70]. Also, type I interferons (IFN) α and B cell factors produced by bone marrow neutrophils have been shown to inhibit early B cell development and expansion in SLE, leading to possibly enhanced recruitment of autoreactive clones into the mature B cell repertoire [71]. Conversely, circulating neutrophils activated with ANCA caused the release of a B lymphocyte stimulator and promoted B cell survival [72]. Recently, it also was shown that LL37-DNA complexes in NETs can directly trigger self-reactive memory B cells to produce anti-LL37 antibodies in SLE [41]. Self-reactive B cells generally do not react to DNA, however, if the DNA originates from NETs in the form of LL37-DNA complex, it can trigger B cell activation in a toll-like receptor 9 (TLR9)-dependent manner [41]. Notably, SLE-immune complexes were found to induce NET formation recently [36]. Thus, it is conceivable that B cell-derived immune complexes may activate neutrophils by binding to the Fc gamma receptor IIIb (FcγRIIIb) and induce further NET formation [73], causing a feedback loop of autoimmune responses and disease progression.

5.2. NETs and Antigen Presenting Cells

IFNs play a key role in the pathogenesis of autoimmune diseases and are described as a hallmark for SLE [74]. Plasmacytoid dendritic cells (pDC), the main producers of IFN, can be activated by NETs [40]. Specifically, proteins LL37 and HMGB1 form complexes with NETs DNA, which further facilitates uptake and recognition of DNA by pDCs and increases production of IFN-α [42]. In g a RA mouse model, it was shown that T cell response in the presence of NETs is mediated through DC activation [75]. Spontaneous mouse and human NETs could directly activate DCs to induce costimulatory molecules CD80 and CD86, and proinflammatory cytokine IL-6. Furthermore, mouse NETs-treated DCs promoted CD4+ Th cell immune response to secrete INF-γ and IL-17. PMA–NETs activated DCs, on the other hand, were unable to activate CD4+ T cells [76].

NETs also can activate another type of antigen presenting cell (APC): macrophages [77]. However, prolonged exposure to NETs led to damage of the mitochondrial membrane of the macrophage, indicating macrophage death [77] Remarkably, the presence of LL37 and C1q on NETs increased activation of macrophages by RA NETs, leading to secretion of pro-inflammatory IL-8, IL-6 and TNF-α [7]. Activation of inflammatory macrophages also was seen in adult-onset Still's disease [59]. Contrary, strongly activated macrophages exposed to NETs mediated an anti-inflammatory response with increased IL-10 secretion and inhibited IL-6 secretion [7].

5.3. NETs and T Cells

Recently, an indirect interaction between NETs and T cells was found in the joint of an RA patient [78]. Specifically, NETs were shown to be taken up by fibroblasts, which then presented NET-associated citrullinated peptides to T cells. Also, a direct interaction between PMA–NETs and T cells was proposed [76]. NETs directly prime CD4$^+$ T cells and lower the activation threshold. Therefore, T cell response to specific antigens and suboptimal stimuli is increased, which would otherwise not lead to activation of resting T cells. Interestingly, this T cell priming by NETs seems to involve T cell receptor (TCR) mediation, but is not TLR9-dependent [76]. Direct interaction also was found between SLE low-density granulocytes (LDGs) and T cells [79]. Activation of T cells by SLE LDGs induced the release of proinflammatory cytokines INF-γ and TNF-α. This induction of proinflammatory cytokines was not detected by normal density granulocytes [79]. The study investigated in vitro activation of T cells by LDGs, not NETs. Considering that LDGs in SLE are known to form NETs [5], possibly NETs could play a role in the T cell activation.

6. Neutrophil Extracellular Traps (NETs) in Various Autoimmune Diseases

6.1. Rheumatoid Arthritis (RA)

RA is a chronic systemic disease characterized by joint inflammation and bone destruction. Being an autoimmune disease, a distinct feature of RA is the presence of specific autoantibodies against post-translationally modified proteins known as anti-modified protein antibodies (AMPA) in serum and synovial fluid samples of RA patients [80] Examples of AMPA include antibodies against post-translationally modified proteins like citrullinated proteins (ACPA), antibodies against protein carbamylation (anti-CarP), and antibodies against acetylated proteins (AAPA) [81–83] The presence of autoantibodies has been associated with disease progression and pathogenesis. ACPA can bind to citrullinate proteins to form immune complexes, inducing a pro-inflammatory response which further includes complement activation [84,85], for example. Interestingly, AMPA (for example ACPA) can be present in circulation for several years before RA onset [86]. These clinical observations indicate that systemic autoimmunity and development of autoimmune disease are not coupled, and factors driving the transition from pre-existing autoimmunity to RA pathogenesis need to be determined.

NET formation is strongly associated with inflammatory RA [18]. NETs extrude novel autoantigens, such as citrullinated histones, which can promote the autoimmune response in RA [18,32]. Certainly ACPAs are reported to recognize autoantigens on NETs [7,30]; in particular citrullinated histones [31]. The NET-protein MPO was found elevated in RA synovial fluid (SF), skin and rheumatoid nodules, indicating that NETs are present in these inflamed areas (joint/synovium). Neutrophils of RA patients show increased spontaneous NET propensity, compared to healthy control neutrophils in vitro [18,87]. NET propensity increases when neutrophils are stimulated with RA SF and ACPA RA serum [18,87]. Several research groups also have reported the potential of ACPA to drive NET formation in vitro, demonstrating the inflammatory potential of ACPA [18,87]. Elevated MPO–DNA complexes [88] and cell-free nucleosome levels [89] are detected in RA serum. These serum levels of cell-free nucleosome in RA patients also correlate with clinical parameters, such as C-reactive protein (CRP) and positivity for rheumatoid factor (RF) and ACPA [89]. The MPO–DNA complex level also correlated with the ACPA level in RA patient sera samples [88]. Thus, NETs and NET-derived products could serve as a biomarker for RA disease activity. Besides potential biomarkers, NET and NET-derived products also may be promising therapeutic targets for inflammatory RA (Table 2).

6.2. Anti-Neutrophil Cytoplasmic Antibodies (ANCA) Vasculitis (AAV)

AAV is a systemic autoimmune disorder, characterized by inflammation and destruction of small vessels in various organs. Presence of autoantibodies against MPO and PR3 are the key hallmarks that are believed to trigger the disease response.

PR3 is expressed on the membrane of resting neutrophils while MPO is stored within the granules of the neutrophils [122]. Their expression increases when neutrophils are activated by cytokines [123]. NETs also are decorated with MPO and PR3, as shown by several immunofluorescence studies on in vitro NETs and in vivo NETs in necrotizing lesions of AAV [17]. Colocalization of DNA, MPO and PR3 in kidney tissue of small-vessel vasculitis (SVV) glomerulonephritis patients, for example, indicates the presence of NETs and ANCA antigens in inflamed tissue [17]. MPO release in the presence of NETs also was found in kidney biopsies of MPO–ANCA-associated glomerulonephritis patients [49,50]. NETs not only were found in the kidneys of AAV patients, but in other types of vasculitis as well. Nerve samples of ANCA-associated vasculitic neuropathy, for instance, had citrullinated histones and MPO identified as NETs [47]. One recent study suggests that NET-protein neutrophil elastase can digest ANCA in a time-dependent manner, leading to pauci-immune lesions [124].

Table 2. Potential drug interventions targeting neutrophil extracellular traps (NETs) in autoimmune diseases (in vitro and in vivo evidences).

Potential Drug Interventions	Mechanism	Study Design	Effect on Neutrophil Extracellular Traps (NET)	Autoimmune Disease	Effect on Disease Clinical Endpoint	References
			PAD4			
Cl-amidine	PAD4 enzymes inhibitor	In vitro PMA-induced NETs	Blocked NET formation	AAV	Not tested	[90]
		Mouse model with MPO–ANCA production	Reduced citrullination and reduced serum MPO–ANCA level	AAV	Not tested	[90]
		SLE mouse model	Decreased histone citrullination and reduced release of NETs	SLE	Not tested	[91,92]
		pGIA mouse model	Reduced citrullinated proteins	RA	Reduced arthritis severity, but not significantly	[93]
GSK199	Low-calcium PAD4 enzymes inhibitor	In vitro ionomycin-induced mouse neutrophils	Inhibition mouse NETs	-	-	[94]
		In vitro *S. aureus*-induced human neutrophils	Partial NET formation remained	-	-	[94]
		Collagen-induced arthritis mouse model	Unknown	RA	Prevented clinical and histological disease severity	[95,96]
			DNase			
DNase	DNA degradation	SLE mouse model	Unknown	SLE	Prolongation of survival	[97]
		Phase Ib study	Unknown	SLE	Unaffected disease activity	[14,98]
		APS IgG treated mice	Decreased NET formation	APS	Decrease in thrombus formation	[99]
		Anti-β2-GP1/β2-GP1 treated rats	Decreased NET formation	APS	Decrease in thrombus formation	[100]
			ROS			
PRAK inhibitor	Inhibition of ROS-regulating PRAK	In vitro PMA-induced NETs	Increased neutrophil apoptosis over NET formation	-	-	[101]
Trolox	Antioxidant	In vitro PMA-induced NETs	Inhibited ROS-dependent NET formation	-	-	[102]
Tiron	Antioxidant	In vitro PMA-induced NETs	Remained NET formation	-	-	[102]
Tempol	Antioxidant	In vitro PMA-induced NETs	Inhibited ROS-dependent NET formation	-	-	[102]
Vitamin C	Unknown	In vitro PMA-induced NETs	Decreased NET formation	-	-	[103]
			IFN-alpha			
Sifalimumab	Blocks IFN-α NETs stimulation	Phase I study	Unknown	SLE	Inhibited type I IFN signature and trend in improved SLEDAI	[104,105]
		Phase IIb study	Unknown	SLE	Improved SLE responder rate	[106]
Rontalizumab	Blocks IFN-α NETs stimulation	Phase I study	Unknown	SLE	No effect on IFN and anti-dsDNA levels	[107]
Anifrolumab	Blocks IFN-α NETs stimulation	Phase IIb study	Reduced plasma NETs complexes	SLE	Improved cholesterol efflux capacity	White et al., 2018 (unpublished, conference abstract)
		Phase IIb study	Unknown	SLE	Reduced SLE disease activity	[108]
			Complement			
PA-dPEG24	C1 inhibitor	In vitro PMA, MPO or immune complex activated human sera	Inhibited complement activation and inhibited NET formation	-	-	[109]
Eculizumab	Antibody against c5a	PNH patients	Decreased neutrophil activation	-	Unknown	[110]
			Proteases			
IcatC	CatC inhibition blocks PR3 activity and NET formation	Neutrophil differentiated CD34+ HSC	IcatC leads to absence of PR3 and suppression of PR3-ANCA antigen	-	-	[111,112]
Chloroquine	Inhibits autophagy	AP patients NETs	Decreased NET formation	-	-	[113]
		AP mouse model	Decreased NET formation and improved survival	-	-	[113]

Table 2. Potential drug interventions targeting neutrophil extracellular traps (NETs) in autoimmune diseases (in vitro and in vivo evidences).

Potential Drug Interventions	Mechanism	Study Design	Effect on Neutrophil Extracellular Traps (NET)	Autoimmune Disease	Effect on Disease Clinical Endpoint	References
Vitamin D						
Vitamin D	Unknown	In vitro PMA-induced NETs and endothelial cells	Reduced NET formation	SLE	Reduced endothelial apoptosis	[114]
Vitamin D	Unknown	SLE patients with low vitamin D	Unknown	SLE	Improved endothelial function	[115]
Nanoparticles						
A2,8-sialylated nanoparticles	Reduce PMA-initiated ROS production	In vitro PMA-induced NETs	Inhibited NET release	-	-	[116]
Polysialylated vesicles	Counteract cytotoxic characteristic of extracellular histones, possibly through lactoferrin	5B8 cells in presence of histones	Reduced cytotoxicity reduced in 5B8 cells. Vesicles bind to PMA–NETs	-	-	[117,118]
Existing autoimmune disease therapies and their effects on NETs						
-Tocilizumab	Antibody against IL-6 receptor	In vitro IL-6 and PMA-induced NETs	Blocked NET formation	RA	Unknown	[119]
Rituximab and belimumab	Blocking IC formation	Phase IIa study	Reduced NET formation	RA	Decreased lupus disease activity	[120]
IVIG-S	Mechanisms unknown	MPO-AAV rat model	Reduced NET formation and ANCA titers	AAV	Unknown	[121]

Abbreviations: AAV: Anti-neutrophil cytoplasmic antibodies associated vasculitis, ANCA: Anti-neutrophil cytoplasmic antibodies, AP: acute pancreatitis, APS: antiphospholipid syndrome, CatC: cathepsin C, CI-amidine: chloramidine, dsDNA: double strand DNA, EA: elastase-alpha1-antitrypsin, GSK199: hydrochloride, HSC: hematopoietic stem cells, IC: immune complex, IcatC: inhibitor cathepsin C, IFN: interferon, IVIG-S: sulfo-immunoglobulins, MPO: myeloperoxidase, NAC: n-acetylcysteine, NETs: neutrophil extracellular traps, PAD4: peptidylarginine deiminase 4, pGIA: glucose 6-phosphate isomerase induced arthritis, PMA: phorbol myristate acetate, PNH: paroxysmal nocturnal haemoglobinuria, PR3: proteinase 3, PRAK: p38-regulated/activated protein kinase, RA: rheumatoid arthritis, SLE: systemic lupus erythematosus, SLEDAI: systemic lupus erythematosus disease activity index, β2-GP1: β2-glycoprotein.

The presence of NETs in AAV patients is evident, however their potential as biomarkers for AAV disease activity is inconclusive. Regarding the serum of active AAV patients, higher MPO–DNA levels were detected compared to AAV patients in remission [125]. Another study, however, did not find a difference between the serum MPO–DNA levels in active and remissive AAV [126].

While it is becoming clear that NETs may be a crucial source of ANCA-autoantigens, some studies suggest that binding of ANCA to their target antigens, PR3 and MPO, further activate the neutrophils. NETs are released in response to ANCA stimulation [17]. A recent study, however, contrasts these findings. NET formation in vitro, through stimulation of healthy neutrophils with AAV serum, did not correlate with serum levels of ANCA [127]. Also, after depletion of immunoglobulin (Ig)-G and IgA in serum, NET formation remained unchanged, raising the question whether ANCA actually influences NET formation [127]. Added to being antigenic in nature, NETs also influence AAV disease progression by directly damaging vessels through cytotoxicity of NET-associated histone release [56]. NET-induced endothelial cell damage can be prevented when NETs are degraded with DNase1 [55]. Intravenous immunoglobulin (IVIG) is a potential treatment for AAV patients [121]. Intriguingly, the amount of PMA-induced NETs was significantly lower when neutrophils were pre-treated with IVIG before exposure to PMA [121]. Moreover, the inhibitory effect of IVIG on NETs, as well as decreased ANCA titers and pulmonary haemorrhage, also was seen in peritoneal tissue of MPO–AAV rats treated with IVIG [121]. To conclude, the presence of NETs and their autoantigenic properties in AAV patients is well-demonstrated. Therefore, NETs could represent informative biomarkers for disease diagnosis and targets for future therapeutics (Table 2). Conversely, the role of ANCA-mediated NET induction is not yet fully convincing. Further research is needed in understanding the interplay of ANCA and NETs in the pathophysiology of AAV.

6.3. Systemic Lupus Erythematosus (SLE)

Systemic lupus erythematosus (SLE) is a chronic autoimmune disease attacking healthy tissue across the body. SLE can manifest in milder forms, in skin and joints, while more serious manifestations impair functions of the kidneys and central nervous system. Regarding the kidneys, autoantigens and autoantibodies can deposit as immune complexes causing severe lupus nephritis. SLE progression is a result of autoantibodies against nucleic acids and dsDNA. These autoantigens can be sourced from apoptotic and necrotic material [128]. Clearance of this material is thought to be defective in SLE [129].

NETs are known to be a central source of SLE autoantigens [5,130–133]. The persistence of NETs also could extend the exposure time of autoantigens, due to impaired NET clearance and thereby contribute to SLE pathogenesis [14,133,134]. Removal of NETs by DNase1 was shown to be malfunctioning in in vitro NETs stimulated with SLE serum [14]. This finding indicates that DNase-1 inhibitors may either be present in NETs or (auto) antibodies bound to NETs could inhibit NET-degradation by protecting against proteases. Studies in SLE patients on the relation between NET degradation and disease manifestation support this hypothesis. SLE patients with impaired NET degradation were found more likely to develop lupus nephritis, compared to SLE patients with functioning NET degradation [14,135]. Impaired NET degradation also correlated with high levels of SLE-associated autoantibodies [135]. Other effects of nondegraded NETs are activation of the complement system, thereby driving inflammation forward [26], as well as priming other neutrophils into NET formation [130]. Notably, SLE patients possess a distinct set of neutrophils, called low-density granulocytes (LDGs) [3,136,137]. These specific neutrophils have an increased spontaneous NET propensity, compared to other neutrophils of SLE patients [5,29,134]. Endothelial damage is a common symptom of SLE and may be due to the actions of NETs [5], particularly those formed by LDGs [45]. A recent study characterized two subsets of SLE LDGs, CD10$^+$ LDGs and CD10$^-$ LDGs [138]. The phenotype of CD10$^-$ LDGs display a more immature stage of neutrophil differentiation and is less prone to spontaneous NET formation, as compared to CD10$^+$ LDGs [139]. Together, this points to the importance of NETs in SLE pathogenesis and how impaired clearance of NETs may prolong the (auto)inflammatory effects of NETs.

6.4. Antiphospholipid Syndrome (APS)

Antiphospholipid syndrome (APS) is an autoimmune disease that often occurs together with SLE, but also presents itself as a primary disease. Autoantibodies targeting phospholipids and phospholipid binding proteins, such as β2-glycoprotein 1 (β2-GP1) are the hallmarks of APS [140]. Particularly, APS patients showcase an increased risk of thrombosis. Thrombi consist of platelets and neutrophils, but also NETs, suggesting the possible role of NETs in APS development [141]. Furthermore, neutrophils from APS patients were shown to display enhanced spontaneous NET release [134,142]. NET response might be mediated through activation of TLR4 [100,142], together with reactive oxygen species (ROS) [100,142,143]. Remarkably, IgG purified from APS patients induced NET release from healthy neutrophils [142]. Furthermore, NET release did not correlate with APS disease activity, but rather with the presence of autoantibodies [134]. An increase in NET release in response to autoantibodies could be explained by the presence of β2-GP1 on the surface of neutrophils [142]. Several studies observed anti-β2-GP1 to induce NET formation in healthy neutrophils [100,142,143]. Evidences suggest that NETs may directly mediate APS pathology by featuring as a scaffold for platelets to aggregate [144], possibly by presenting a tissue factor [53,100]. Moreover, activated platelets can stimulate neutrophils to NET formation by releasing HMGB1 [141]. Accordingly, this highlights a central role for NETs in thrombosis and, thereby, APS development.

6.5. Multiple Sclerosis (MS)

Multiple sclerosis (MS) is a disease of the central nervous system with a strong autoimmune character. Few studies have been performed on the role of NETs in MS pathogenesis [145]. However, in a MS rodent model it became apparent that NETs could be of importance in MS, as depletion of MPO, attenuated rodent MS phenotypes and restored the blood–brain barrier integrity [146]. Elevated MPO–DNA complexes also were detected in the MS serum of patients, but these levels did not correlate with disease activity [147]. Within MS patients, differences in MPO–DNA complex levels correlated with the patient's gender, suggesting that NETs may underlie gender-specific differences in MS pathogenesis. Moreover, LDGs, $CD14^-CD15^{high}$, were found in peripheral blood of MS patients, at levels comparable to SLE patients [148]. Whether the propensity of MS LDGs to form NETs differentiates from normal density neutrophils has not been investigated yet.

6.6. Anti-Inflammatory NETs

While NETs clearly enhance the inflammatory response in various ways, recent evidence suggests that they also may have anti-inflammatory properties or induce an anti-inflammatory response. Found in the presence of PMA–NETs, LPS-activated macrophages act in an anti-inflammatory manner [7]. A downregulation of IL-6 and an increase in IL-10 secretion by these macrophages shows the anti-inflammatory potential of NETs. This effect was enhanced in presence of C1q and LL37 [7]. Viable and apoptotic neutrophils also mediate an anti-inflammatory response in macrophages through NF-kB signalling suppression [149], suggesting that an anti-inflammatory response may be mediated by the type of neutrophil cell death. Certain proteases in NETs also could contribute to the anti-inflammatory potential of NETs. Regarding gout, where NETs are aggregated in the synovial joint, monosodium urate crystals (MSU)-induced aggregated NETs were found to degrade inflammatory mediators, such as IL-1β, IL-6 and TNF [150]. NET-proteases also could act on NET-proteins that are autoantigens [151]. Shown in the presence of the neutrophil protease inhibitor phenylmethylsulfonyl fluoride (PMSF), autoantigens in PMA–NETs remain present. While without PMSF, PMA–NET proteases degrade NET autoantigens. More research is needed toward understanding the anti-inflammatory role of NETs and their association with autoimmunity.

7. Conclusions and Future Directions

Neutrophils and NETs are present in abundance at the inflammatory sites of various autoimmune diseases and play an active role during the development and persistence of autoimmune responses. As a potential source of autoantigens and activators of immune-cells, NETs could be crucial attributors to the development of 'autoimmunity' and the breaking of self-tolerance. Further research is required to understand the physiology and responses of NETs in a disease-specific manner. Therefore, the use of physiological disease-specific stimulants to induce NETs in vitro, an improved understanding of the disease-specific NETome, as well as their impact on other immune cells and inflammation will be crucial for future research. These efforts would provide a substantial basis to target NETs as promising biomarkers or therapeutics to treat inflammatory autoimmune diseases.

Author Contributions: R.T. and J.D. designed the concept of the review. E.F. and J.D. wrote and significantly revised the manuscript. All authors have read and agreed to the published version of the manuscript.

Funding: This research was funded by European Union's Horizon 2020 research and innovation programme under the Marie Sklodowska Curie grant agreement No 707404.

Conflicts of Interest: The authors declare no conflict of interest.

References

1. Brinkmann, V.; Reichard, U.; Goosmann, C.; Fauler, B.; Uhlemann, Y.; Weiss, D.S.; Weinrauch, Y.; Zychlinsky, A. Neutrophil extracellular traps kill bacteria. *Science* **2004**, *303*, 1532–1535. [CrossRef]
2. Ng, L.G.; Ostuni, R.; Hidalgo, A. Heterogeneity of neutrophils. *Nat. Rev. Immunol.* **2019**, *19*, 255–265. [CrossRef]
3. Denny, M.F.; Yalavarthi, S.; Zhao, W.; Thacker, S.G.; Anderson, M.; Sandy, A.R.; McCune, W.J.; Kaplan, M.J. A distinct subset of proinflammatory neutrophils isolated from patients with systemic lupus erythematosus induces vascular damage and synthesizes type I IFNs. *J. Immunol.* **2010**, *184*, 3284–3297. [CrossRef] [PubMed]

4. Christoffersson, G.; Phillipson, M. The neutrophil: One cell on many missions or many cells with different agendas? *Cell Tissue Res.* **2018**, *371*, 415–423. [CrossRef] [PubMed]

5. Villanueva, E.; Yalavarthi, S.; Berthier, C.C.; Hodgin, J.B.; Khandpur, R.; Lin, A.M.; Rubin, C.J.; Zhao, W.; Olsen, S.H.; Klinker, M.; et al. Netting Neutrophils Induce Endothelial Damage, Infiltrate Tissues, and Expose Immunostimulatory Molecules in Systemic Lupus Erythematosus. *J. Immunol.* **2011**, *187*, 538–552. [CrossRef] [PubMed]

6. Petretto, A.; Bruschi, M.; Pratesi, F.; Croia, C.; Candiano, G.; Ghiggeri, G.; Migliorini, P. Neutrophil extracellular traps (NET) induced by different stimuli: A comparative proteomic analysis. *PLoS ONE* **2019**, *14*, e0218946. [CrossRef] [PubMed]

7. Ribon, M.; Seninet, S.; Mussard, J.; Sebbag, M.; Clavel, C.; Serre, G.; Boissier, M.-C.; Semerano, L.; Decker, P. Neutrophil extracellular traps exert both pro- and anti-inflammatory actions in rheumatoid arthritis that are modulated by C1q and LL-37. *J. Autoimmun.* **2019**, *98*, 122–131. [CrossRef]

8. Papayannopoulos, V. Neutrophil extracellular traps in immunity and disease. *Nat. Rev. Immunol.* **2018**, *18*, 134–147. [CrossRef]

9. Boeltz, S.; Amini, P.; Anders, H.-J.; Andrade, F.; Bilyy, R.; Chatfield, S.; Cichon, I.; Clancy, D.M.; Desai, J.; Dumych, T.; et al. To NET or not to NET:current opinions and state of the science regarding the formation of neutrophil extracellular traps. *Cell Death Differ.* **2019**, *26*, 395–408. [CrossRef]

10. Chapman, E.A.; Lyon, M.; Simpson, D.; Mason, D.; Beynon, R.J.; Moots, R.J.; Wright, H.L. Caught in a Trap? Proteomic Analysis of Neutrophil Extracellular Traps in Rheumatoid Arthritis and Systemic Lupus Erythematosus. *Front. Immunol.* **2019**, *10*, 423. [CrossRef]

11. Amulic, B.; Cazalet, C.; Hayes, G.L.; Metzler, K.D.; Zychlinsky, A. Neutrophil function: From mechanisms to disease. *Annu. Rev. Immunol.* **2012**, *30*, 459–489. [CrossRef] [PubMed]

12. Martinod, K.; Witsch, T.; Farley, K.; Gallant, M.; Remold-O'Donnell, E.; Wagner, D.D. Neutrophil elastase-deficient mice form neutrophil extracellular traps in an experimental model of deep vein thrombosis. *J. Thromb. Haemost. JTH* **2016**, *14*, 551–558. [CrossRef] [PubMed]

13. Naffah de Souza, C.; Breda, L.C.D.; Khan, M.A.; de Almeida, S.R.; Câmara, N.O.S.; Sweezey, N.; Palaniyar, N. Alkaline pH Promotes NADPH Oxidase-Independent Neutrophil Extracellular Trap Formation: A Matter of Mitochondrial Reactive Oxygen Species Generation and Citrullination and Cleavage of Histone. *Front. Immunol.* **2018**, *8*, 1849. [CrossRef] [PubMed]

14. Hakkim, A.; Fürnrohr, B.G.; Amann, K.; Laube, B.; Abed, U.A.; Brinkmann, V.; Herrmann, M.; Voll, R.E.; Zychlinsky, A. Impairment of neutrophil extracellular trap degradation is associated with lupus nephritis. *Proc. Natl. Acad. Sci. USA* **2010**, *107*, 9813–9818. [CrossRef] [PubMed]

15. Bruschi, M.; Petretto, A.; Santucci, L.; Vaglio, A.; Pratesi, F.; Migliorini, P.; Bertelli, R.; Lavarello, C.; Bartolucci, M.; Candiano, G.; et al. Neutrophil Extracellular Traps protein composition is specific for patients with Lupus nephritis and includes methyl-oxidized αenolase (methionine sulfoxide 93). *Sci. Rep.* **2019**, *9*, 1–13. [CrossRef]

16. Jorch, S.K.; Kubes, P. An emerging role for neutrophil extracellular traps in noninfectious disease. *Nat. Med.* **2017**, *23*, 279–287. [CrossRef]

17. Kessenbrock, K.; Krumbholz, M.; Schönermarck, U.; Back, W.; Gross, W.L.; Werb, Z.; Gröne, H.-J.; Brinkmann, V.; Jenne, D.E. Netting neutrophils in autoimmune small-vessel vasculitis. *Nat. Med.* **2009**, *15*, 623–625. [CrossRef]

18. Khandpur, R.; Carmona-Rivera, C.; Vivekanandan-Giri, A.; Gizinski, A.; Yalavarthi, S.; Knight, J.S.; Friday, S.; Li, S.; Patel, R.M.; Subramanian, V.; et al. NETs are a source of citrullinated autoantigens and stimulate inflammatory responses in rheumatoid arthritis. *Sci. Transl. Med.* **2013**, *5*, 178ra40. [CrossRef]

19. Grayson, P.C.; Kaplan, M.J. At the Bench: Neutrophil extracellular traps (NETs) highlight novel aspects of innate immune system involvement in autoimmune diseases. *J. Leukoc. Biol.* **2016**, *99*, 253–264. [CrossRef]

20. Bonanni, A.; Vaglio, A.; Bruschi, M.; Sinico, R.A.; Cavagna, L.; Moroni, G.; Franceschini, F.; Allegri, L.; Pratesi, F.; Migliorini, P.; et al. Multi-antibody composition in lupus nephritis: Isotype and antigen specificity make the difference. *Autoimmun. Rev.* **2015**, *14*, 692–702. [CrossRef]

21. Bruschi, M.; Sinico, R.A.; Moroni, G.; Pratesi, F.; Migliorini, P.; Galetti, M.; Murtas, C.; Tincani, A.; Madaio, M.; Radice, A.; et al. Glomerular autoimmune multicomponents of human lupus nephritis in vivo: α-enolase and annexin AI. *J. Am. Soc. Nephrol. JASN* **2014**, *25*, 2483–2498. [CrossRef] [PubMed]

22. Iaccarino, L.; Ghirardello, A.; Canova, M.; Zen, M.; Bettio, S.; Nalotto, L.; Punzi, L.; Doria, A. Anti-annexins autoantibodies: Their role as biomarkers of autoimmune diseases. *Autoimmun. Rev.* **2011**, *10*, 553–558. [CrossRef] [PubMed]

23. Kretz, C.C.; Norpo, M.; Abeler-Dörner, L.; Linke, B.; Haust, M.; Edler, L.; Krammer, P.H.; Kuhn, A. Anti-annexin 1 antibodies: A new diagnostic marker in the serum of patients with discoid lupus erythematosus. *Exp. Dermatol.* **2010**, *19*, 919–921. [CrossRef]

24. van Beers, J.J.B.C.; Schwarte, C.M.; Stammen-Vogelzangs, J.; Oosterink, E.; Božič, B.; Pruijn, G.J.M. The rheumatoid arthritis synovial fluid citrullinome reveals novel citrullinated epitopes in apolipoprotein E, myeloid nuclear differentiation antigen, and β-actin. *Arthritis Rheum.* **2013**, *65*, 69–80. [CrossRef] [PubMed]

25. Wang, H.; Wang, C.; Zhao, M.-H.; Chen, M. Neutrophil extracellular traps can activate alternative complement pathways. *Clin. Exp. Immunol.* **2015**, *181*, 518–527. [CrossRef]

26. Leffler, J.; Martin, M.; Gullstrand, B.; Tydén, H.; Lood, C.; Truedsson, L.; Bengtsson, A.A.; Blom, A.M. Neutrophil extracellular traps that are not degraded in systemic lupus erythematosus activate complement exacerbating the disease. *J. Immunol. Baltim. Md 1950* **2012**, *188*, 3522–3531. [CrossRef]

27. Schaller, M.; Bigler, C.; Danner, D.; Ditzel, H.J.; Trendelenburg, M. Autoantibodies against C1q in systemic lupus erythematosus are antigen-driven. *J. Immunol.* **2009**, *183*, 8225–8231. [CrossRef]

28. Mansour, R.B.; Lassoued, S.; Gargouri, B.; El Gaïd, A.; Attia, H.; Fakhfakh, F. Increased levels of autoantibodies against catalase and superoxide dismutase associated with oxidative stress in patients with rheumatoid arthritis and systemic lupus erythematosus. *Scand. J. Rheumatol.* **2008**, *37*, 103–108. [CrossRef]

29. Carmona-Rivera, C.; Kaplan, M.J. Low density granulocytes: A distinct class of neutrophils in systemic autoimmunity. *Semin. Immunopathol.* **2013**, *35*, 455–463. [CrossRef]

30. Corsiero, E.; Bombardieri, M.; Carlotti, E.; Pratesi, F.; Robinson, W.; Migliorini, P.; Pitzalis, C. Single cell cloning and recombinant monoclonal antibodies generation from RA synovial B cells reveal frequent targeting of citrullinated histones of NETs. *Ann. Rheum. Dis.* **2016**, *75*, 1866–1875. [CrossRef]

31. Lloyd, K.A.; Wigerblad, G.; Sahlström, P.; Garimella, M.G.; Chemin, K.; Steen, J.; Titcombe, P.J.; Marklein, B.; Zhou, D.; Stålesen, R.; et al. Differential ACPA Binding to Nuclear Antigens Reveals a PAD-Independent Pathway and a Distinct Subset of Acetylation Cross-Reactive Autoantibodies in Rheumatoid Arthritis. *Front. Immunol.* **2018**, *9*, 3033. [CrossRef] [PubMed]

32. Pratesi, F.; Dioni, I.; Tommasi, C.; Alcaro, M.C.; Paolini, I.; Barbetti, F.; Boscaro, F.; Panza, F.; Puxeddu, I.; Rovero, P.; et al. Antibodies from patients with rheumatoid arthritis target citrullinated histone 4 contained in neutrophils extracellular traps. *Ann. Rheum. Dis.* **2014**, *73*, 1414–1422. [CrossRef] [PubMed]

33. Yaniv, G.; Twig, G.; Shor, D.B.-A.; Furer, A.; Sherer, Y.; Mozes, O.; Komisar, O.; Slonimsky, E.; Klang, E.; Lotan, E.; et al. A volcanic explosion of autoantibodies in systemic lupus erythematosus: A diversity of 180 different antibodies found in SLE patients. *Autoimmun. Rev.* **2015**, *14*, 75–79. [CrossRef] [PubMed]

34. Isenberg, D.A.; Manson, J.J.; Ehrenstein, M.R.; Rahman, A. Fifty years of anti-ds DNA antibodies: Are we approaching journey's end? *Rheumatol. Oxf. Engl.* **2007**, *46*, 1052–1056. [CrossRef]

35. Gripenberg, M.; Helve, T.; Kurki, P. Profiles of antibodies to histones, DNA and IgG in patients with systemic rheumatic diseases determined by ELISA. *J. Rheumatol.* **1985**, *12*, 934–939.

36. van Dam, L.S.; Kraaij, T.; Kamerling, S.W.A.; Bakker, J.A.; Scherer, U.H.; Rabelink, T.J.; van Kooten, C.; Teng, Y.K.O. Intrinsically Distinct Role of Neutrophil Extracellular Trap Formation in Antineutrophil Cytoplasmic Antibody-Associated Vasculitis Compared to Systemic Lupus Erythematosus. *Arthritis Rheumatol. Hoboken NJ* **2019**.

37. Whittall-García, L.P.; Torres-Ruiz, J.; Zentella-Dehesa, A.; Tapia-Rodríguez, M.; Alcocer-Varela, J.; Mendez-Huerta, N.; Gómez-Martín, D. Neutrophil extracellular traps are a source of extracellular HMGB1 in lupus nephritis: Associations with clinical and histopathological features. *Lupus* **2019**, *28*, 1549–1557. [CrossRef]

38. Tang, S.; Zhang, Y.; Yin, S.-W.; Gao, X.-J.; Shi, W.-W.; Wang, Y.; Huang, X.; Wang, L.; Zou, L.-Y.; Zhao, J.-H.; et al. Neutrophil extracellular trap formation is associated with autophagy-related signalling in ANCA-associated vasculitis. *Clin. Exp. Immunol.* **2015**, *180*, 408–418. [CrossRef]

39. Kain, R.; Tadema, H.; McKinney, E.F.; Benharkou, A.; Brandes, R.; Peschel, A.; Hubert, V.; Feenstra, T.; Sengölge, G.; Stegeman, C.; et al. High prevalence of autoantibodies to hLAMP-2 in anti-neutrophil cytoplasmic antibody-associated vasculitis. *J. Am. Soc. Nephrol. JASN* **2012**, *23*, 556–566. [CrossRef]

40. Garcia-Romo, G.S.; Caielli, S.; Vega, B.; Connolly, J.; Allantaz, F.; Xu, Z.; Punaro, M.; Baisch, J.; Guiducci, C.; Coffman, R.L.; et al. Netting neutrophils are major inducers of type I IFN production in pediatric systemic lupus erythematosus. *Sci. Transl. Med.* **2011**, *3*, 73ra20. [CrossRef]

41. Gestermann, N.; Di Domizio, J.; Lande, R.; Demaria, O.; Frasca, L.; Feldmeyer, L.; Di Lucca, J.; Gilliet, M. Netting Neutrophils Activate Autoreactive B Cells in Lupus. *J. Immunol. Baltim. Md 1950* **2018**, *200*, 3364–3371. [CrossRef] [PubMed]

42. Lande, R.; Ganguly, D.; Facchinetti, V.; Frasca, L.; Conrad, C.; Gregorio, J.; Meller, S.; Chamilos, G.; Sebasigari, R.; Riccieri, V.; et al. Neutrophils activate plasmacytoid dendritic cells by releasing self-DNA-peptide complexes in systemic lupus erythematosus. *Sci. Transl. Med.* **2011**, *3*, 73ra19. [CrossRef]

43. Frasca, L.; Palazzo, R.; Chimenti, M.S.; Alivernini, S.; Tolusso, B.; Bui, L.; Botti, E.; Giunta, A.; Bianchi, L.; Petricca, L.; et al. Anti-LL37 Antibodies Are Present in Psoriatic Arthritis (PsA) Patients: New Biomarkers in PsA. *Front. Immunol.* **2018**, *9*. [CrossRef] [PubMed]

44. Mattey, D.L.; Nixon, N.B.; Dawes, P.T. Association of circulating levels of MMP-8 with mortality from respiratory disease in patients with rheumatoid arthritis. *Arthritis Res. Ther.* **2012**, *14*, R204. [CrossRef] [PubMed]

45. Carmona-Rivera, C.; Zhao, W.; Yalavarthi, S.; Kaplan, M.J. Neutrophil extracellular traps induce endothelial dysfunction in systemic lupus erythematosus through the activation of matrix metalloproteinase-2. *Ann. Rheum. Dis.* **2015**, *74*, 1417–1424. [CrossRef]

46. Nakazawa, D.; Shida, H.; Tomaru, U.; Yoshida, M.; Nishio, S.; Atsumi, T.; Ishizu, A. Enhanced formation and disordered regulation of NETs in myeloperoxidase-ANCA-associated microscopic polyangiitis. *J. Am. Soc. Nephrol. JASN* **2014**, *25*, 990–997. [CrossRef] [PubMed]

47. Takeuchi, H.; Kawasaki, T.; Shigematsu, K.; Kawamura, K.; Oka, N. Neutrophil extracellular traps in neuropathy with anti-neutrophil cytoplasmic autoantibody-associated microscopic polyangiitis. *Clin. Rheumatol.* **2017**, *36*, 913–917. [CrossRef]

48. Urban, C.F.; Ermert, D.; Schmid, M.; Abu-Abed, U.; Goosmann, C.; Nacken, W.; Brinkmann, V.; Jungblut, P.R.; Zychlinsky, A. Neutrophil extracellular traps contain calprotectin, a cytosolic protein complex involved in host defense against Candida albicans. *PLoS Pathog.* **2009**, *5*, e1000639. [CrossRef]

49. Yoshida, M.; Sasaki, M.; Sugisaki, K.; Yamaguchi, Y.; Yamada, M. Neutrophil extracellular trap components in fibrinoid necrosis of the kidney with myeloperoxidase-ANCA-associated vasculitis. *Clin. Kidney J.* **2013**, *6*, 308–312. [CrossRef] [PubMed]

50. O'Sullivan, K.M.; Lo, C.Y.; Summers, S.A.; Elgass, K.D.; McMillan, P.J.; Longano, A.; Ford, S.L.; Gan, P.-Y.; Kerr, P.G.; Kitching, A.R.; et al. Renal participation of myeloperoxidase in antineutrophil cytoplasmic antibody (ANCA)-associated glomerulonephritis. *Kidney Int.* **2015**, *88*, 1030–1046. [CrossRef]

51. Schultz, D.R.; Tozman, E.C. Antineutrophil cytoplasmic antibodies: Major autoantigens, pathophysiology, and disease associations. *Semin. Arthritis Rheum.* **1995**, *25*, 143–159. [CrossRef]

52. Kambas, K.; Mitroulis, I.; Apostolidou, E.; Girod, A.; Chrysanthopoulou, A.; Pneumatikos, I.; Skendros, P.; Kourtzelis, I.; Koffa, M.; Kotsianidis, I.; et al. Autophagy Mediates the Delivery of Thrombogenic Tissue Factor to Neutrophil Extracellular Traps in Human Sepsis. *PLoS ONE* **2012**, *7*, e45427. [CrossRef] [PubMed]

53. Frangou, E.; Chrysanthopoulou, A.; Mitsios, A.; Kambas, K.; Arelaki, S.; Angelidou, I.; Arampatzioglou, A.; Gakiopoulou, H.; Bertsias, G.K.; Verginis, P.; et al. REDD1/autophagy pathway promotes thromboinflammation and fibrosis in human systemic lupus erythematosus (SLE) through NETs decorated with tissue factor (TF) and interleukin-17A (IL-17A). *Ann. Rheum. Dis.* **2019**, *78*, 238–248. [CrossRef] [PubMed]

54. Ramsey-Goldman, R.; Alexander, R.V.; Massarotti, E.M.; Wallace, D.J.; Narain, S.; Arriens, C.; Collins, C.E.; Saxena, A.; Putterman, C.; Kalunian, K.C.; et al. Complement activation occurs in patients with probable systemic lupus erythematosus and may predict progression to ACR classified SLE. *Arthritis Rheumatol.* **2020**, *72*, 78–88. [CrossRef]

55. Schreiber, A.; Rousselle, A.; Becker, J.U.; von Mässenhausen, A.; Linkermann, A.; Kettritz, R. Necroptosis controls NET generation and mediates complement activation, endothelial damage, and autoimmune vasculitis. *Proc. Natl. Acad. Sci. USA* **2017**, *114*, E9618–E9625. [CrossRef]

56. Kumar, S.V.R.; Kulkarni, O.P.; Mulay, S.R.; Darisipudi, M.N.; Romoli, S.; Thomasova, D.; Scherbaum, C.R.; Hohenstein, B.; Hugo, C.; Müller, S.; et al. Neutrophil Extracellular Trap-Related Extracellular Histones Cause Vascular Necrosis in Severe GN. *J. Am. Soc. Nephrol. JASN* **2015**, *26*, 2399–2413. [CrossRef]

57. Ma, Y.-H.; Ma, T.; Wang, C.; Wang, H.; Chang, D.-Y.; Chen, M.; Zhao, M.-H. High-mobility group box 1 potentiates antineutrophil cytoplasmic antibody-inducing neutrophil extracellular traps formation. *Arthritis Res. Ther.* **2016**, *18*, 2. [CrossRef]

58. Kahlenberg, J.M.; Carmona-Rivera, C.; Smith, C.K.; Kaplan, M.J. Neutrophil extracellular trap-associated protein activation of the NLRP3 inflammasome is enhanced in lupus macrophages. *J. Immunol. Baltim. Md 1950* **2013**, *190*, 1217–1226. [CrossRef]

59. Hu, Q.; Shi, H.; Zeng, T.; Liu, H.; Su, Y.; Cheng, X.; Ye, J.; Yin, Y.; Liu, M.; Zheng, H.; et al. Increased neutrophil extracellular traps activate NLRP3 and inflammatory macrophages in adult-onset Still's disease. *Arthritis Res. Ther.* **2019**, *21*, 9. [CrossRef]

60. Chen, K.W.; Monteleone, M.; Boucher, D.; Sollberger, G.; Ramnath, D.; Condon, N.D.; von Pein, J.B.; Broz, P.; Sweet, M.J.; Schroder, K. Noncanonical inflammasome signaling elicits gasdermin D-dependent neutrophil extracellular traps. *Sci. Immunol.* **2018**, *3*, eaar6676. [CrossRef]

61. Sollberger, G.; Choidas, A.; Burn, G.L.; Habenberger, P.; Di Lucrezia, R.; Kordes, S.; Menninger, S.; Eickhoff, J.; Nussbaumer, P.; Klebl, B.; et al. Gasdermin D plays a vital role in the generation of neutrophil extracellular traps. *Sci. Immunol.* **2018**, *3*, eaar6689. [CrossRef] [PubMed]

62. Lazzaretto, B.; Fadeel, B. Intra- and Extracellular Degradation of Neutrophil Extracellular Traps by Macrophages and Dendritic Cells. *J. Immunol.* **2019**, *203*, 2276–2290. [CrossRef] [PubMed]

63. Farrera, C.; Fadeel, B. Macrophage clearance of neutrophil extracellular traps is a silent process. *J. Immunol.* **2013**, *191*, 2647–2656. [CrossRef] [PubMed]

64. Mahajan, A.; Herrmann, M.; Muñoz, L.E. Clearance Deficiency and Cell Death Pathways: A Model for the Pathogenesis of SLE. *Front. Immunol.* **2016**, *7*, 35. [CrossRef]

65. Nakazawa, D.; Tomaru, U.; Suzuki, A.; Masuda, S.; Hasegawa, R.; Kobayashi, T.; Nishio, S.; Kasahara, M.; Ishizu, A. Abnormal conformation and impaired degradation of propylthiouracil-induced neutrophil extracellular traps: Implications of disordered neutrophil extracellular traps in a rat model of myeloperoxidase antineutrophil cytoplasmic antibody-associated vasculitis. *Arthritis Rheum.* **2012**, *64*, 3779–3787. [CrossRef]

66. Al-Mayouf, S.M.; Sunker, A.; Abdwani, R.; Abrawi, S.A.; Almurshedi, F.; Alhashmi, N.; Al Sonbul, A.; Sewairi, W.; Qari, A.; Abdallah, E.; et al. Loss-of-function variant in DNASE1L3 causes a familial form of systemic lupus erythematosus. *Nat. Genet.* **2011**, *43*, 1186–1188. [CrossRef]

67. Nakazawa, D.; Shida, H.; Kusunoki, Y.; Miyoshi, A.; Nishio, S.; Tomaru, U.; Atsumi, T.; Ishizu, A. The responses of macrophages in interaction with neutrophils that undergo NETosis. *J. Autoimmun.* **2016**, *67*, 19–28. [CrossRef]

68. Barrera-Vargas, A.; Gómez-Martín, D.; Carmona-Rivera, C.; Merayo-Chalico, J.; Torres-Ruiz, J.; Manna, Z.; Hasni, S.; Alcocer-Varela, J.; Kaplan, M.J. Differential ubiquitination in NETs regulates macrophage responses in systemic lupus erythematosus. *Ann. Rheum. Dis.* **2018**, *77*, 944–950. [CrossRef]

69. Lee, K.H.; Kronbichler, A.; Park, D.D.-Y.; Park, Y.; Moon, H.; Kim, H.; Choi, J.H.; Choi, Y.; Shim, S.; Lyu, I.S.; et al. Neutrophil extracellular traps (NETs) in autoimmune diseases: A comprehensive review. *Autoimmun. Rev.* **2017**, *16*, 1160–1173. [CrossRef]

70. Puga, I.; Cols, M.; Barra, C.M.; He, B.; Cassis, L.; Gentile, M.; Comerma, L.; Chorny, A.; Shan, M.; Xu, W.; et al. B cell-helper neutrophils stimulate the diversification and production of immunoglobulin in the marginal zone of the spleen. *Nat. Immunol.* **2011**, *13*, 170–180. [CrossRef]

71. Palanichamy, A.; Bauer, J.W.; Yalavarthi, S.; Meednu, N.; Barnard, J.; Owen, T.; Cistrone, C.; Bird, A.; Rabinovich, A.; Nevarez, S.; et al. Neutrophil-mediated IFN activation in the bone marrow alters B cell development in human and murine systemic lupus erythematosus. *J. Immunol.* **2014**, *192*, 906–918. [CrossRef] [PubMed]

72. Holden, N.J.; Williams, J.M.; Morgan, M.D.; Challa, A.; Gordon, J.; Pepper, R.J.; Salama, A.D.; Harper, L.; Savage, C.O.S. ANCA-stimulated neutrophils release BLyS and promote B cell survival: A clinically relevant cellular process. *Ann. Rheum. Dis.* **2011**, *70*, 2229–2233. [CrossRef] [PubMed]

73. Behnen, M.; Leschczyk, C.; Möller, S.; Batel, T.; Klinger, M.; Solbach, W.; Laskay, T. Immobilized immune complexes induce neutrophil extracellular trap release by human neutrophil granulocytes via FcγRIIIB and Mac-1. *J. Immunol.* **2014**, *193*, 1954–1965. [CrossRef] [PubMed]

74. Crow, M.K. Type I Interferon in the Pathogenesis of Lupus. *J. Immunol.* **2014**, *192*, 5459–5468. [CrossRef]

75. Papadaki, G.; Kambas, K.; Choulaki, C.; Vlachou, K.; Drakos, E.; Bertsias, G.; Ritis, K.; Boumpas, D.T.; Thompson, P.R.; Verginis, P.; et al. Neutrophil extracellular traps exacerbate Th1-mediated autoimmune

responses in rheumatoid arthritis by promoting DC maturation. *Eur. J. Immunol.* **2016**, *46*, 2542–2554. [CrossRef]

76. Tillack, K.; Breiden, P.; Martin, R.; Sospedra, M. T lymphocyte priming by neutrophil extracellular traps links innate and adaptive immune responses. *J. Immunol.* **2012**, *188*, 3150–3159. [CrossRef]

77. Donis-Maturano, L.; Sánchez-Torres, L.E.; Cerbulo-Vázquez, A.; Chacón-Salinas, R.; García-Romo, G.S.; Orozco-Uribe, M.C.; Yam-Puc, J.C.; González-Jiménez, M.A.; Paredes-Vivas, Y.L.; Calderón-Amador, J.; et al. Prolonged exposure to neutrophil extracellular traps can induce mitochondrial damage in macrophages and dendritic cells. *SpringerPlus* **2015**, *4*, 161. [CrossRef]

78. Carmona-Rivera, C.; Carlucci, P.M.; Moore, E.; Lingampalli, N.; Uchtenhagen, H.; James, E.; Liu, Y.; Bicker, K.L.; Wahamaa, H.; Hoffmann, V.; et al. Synovial fibroblast-neutrophil interactions promote pathogenic adaptive immunity in rheumatoid arthritis. *Sci. Immunol.* **2017**, *2*, eaag3358. [CrossRef]

79. Rahman, S.; Sagar, D.; Hanna, R.N.; Lightfoot, Y.L.; Mistry, P.; Smith, C.K.; Manna, Z.; Hasni, S.; Siegel, R.M.; Sanjuan, M.A.; et al. Low-density granulocytes activate T cells and demonstrate a non-suppressive role in systemic lupus erythematosus. *Ann. Rheum. Dis.* **2019**, *78*, 957–966. [CrossRef]

80. Scott, D.L.; Wolfe, F.; Huizinga, T.W. Rheumatoid arthritis. *Lancet* **2010**, *376*, 1094–1108. [CrossRef]

81. Juarez, M.; Bang, H.; Hammar, F.; Reimer, U.; Dyke, B.; Sahbudin, I.; Buckley, C.D.; Fisher, B.; Filer, A.; Raza, K. Identification of novel antiacetylated vimentin antibodies in patients with early inflammatory arthritis. *Ann. Rheum. Dis.* **2016**, *75*, 1099–1107. [CrossRef] [PubMed]

82. Schellekens, G.A.; De Jong, B.A.; Van den Hoogen, F.H.; Van de Putte, L.B.; van Venrooij, W.J. Citrulline is an essential constituent of antigenic determinants recognized by rheumatoid arthritis-specific autoantibodies. *J. Clin. Investig.* **1998**, *101*, 273–281. [CrossRef] [PubMed]

83. Shi, J.; Knevel, R.; Suwannalai, P.; van der Linden, M.P.; Janssen, G.M.C.; van Veelen, P.A.; Levarht, N.E.W.; van Mil, A.H.M.v.d.H.; Cerami, A.; Huizinga, T.W.J.; et al. Autoantibodies recognizing carbamylated proteins are present in sera of patients with rheumatoid arthritis and predict joint damage. *Proc. Natl. Acad. Sci. USA* **2011**, *108*, 17372–17377. [CrossRef] [PubMed]

84. Trouw, L.A.; Haisma, E.M.; Levarht, E.W.N.; van der Woude, D.; Ioan-Facsinay, A.; Daha, M.R.; Huizinga, T.W.J.; Toes, R.E. Anti-cyclic citrullinated peptide antibodies from rheumatoid arthritis patients activate complement via both the classical and alternative pathways. *Arthritis Rheum.* **2009**, *60*, 1923–1931. [CrossRef] [PubMed]

85. Toes, R.; Pisetsky, D.S. Pathogenic effector functions of ACPA: Where do we stand? *Ann. Rheum. Dis.* **2019**, *78*, 716–721. [CrossRef] [PubMed]

86. Nielen, M.M.J.; van Schaardenburg, D.; Reesink, H.W.; van de Stadt, R.J.; van der Horst-Bruinsma, I.E.; de Koning, M.H.M.T.; Habibuw, M.R.; Vandenbroucke, J.P.; Dijkmans, B.A.C. Specific autoantibodies precede the symptoms of rheumatoid arthritis: A study of serial measurements in blood donors. *Arthritis Rheum.* **2004**, *50*, 380–386. [CrossRef] [PubMed]

87. Sur Chowdhury, C.; Giaglis, S.; Walker, U.A.; Buser, A.; Hahn, S.; Hasler, P. Enhanced neutrophil extracellular trap generation in rheumatoid arthritis: Analysis of underlying signal transduction pathways and potential diagnostic utility. *Arthritis Res. Ther.* **2014**, *16*, R122. [CrossRef]

88. Wang, W.; Peng, W.; Ning, X. Increased levels of neutrophil extracellular trap remnants in the serum of patients with rheumatoid arthritis. *Int. J. Rheum. Dis.* **2018**, *21*, 415–421. [CrossRef]

89. Pérez-Sánchez, C.; Ruiz-Limón, P.; Aguirre, M.A.; Jiménez-Gómez, Y.; Arias-de la Rosa, I.; Ábalos-Aguilera, M.C.; Rodriguez-Ariza, A.; Castro-Villegas, M.C.; Ortega-Castro, R.; Segui, P.; et al. Diagnostic potential of NETosis-derived products for disease activity, atherosclerosis and therapeutic effectiveness in Rheumatoid Arthritis patients. *J. Autoimmun.* **2017**, *82*, 31–40. [CrossRef]

90. Kusunoki, Y.; Nakazawa, D.; Shida, H.; Hattanda, F.; Miyoshi, A.; Masuda, S.; Nishio, S.; Tomaru, U.; Atsumi, T.; Ishizu, A. Peptidylarginine Deiminase Inhibitor Suppresses Neutrophil Extracellular Trap Formation and MPO-ANCA Production. *Front. Immunol.* **2016**, *7*, 227. [CrossRef]

91. Knight, J.S.; Subramanian, V.; O'Dell, A.A.; Yalavarthi, S.; Zhao, W.; Smith, C.K.; Hodgin, J.B.; Thompson, P.R.; Kaplan, M.J. Peptidylarginine deiminase inhibition disrupts NET formation and protects against kidney, skin and vascular disease in lupus-prone MRL/lpr mice. *Ann. Rheum. Dis.* **2015**, *74*, 2199–2206. [CrossRef] [PubMed]

92. Knight, J.S.; Zhao, W.; Luo, W.; Subramanian, V.; O'Dell, A.A.; Yalavarthi, S.; Hodgin, J.B.; Eitzman, D.T.; Thompson, P.R.; Kaplan, M.J. Peptidylarginine deiminase inhibition is immunomodulatory and vasculoprotective in murine lupus. *J. Clin. Investig.* **2013**, *123*, 2981–2993. [CrossRef] [PubMed]

93. Kawaguchi, H.; Matsumoto, I.; Osada, A.; Kurata, I.; Ebe, H.; Tanaka, Y.; Inoue, A.; Umeda, N.; Kondo, Y.; Tsuboi, H.; et al. Peptidyl arginine deiminase inhibition suppresses arthritis via decreased protein citrullination in joints and serum with the downregulation of interleukin-6. *Mod. Rheumatol.* **2019**, *29*, 964–969. [CrossRef] [PubMed]

94. Lewis, H.D.; Liddle, J.; Coote, J.E.; Atkinson, S.J.; Barker, M.D.; Bax, B.D.; Bicker, K.L.; Bingham, R.P.; Campbell, M.; Chen, Y.H.; et al. Inhibition of PAD4 activity is sufficient to disrupt mouse and human NET formation. *Nat. Chem. Biol.* **2015**, *11*, 189–191. [CrossRef] [PubMed]

95. Willis, V.C.; Banda, N.K.; Cordova, K.N.; Chandra, P.E.; Robinson, W.H.; Cooper, D.C.; Lugo, D.; Mehta, G.; Taylor, S.; Tak, P.P.; et al. Protein arginine deiminase 4 inhibition is sufficient for the amelioration of collagen-induced arthritis. *Clin. Exp. Immunol.* **2017**, *188*, 263–274. [CrossRef]

96. Willis, V.C.; Gizinski, A.M.; Banda, N.K.; Causey, C.P.; Knuckley, B.; Cordova, K.N.; Luo, Y.; Levitt, B.; Glogowska, M.; Chandra, P.; et al. N-α-benzoyl-N5-(2-chloro-1-iminoethyl)-L-ornithine amide, a protein arginine deiminase inhibitor, reduces the severity of murine collagen-induced arthritis. *J. Immunol.* **2011**, *186*, 4396–4404. [CrossRef]

97. Macanovic, M.; Sinicropi, D.; Shak, S.; Baughman, S.; Thiru, S.; Lachmann, P.J. The treatment of systemic lupus erythematosus (SLE) in NZB/W F1 hybrid mice; studies with recombinant murine DNase and with dexamethasone. *Clin. Exp. Immunol.* **1996**, *106*, 243–252. [CrossRef]

98. Davis, J.C.; Manzi, S.; Yarboro, C.; Rairie, J.; Mcinnes, I.; Averthelyi, D.; Sinicropi, D.; Hale, V.G.; Balow, J.; Austin, H.; et al. Recombinant human Dnase I (rhDNase) in patients with lupus nephritis. *Lupus* **1999**, *8*, 68–76. [CrossRef]

99. Meng, H.; Yalavarthi, S.; Kanthi, Y.; Mazza, L.F.; Elfline, M.A.; Luke, C.E.; Pinsky, D.J.; Henke, P.K.; Knight, J.S. In Vivo Role of Neutrophil Extracellular Traps in Antiphospholipid Antibody–Mediated Venous Thrombosis. *Arthritis Rheumatol.* **2017**, *69*, 655–667. [CrossRef]

100. Zha, C.; Zhang, W.; Gao, F.; Xu, J.; Jia, R.; Cai, J.; Liu, Y. Anti-β2GPI/β2GPI induces neutrophil extracellular traps formation to promote thrombogenesis via the TLR4/MyD88/MAPKs axis activation. *Neuropharmacology* **2018**, *138*, 140–150. [CrossRef]

101. Wang, Y.; Wang, Y.; Wu, J.; Liu, C.; Zhou, Y.; Mi, L.; Zhang, Y.; Wang, W. PRAK Is Required for the Formation of Neutrophil Extracellular Traps. *Front. Immunol.* **2019**, *10*, 1252. [CrossRef] [PubMed]

102. Vorobjeva, N.V.; Pinegin, B.V. Effects of the antioxidants Trolox, Tiron and Tempol on neutrophil extracellular trap formation. *Immunobiology* **2016**, *221*, 208–219. [CrossRef] [PubMed]

103. Mohammed, B.M.; Fisher, B.J.; Kraskauskas, D.; Farkas, D.; Brophy, D.F.; Fowler, A.A.; Natarajan, R. Vitamin C: A novel regulator of neutrophil extracellular trap formation. *Nutrients* **2013**, *5*, 3131–3151. [CrossRef] [PubMed]

104. Merrill, J.T.; Wallace, D.J.; Petri, M.; Kirou, K.A.; Yao, Y.; White, W.I.; Robbie, G.; Levin, R.; Berney, S.M.; Chindalore, V.; et al. Safety profile and clinical activity of sifalimumab, a fully human anti-interferon α monoclonal antibody, in systemic lupus erythematosus: A phase I, multicentre, double-blind randomised study. *Ann. Rheum. Dis.* **2011**, *70*, 1905–1913. [CrossRef]

105. Petri, M.; Wallace, D.J.; Spindler, A.; Chindalore, V.; Kalunian, K.; Mysler, E.; Neuwelt, C.M.; Robbie, G.; White, W.I.; Higgs, B.W.; et al. Sifalimumab, a human anti-interferon-α monoclonal antibody, in systemic lupus erythematosus: A phase I randomized, controlled, dose-escalation study. *Arthritis Rheum.* **2013**, *65*, 1011–1021. [CrossRef]

106. Khamashta, M.; Merrill, J.T.; Werth, V.P.; Furie, R.; Kalunian, K.; Illei, G.G.; Drappa, J.; Wang, L.; Greth, W.; CD1067 study investigators. Sifalimumab, an anti-interferon-α monoclonal antibody, in moderate to severe systemic lupus erythematosus: A randomised, double-blind, placebo-controlled study. *Ann. Rheum. Dis.* **2016**, *75*, 1909–1916. [CrossRef]

107. McBride, J.M.; Jiang, J.; Abbas, A.R.; Morimoto, A.; Li, J.; Maciuca, R.; Townsend, M.; Wallace, D.J.; Kennedy, W.P.; Drappa, J. Safety and pharmacodynamics of rontalizumab in patients with systemic lupus erythematosus: Results of a phase I, placebo-controlled, double-blind, dose-escalation study. *Arthritis Rheum.* **2012**, *64*, 3666–3676. [CrossRef]

108. Furie, R.; Khamashta, M.; Merrill, J.T.; Werth, V.P.; Kalunian, K.; Brohawn, P.; Illei, G.G.; Drappa, J.; Wang, L.; Yoo, S.; et al. Anifrolumab, an Anti-Interferon-α Receptor Monoclonal Antibody, in Moderate-to-Severe Systemic Lupus Erythematosus. *Arthritis Rheumatol. Hoboken NJ* **2017**, *69*, 376–386. [CrossRef]

109. Hair, P.S.; Enos, A.I.; Krishna, N.K.; Cunnion, K.M. Inhibition of Immune Complex Complement Activation and Neutrophil Extracellular Trap Formation by Peptide Inhibitor of Complement C1. *Front. Immunol.* **2018**, *9*, 558. [CrossRef]

110. van Bijnen, S.T.A.; Wouters, D.; van Mierlo, G.J.; Muus, P.; Zeerleder, S. Neutrophil activation and nucleosomes as markers of systemic inflammation in paroxysmal nocturnal hemoglobinuria: Effects of eculizumab. *J. Thromb. Haemost. JTH* **2015**, *13*, 2004–2011. [CrossRef]

111. Roberts, H.; White, P.; Dias, I.; McKaig, S.; Veeramachaneni, R.; Thakker, N.; Grant, M.; Chapple, I. Characterization of neutrophil function in Papillon-Lefèvre syndrome. *J. Leukoc. Biol.* **2016**, *100*, 433–444. [CrossRef] [PubMed]

112. Seren, S.; Rashed Abouzaid, M.; Eulenberg-Gustavus, C.; Hirschfeld, J.; Nasr Soliman, H.; Jerke, U.; N'Guessan, K.; Dallet-Choisy, S.; Lesner, A.; Lauritzen, C.; et al. Consequences of cathepsin C inactivation for membrane exposure of proteinase 3, the target antigen in autoimmune vasculitis. *J. Biol. Chem.* **2018**, *293*, 12415–12428. [CrossRef] [PubMed]

113. Murthy, P.; Singhi, A.D.; Ross, M.A.; Loughran, P.; Paragomi, P.; Papachristou, G.I.; Whitcomb, D.C.; Zureikat, A.H.; Lotze, M.T.; Zeh III, H.J.; et al. Enhanced Neutrophil Extracellular Trap Formation in Acute Pancreatitis Contributes to Disease Severity and Is Reduced by Chloroquine. *Front. Immunol.* **2019**, *10*, 28. [CrossRef]

114. Handono, K.; Sidarta, Y.O.; Pradana, B.A.; Nugroho, R.A.; Hartono, I.A.; Kalim, H.; Endharti, A.T. Vitamin D prevents endothelial damage induced by increased neutrophil extracellular traps formation in patients with systemic lupus erythematosus. *Acta Medica Indones.* **2014**, *46*, 189–198.

115. Reynolds, J.; Ray, D.; Alexander, M.Y.; Bruce, I. Role of vitamin D in endothelial function and endothelial repair in clinically stable systemic lupus erythematosus. *Lancet Lond. Engl.* **2015**, *385* (Suppl. 1), S83. [CrossRef]

116. Bornhöfft, K.F.; Viergutz, T.; Kühnle, A.; Galuska, S.P. Nanoparticles Equipped with α2,8-Linked Sialic Acid Chains Inhibit the Release of Neutrophil Extracellular Traps. *Nanomaterials* **2019**, *9*, E610.

117. Galuska, C.E.; Dambon, J.A.; Kühnle, A.; Bornhöfft, K.F.; Prem, G.; Zlatina, K.; Lütteke, T.; Galuska, S.P. Artificial Polysialic Acid Chains as Sialidase-Resistant Molecular-Anchors to Accumulate Particles on Neutrophil Extracellular Traps. *Front. Immunol.* **2017**, *8*, 1229. [CrossRef] [PubMed]

118. Kühnle, A.; Lütteke, T.; Bornhöfft, K.F.; Galuska, S.P. Polysialic Acid Modulates the Binding of External Lactoferrin in Neutrophil Extracellular Traps. *Biology* **2019**, *8*, 20. [CrossRef]

119. Ruiz-Limón, P.; Ortega, R.; de la Rosa, I.A.; del Carmen Abalos-Aguilera, M.; Perez-Sanchez, C.; Jimenez-Gomez, Y.; Peralbo-Santaella, E.; Font, P.; Ruiz-Vilches, D.; Ferrin, G.; et al. Tocilizumab improves the proatherothrombotic profile of rheumatoid arthritis patients modulating endothelial dysfunction, NETosis, and inflammation. *Transl. Res.* **2017**, *183*, 87–103. [CrossRef]

120. Kraaij, T.; Kamerling, S.W.A.; de Rooij, E.N.M.; van Daele, P.L.A.; Bredewold, O.W.; Bakker, J.A.; Bajema, I.M.; Scherer, H.U.; Toes, R.E.M.; Huizinga, T.J.W.; et al. The NET-effect of combining rituximab with belimumab in severe systemic lupus erythematosus. *J. Autoimmun.* **2018**, *91*, 45–54. [CrossRef]

121. Uozumi, R.; Iguchi, R.; Masuda, S.; Nishibata, Y.; Nakazawa, D.; Tomaru, U.; Ishizu, A. Pharmaceutical immunoglobulins reduce neutrophil extracellular trap formation and ameliorate the development of MPO-ANCA-associated vasculitis. *Mod. Rheumatol.* **2019**, 1–7. [CrossRef]

122. Cornec, D.; Cornec-Le Gall, E.; Fervenza, F.C.; Specks, U. ANCA-associated vasculitis—Clinical utility of using ANCA specificity to classify patients. *Nat. Rev. Rheumatol.* **2016**, *12*, 570–579. [CrossRef] [PubMed]

123. Csernok, E.; Ernst, M.; Schmitt, W.; Bainton, D.F.; Gross, W.L. Activated neutrophils express proteinase 3 on their plasma membrane in vitro and in vivo. *Clin. Exp. Immunol.* **1994**, *95*, 244–250. [CrossRef] [PubMed]

124. Futamata, E.; Masuda, S.; Nishibata, Y.; Tanaka, S.; Tomaru, U.; Ishizu, A. Vanishing Immunoglobulins: The Formation of Pauci-Immune Lesions in Myeloperoxidase-Antineutrophil Cytoplasmic Antibody-Associated Vasculitis. *Nephron* **2018**, *138*, 328–330. [CrossRef] [PubMed]

125. Söderberg, D.; Kurz, T.; Motamedi, A.; Hellmark, T.; Eriksson, P.; Segelmark, M. Increased levels of neutrophil extracellular trap remnants in the circulation of patients with small vessel vasculitis, but an inverse correlation

to anti-neutrophil cytoplasmic antibodies during remission. *Rheumatol. Oxf. Engl.* **2015**, *54*, 2085–2094. [CrossRef] [PubMed]

126. Wang, H.; Sha, L.-L.; Ma, T.-T.; Zhang, L.-X.; Chen, M.; Zhao, M.-H. Circulating Level of Neutrophil Extracellular Traps Is Not a Useful Biomarker for Assessing Disease Activity in Antineutrophil Cytoplasmic Antibody-Associated Vasculitis. *PLoS ONE* **2016**, *11*, e0148197. [CrossRef]

127. Kraaij, T.; Kamerling, S.W.A.; van Dam, L.S.; Bakker, J.A.; Bajema, I.M.; Page, T.; Brunini, F.; Pusey, C.D.; Toes, R.E.M.; Scherer, H.U.; et al. Excessive neutrophil extracellular trap formation in ANCA-associated vasculitis is independent of ANCA. *Kidney Int.* **2018**, *94*, 139–149. [CrossRef]

128. Midgley, A.; Beresford, M. Cellular localization of nuclear antigen during neutrophil apoptosis: Mechanism for autoantigen exposure? *Lupus* **2011**, *20*, 641–646. [CrossRef]

129. Ren, Y.; Tang, J.; Mok, M.Y.; Chan, A.W.K.; Wu, A.; Lau, C.S. Increased apoptotic neutrophils and macrophages and impaired macrophage phagocytic clearance of apoptotic neutrophils in systemic lupus erythematosus. *Arthritis Rheum.* **2003**, *48*, 2888–2897. [CrossRef]

130. Dieker, J.; Tel, J.; Pieterse, E.; Thielen, A.; Rother, N.; Bakker, M.; Fransen, J.; Dijkman, H.B.P.M.; Berden, J.H.; de Vries, J.M.; et al. Circulating Apoptotic Microparticles in Systemic Lupus Erythematosus Patients Drive the Activation of Dendritic Cell Subsets and Prime Neutrophils for NETosis. *Arthritis Rheumatol. Hoboken NJ* **2016**, *68*, 462–472. [CrossRef]

131. Liu, C.L.; Tangsombatvisit, S.; Rosenberg, J.M.; Mandelbaum, G.; Gillespie, E.C.; Gozani, O.P.; Alizadeh, A.A.; Utz, P.J. Specific post-translational histone modifications of neutrophil extracellular traps as immunogens and potential targets of lupus autoantibodies. *Arthritis Res. Ther.* **2012**, *14*, R25. [CrossRef] [PubMed]

132. Lood, C.; Blanco, L.P.; Purmalek, M.M.; Carmona-Rivera, C.; De Ravin, S.S.; Smith, C.K.; Malech, H.L.; Ledbetter, J.A.; Elkon, K.B.; Kaplan, M.J. Neutrophil extracellular traps enriched in oxidized mitochondrial DNA are interferogenic and contribute to lupus-like disease. *Nat. Med.* **2016**, *22*, 146–153. [CrossRef] [PubMed]

133. Wang, H.; Li, T.; Chen, S.; Gu, Y.; Ye, S. Neutrophil Extracellular Trap Mitochondrial DNA and Its Autoantibody in Systemic Lupus Erythematosus and a Proof-of-Concept Trial of Metformin. *Arthritis Rheumatol. Hoboken NJ* **2015**, *67*, 3190–3200. [CrossRef]

134. van der Linden, M.; van den Hoogen, L.L.; Westerlaken, G.H.A.; Fritsch-Stork, R.D.E.; van Roon, J.A.G.; Radstake, T.R.D.J.; Meyaard, L. Neutrophil extracellular trap release is associated with antinuclear antibodies in systemic lupus erythematosus and anti-phospholipid syndrome. *Rheumatol. Oxf. Engl.* **2018**, *57*, 1228–1234. [CrossRef]

135. Leffler, J.; Gullstrand, B.; Jönsen, A.; Nilsson, J.-Å.; Martin, M.; Blom, A.M.; Bengtsson, A.A. Degradation of neutrophil extracellular traps co-varies with disease activity in patients with systemic lupus erythematosus. *Arthritis Res. Ther.* **2013**, *15*, R84. [CrossRef]

136. Hacbarth, E.; Kajdacsy-Balla, A. Low density neutrophils in patients with systemic lupus erythematosus, rheumatoid arthritis, and acute rheumatic fever. *Arthritis Rheum.* **1986**, *29*, 1334–1342. [CrossRef]

137. Yang, P.; Li, Y.; Xie, Y.; Liu, Y. Different Faces for Different Places: Heterogeneity of Neutrophil Phenotype and Function. *J. Immunol. Res.* **2019**, *2019*, 8016254. [CrossRef] [PubMed]

138. Mistry, P.; Nakabo, S.; O'Neil, L.; Goel, R.R.; Jiang, K.; Carmona-Rivera, C.; Gupta, S.; Chan, D.W.; Carlucci, P.M.; Wang, X.; et al. Transcriptomic, epigenetic, and functional analyses implicate neutrophil diversity in the pathogenesis of systemic lupus erythematosus. *Proc. Natl. Acad. Sci. USA* **2019**, *116*, 25222–25228. [CrossRef]

139. Odqvist, L.; Jevnikar, Z.; Riise, R.; Öberg, L.; Rhedin, M.; Leonard, D.; Yrlid, L.; Jackson, S.; Mattsson, J.; Nanda, S.; et al. Genetic variations in A20 DUB domain provide a genetic link to citrullination and neutrophil extracellular traps in systemic lupus erythematosus. *Ann. Rheum. Dis.* **2019**, *78*, 1363–1370. [CrossRef]

140. Radic, M.; Pattanaik, D. Cellular and Molecular Mechanisms of Anti-Phospholipid Syndrome. *Front. Immunol.* **2018**, *9*, 969. [CrossRef]

141. Maugeri, N.; Campana, L.; Gavina, M.; Covino, C.; De Metrio, M.; Panciroli, C.; Maiuri, L.; Maseri, A.; D'Angelo, A.; Bianchi, M.E.; et al. Activated platelets present high mobility group box 1 to neutrophils, inducing autophagy and promoting the extrusion of neutrophil extracellular traps. *J. Thromb. Haemost.* **2014**, *12*, 2074–2088. [CrossRef] [PubMed]

142. Yalavarthi, S.; Gould, T.J.; Rao, A.N.; Mazza, L.F.; Morris, A.E.; Núñez-Álvarez, C.; Hernández-Ramírez, D.; Bockenstedt, P.L.; Liaw, P.C.; Cabral, A.R.; et al. Release of Neutrophil Extracellular Traps by Neutrophils Stimulated With Antiphospholipid Antibodies: A Newly Identified Mechanism of Thrombosis in the Antiphospholipid Syndrome. *Arthritis Rheumatol.* **2015**, *67*, 2990–3003. [CrossRef] [PubMed]

143. You, Y.; Liu, Y.; Li, F.; Mu, F.; Zha, C. Anti-β2GPI/β2GPI induces human neutrophils to generate NETs by relying on ROS. *Cell Biochem. Funct.* **2019**, *37*, 56–61. [CrossRef] [PubMed]

144. Fuchs, T.A.; Brill, A.; Duerschmied, D.; Schatzberg, D.; Monestier, M.; Myers, D.D.; Wrobleski, S.K.; Wakefield, T.W.; Hartwig, J.H.; Wagner, D.D. Extracellular DNA traps promote thrombosis. *Proc. Natl. Acad. Sci. USA* **2010**, *107*, 15880. [CrossRef] [PubMed]

145. Woodberry, T.; Bouffler, S.E.; Wilson, A.S.; Buckland, R.L.; Brüstle, A. The Emerging Role of Neutrophil Granulocytes in Multiple Sclerosis. *J. Clin. Med.* **2018**, *7*, 511. [CrossRef] [PubMed]

146. Yu, G.; Zheng, S.; Zhang, H. Inhibition of myeloperoxidase by N-acetyl lysyltyrosylcysteine amide reduces experimental autoimmune encephalomyelitis-induced injury and promotes oligodendrocyte regeneration and neurogenesis in a murine model of progressive multiple sclerosis. *Neuroreport* **2018**, *29*, 208–213. [CrossRef]

147. Tillack, K.; Naegele, M.; Haueis, C.; Schippling, S.; Wandinger, K.-P.; Martin, R.; Sospedra, M. Gender differences in circulating levels of neutrophil extracellular traps in serum of multiple sclerosis patients. *J. Neuroimmunol.* **2013**, *261*, 108–119. [CrossRef]

148. Ostendorf, L.; Mothes, R.; van Koppen, S.; Lindquist, R.L.; Bellmann-Strobl, J.; Asseyer, S.; Ruprecht, K.; Alexander, T.; Niesner, R.A.; Hauser, A.E.; et al. Low-Density Granulocytes Are a Novel Immunopathological Feature in Both Multiple Sclerosis and Neuromyelitis Optica Spectrum Disorder. *Front. Immunol.* **2019**, *10*. [CrossRef]

149. Marwick, J.A.; Mills, R.; Kay, O.; Michail, K.; Stephen, J.; Rossi, A.G.; Dransfield, I.; Hirani, N. Neutrophils induce macrophage anti-inflammatory reprogramming by suppressing NF-κB activation. *Cell Death Dis.* **2018**, *9*, 665. [CrossRef]

150. Schauer, C.; Janko, C.; Munoz, L.E.; Zhao, Y.; Kienhöfer, D.; Frey, B.; Lell, M.; Manger, B.; Rech, J.; Naschberger, E.; et al. Aggregated neutrophil extracellular traps limit inflammation by degrading cytokines and chemokines. *Nat. Med.* **2014**, *20*, 511–517. [CrossRef]

151. de Bont, C.M.; Eerden, N.; Boelens, W.C.; Pruijn, G.J.M. Neutrophil proteases degrade autoepitopes of NET-associated proteins. *Clin. Exp. Immunol.* **2020**, *199*, 1–8. [CrossRef] [PubMed]

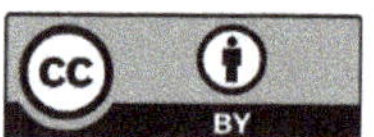

MDPI

St. Alban-Anlage 66

4052 Basel

Switzerland

Tel. +41 61 683 77 34

Fax +41 61 302 89 18

www.mdpi.com

Cells Editorial Office

E-mail: cells@mdpi.com

www.mdpi.com/journal/cells